COSMETICS BUYING GUIDE

ANDREW J. SCHEMAN, M.D.
DAVID L. SEVERSON

COSMETICS BUYING GUIDE

Consumer Reports Books
A Division of Consumers Union
Yonkers, New York

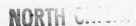

To Cathy Small-Scheman and Kathleen Severson,
without whose love and support
this book would not have been possible.

Copyright © 1993 by Andrew J. Scheman, M.D., and David L. Severson.
Published by Consumers Union of United States, Inc., Yonkers, New York 10703.

Library of Congress Cataloging-in-Publication Data

Scheman, Andrew J.

    Cosmetics buying guide / Andrew J. Scheman, David L. Severson.
      p.   cm.
    Includes bibliographical references and index.
    ISBN 0-89043-581-2 (pbk.)
      1. Skin—Care and hygiene. 2. Cosmetics. 3. Consumer education.
I. Severson, David L. II. Title.
RL87.S33   1993
646.7'26—dc20   93-11552
                                        CIP

Design by Jacqueline Schuman
First printing, September 1993
This book is printed on recycled paper ♲
Manufactured in the United States of America

Cosmetics Buying Guide is a Consumer Reports Book published by Consumers Union, the nonprofit organization that publishes *Consumer Reports*, the monthly magazine of test reports, product Ratings, and buying guidance. Established in 1936, Consumers Union is chartered under the Not-For-Profit Corporation Law of the State of New York. The purposes of Consumers Union, as stated in its charter, are to provide consumers with information and counsel on consumer goods and services, to give information on all matters relating to the expenditure of the family income, and to initiate and to cooperate with individual and group efforts seeking to create and maintain decent living standards.

   Consumers Union derives its income solely from the sale of *Consumer Reports* and other publications. In addition, expenses of occasional public service efforts may be met, in part, by nonrestrictive, noncommercial contributions, grants, and fees. Consumers Union accepts no advertising or product samples and is not beholden in any way to any commercial interest. Its Ratings and reports are solely for the use of the readers of its publications. Neither the Ratings, nor the reports, nor any Consumers Union publication, including this book, may be used in advertising or for any commercial purpose. Consumers Union will take all steps open to it to prevent such uses of its material, its name, or the name of *Consumer Reports*.

ACKNOWLEDGMENTS

The authors would like to acknowledge Kathleen Severson for the tremendous amount of time she so generously offered meticulously collecting product data. Also, Mona Ramsey for her efforts in verifying and updating older product information. We are grateful for the assistance of Dr. Alexander Fisher, who clarified several issues regarding contact allergy of cosmetics. We appreciate the assistance of Sandy Cohen, Denise Limauro, and Gerri Kelly, who gathered pricing information; Marge Florman, who researched prices and devised the price-coding system used in the book; and Deborah Wallace, who contributed packaging information.

We are grateful for the advice, encouragement, and editing skills provided by Roslyn Siegel, whose efforts substantially improved this book.

CONTENTS

PART FOUR
THE EYES

PART FIVE
THE LIPS

PART SIX
THE NAILS

LIST OF CHARTS

INTRODUCTION

Since the beginning of time, people have used substances to color or highlight their skin and enhance their features.

Over the centuries, cosmetic products have evolved from very primitive to very sophisticated. Not only do cosmetics have a higher price tag, but they also have created the need for more knowledge and research into their safe use.

This comprehensive guide tells you how to choose the cosmetic products best for your skin type, and how to avoid potentially harmful reactions to these products. It contains charts that list most of the available products, indicating the type, manufacturer, and potentially harmful ingredients of each and allowing for easy comparison of products.

At a time when allergies and skin irritations seem on the increase, and the numbers of products and claims have proliferated, this book may save you from serious skin problems that can affect your appearance and your health.

If you are like most people, buying cosmetics is very much like going to a gambling casino: Your money is on the line, you are woefully uninformed, and the odds are with the house. Without a guide you will be confused and destined to purchase, through trial and error, many products that are irritating, expensive, or inappropriate for your skin.

You will find within this book a wealth of useful information about cosmetics. The confusing array of available cosmetics is divided into product types, and information is provided on the proper use of each. Cautionary advice is offered for people who tend to have allergies or skin reactions, and attention is focused on the products found to be safest and most helpful for enhancing your appearance. Price codes have been established to help you select the best products for the money. Whether you are age 14 or 50, this book will help you choose cosmetics that are safe, effective, and reasonably priced.

PART ONE

BUYING COSMETICS: WHAT'S SO DIFFICULT?

CHAPTER 1

Cosmetics and Consumer Protection

Although most cosmetics correctly chosen and applied will enhance appearance, cosmetics advertising often exaggerates how much they can actually achieve. Women are therefore frequently vulnerable to the temptation to buy new cosmetics because their expectations are never fully met by the products they are using. Moreover, some products will not only be ineffective, they may also be dangerous.

THE FEDERAL FOOD, DRUG AND COSMETIC ACT

In order to protect the consumer, in 1938 the government passed a set of laws, the Federal Food, Drug and Cosmetic Act, that created legal definitions for cosmetics and drugs. Drugs are defined as products that "affect the structure or any function of the body of man." In contrast, cosmetics are defined as products for "cleansing, beautifying, promoting attractiveness, or altering the appearance." These definitions have been used for classifying individual skin-care products as either cosmetics or drugs.

Drugs and Government Regulation
There is much more stringent regulation of the manufacture of drugs than of cosmetics. A new drug must go through rigorous examination before it is sold to the public. The Food and Drug Administration (FDA) must review and approve data provided by the manufacturer demonstrating that the drug is safe and effective. Alternatively, a product can be formulated using only active ingredients previously approved by the FDA. Once approved, a drug must indicate all active ingredients on the label. Advertising of drugs is carefully regulated and manufacturing facilities must meet strict quality standards.

Cosmetics and Unregulated Ingredients
In contrast, most cosmetic ingredients are unregulated. Cosmetics testing is not reviewed by the FDA, and products do not need to be FDA approved. Furthermore, cosmetics companies do not need to register with the FDA, release their formulas to the FDA, or report adverse effects caused by the use of their products. Some cosmetic ingredients have not been thoroughly

> Most cosmetic ingredients are unregulated. Cosmetics testing is not reviewed by the FDA, and products do not need to be FDA approved.

tested for safety. Long-term adverse effects of cosmetic ingredients are infrequently known, because this kind of research is costly and voluntary. This lack of information makes it difficult to tell the consumer which ingredients and products are unsafe and should be avoided. In some cases, the medical community is aware of potential problems with some cosmetic ingredients, for example, those causing allergic reactions or contributing to acne. On the other hand, ingredients causing other problems may only be discovered years after the product enters the market.

SELF-REGULATION BY COSMETICS COMPANIES

Despite the relative lack of external regulation of the cosmetics industry, many manufacturers make substantial efforts to self-regulate their own performance. Approximately 50 percent of cosmetics companies, mostly larger firms, are registered with the FDA (cosmetics establishment registration program). Many firms voluntarily release their formulas to the FDA (cosmetics product ingredients statement), test their products and ingredients, and report adverse effects that have occurred (products experience report). In addition, an independent panel of expert scientists performs ingredients reviews of cosmetics based on available data and prepares safety

monographs on cosmetics ingredients. The Cosmetic Toiletries and Fragrances Association (CTFA) has also published suggested guidelines for the industry that many companies follow voluntarily. Although these efforts at self-regulation are commendable, unfortunately the consumer has no easy way to determine which companies have been stringent about self-regulation and which products have been tested most thoroughly for safety.

OTHER COSMETICS LAWS

Some additional regulation of cosmetics is provided by laws other than the Federal Food, Drug and Cosmetic Act. The Color Additive Amendment of 1960 requires that coloring ingredients must be tested for safety and approved by the FDA. Because of this law, some color additives were found to be carcinogens (i.e., capable of causing cancer) and were removed from the market. Other color additives found to be potential carcinogens in the laboratory are restricted so that they cannot be used on areas where they will be readily absorbed through the skin, such as the eye area and lips.

Most notably, color additives made from coal tar have been found unsafe to use around the eyes. Coal tar colors will be listed on cosmetics ingredients labels and will begin with the abbreviation FD&C (e.g., FD&C Red #3) or D&C (e.g., D&C Red #7). Each batch of coal tar dyes must be certified and must carry its registration batch number.

In addition, certain coal tar colors should not be used on the lips. Specifically, products designated for "external use only" should not be used on the lips or eyelids. These products contain the abbreviations D&C and Ext. (e.g., Ext. D&C Violet #2).

The consumer must be careful because a foundation makeup for the face may contain coal tar–derived color additives that make the product unsuitable for use on the lips or eyelids. Moreover, while use on other parts of the body might still be permitted, there may not be conclusive evidence that it is actually safe.

Another law, the Fair Packaging and Labelling Act of 1977, requires that ingredients over 1 percent by weight (except color additives and fragrance ingredients) must be listed in descending order of amount on the label of a cosmetic product. The net weight of the product and the name and address of the manufacturer must also be listed on the label. This helpful law makes it possible to determine which ingredients are most dominant in a cosmetic product.

UNLABELED INGREDIENTS

"Fragrance" or "perfume" ingredients may or may not be listed on the labels of cosmetics since the manufacturer is not required to list them. Many fragrance ingredients are known to cause allergic skin reactions and are the most likely components of cosmetics to do so.

Moreover, companies can apply to register certain ingredients as "trade secrets." If approved, these ingredients are not listed separately but come under the heading "and other ingredients." When a label contains the expression "and other ingredients," it is impossible to know whether or not the cosmetic contains a particular ingredient suspected of causing allergic reactions, or whether the cosmetic is oil-free or fragrance-free. Consequently, women who experience problems with cosmetics should avoid products whose packages read "and other ingredients."

ANIMAL TESTING AND "CRUELTY-FREE" PRODUCTS

The issue of animal testing is scientifically and ethically quite complex. No thinking person endorses inflicting needless pain on animals. But manufacturers who have made judicious use of animal tests to assess the safety of their products for consumers may arguably be acting more responsibly than ones who eschew such tests.

Deciphering "cruelty-free" claims is not easy for consumers. While manufacturers themselves may not test their formulated products on animals, their suppliers—the companies that produce the ingredients—may have tested those materials on animals. Or some manufacturers may be relying on information gained from animal testing done by other manufacturers.

Unfortunately, there is no simple way to verify a manufacturer's claim. Like "green" claims, the statement "not tested on animals" is likely to appear on more and more products. But do the same words mean the same thing when used on different products? More important, is the claim true? Marketers have been known to shade the truth with label claims that boost sales. We suggest a skeptical attitude toward such product claims.

For information about which cosmetics companies currently claim they manufacture "cruelty-free" products, contact either of the following organizations:

People for the Ethical Treatment of Animals
(PETA)
P.O. Box 42516
Washington, DC 20015-0516
301-770-PETA

The Humane Society
2100 L Street, N.W.
Washington, DC 20037
202-452-1100

ENFORCEMENT OF COSMETICS LAWS

The FDA enforces the provisions of the Fair Packaging and Labelling Act. The FDA also monitors the industry to ensure that cosmetics do not contain known harmful or unsanitary ingredients and conducts inspections to ensure that manufacturing is not unsanitary. However, the resources of the FDA are limited and some products probably escape these policing efforts. Products with dangerous color additives have been found for sale after the date they were banned by the FDA.

ADVERSE REACTIONS

If it comes to the FDA's attention that a person has been injured by a cosmetic, and it's found that safety hasn't been adequately substantiated, the product may be deemed misbranded and subject to regulatory action.

Manufacturers can avoid regulatory action by putting a caveat on the cosmetic label: "Warning: The safety of this product has not been determined." Of course, cosmetics labels say no such thing. Instead, they state that the product is ophthalmologist tested, dermatologist tested, nonallergenic, and so on. The results of such tests may be kept private until an injured user's lawsuit comes to court or until a third party challenges a formula or ingredient in court.

What about adverse reactions to cosmetics? It's likely that many people who have reactions don't bother to report them to the manufacturer. And cosmetics companies are under no obligation to report the reactions they do hear about to the FDA. However, most large companies (covering 60 to 80 percent of cosmetics sales) do voluntarily keep the FDA informed about adverse reactions.

THE CAREFUL CONSUMER

The inadequacies of the various laws regulating cosmetics suggest that the consumer must still be vigilant. Read the labels carefully on the products you are considering. The information in this book should be helpful in noting which ingredients should be avoided if you tend to suffer from skin irritation, allergies, or other adverse reactions to cosmetics. If you happen to choose a product that does cause an adverse reaction, stop using it immediately.

CHAPTER 2

Fraud, Hype, and Wishful Thinking: What Doesn't Work and Why

Although some policing has been done in the area of exaggerated claims, the consumer must be careful. The FDA has difficulty preventing companies from making exaggerated, and sometimes even fraudulent, claims for certain cosmetics. For example, in 1987 and 1988 the FDA took action against companies promoting skin-care products claiming to retard, control, or counteract skin aging or to rejuvenate, repair, or renew the skin. Because these claims "affect the structure or a function of the body of man," the FDA declared that these products should be considered drugs and the companies producing them be required to prove their claims with testing data. To avoid FDA action, the companies simply diluted their claims; for example, product X "helps to" repair the skin or "promotes" renewal of the skin. The consumer should be aware that it is unlikely that most cosmetics cause alteration of anything other than skin appearance. Otherwise, these products would be regulated as drugs by the FDA. The consumer must

also be aware of potentially misleading qualifiers such as "promotes," "aids," or "helps," which imply the product will deliver a more profound effect on the skin than it can actually produce.

INGREDIENTS THAT MAY REVERSE SKIN AGING

It has now been well established that many changes seen in the skin previously believed to be an unavoidable part of aging are instead caused by the additive effects of exposure to the sun. Only two types of ingredients currently show substantial promise for reversing the signs of skin aging related to the sun—alpha-hydroxy acids and Retin-A (when used along with sunscreen or careful avoidance of the sun).

Alpha-hydroxy Acids

Some physicians believe that alpha-hydroxy acids, such as lactic or glycolic acids, can act to reverse sun-related skin aging. Although the preliminary evidence is promising, this has not yet been proved conclusively. Nevertheless, products containing high amounts of these ingredients may have significant effects. These products are classified as drugs, available only by prescription, and are not yet FDA approved for this purpose. A significant number of skin-care products containing small amounts of alpha-hydroxy acids are available without a prescription, but it is not known if these products contain enough alpha-hydroxy acids to have a substantial effect on sun-related skin aging.

Retin-A

Retin-A (vitamin A acid or tretinoin) is another prescription drug that seems to combat the effects of sun damage. It is not yet FDA approved for this purpose but is currently being reviewed. In addition, preliminary studies on a new related prescription drug, Isotrex (isotretinoin), show similar effects. These ingredients will not prevent further sun damage and must be used with sunscreens or sun avoidance for optimum results. Although these ingredients may deliver what they promise, this is not the case with other ingredients sold as cosmetics and making the same claims as prescription drugs.

Retinyl Palmitate

Some cosmetics contain retinyl palmitate, a vitamin A derivative that is converted to vitamin A acid when applied to the skin. However, it is unlikely that enough vitamin A acid is formed to have a therapeutic effect. Vitamin A itself is not converted to vitamin A acid when applied to the skin and has no effect on sun-related skin aging.

People often mistakenly believe these products will decrease existing sun damage.

Sunscreens

Consumers should also be wary of a potentially misleading claim commonly made by manufacturers of products that purport to "prevent premature skin aging." This is merely an impressive way of saying that these products contain sunscreen ingredients that slow down the development of cumulative sun-related damage to the skin. Buying and applying an inexpensive yet effective sunscreen under makeup will work just as well.

"MIRACLE" INGREDIENTS

Some moisturizers and other cosmetics contain special ingredients that the manufacturer promises will produce miraculous results. Although many of these ingredients probably do not deliver as much as promised, many are still useful as humectants (ingredients that hold water in the skin) or as moisturizing agents.

Phospholipids, Collagen, Hyaluronic Acid, Mucopolysaccharides, Elastin, Amino Acids, and Hydrolyzed Animal Protein

Certain skin components and other structural molecules have been added to some moisturizers. In general these substances are large molecules that will not penetrate the skin and therefore will not "refortify" or "replenish" the structure of the skin. However, most of these do act as humectants (non-oily moisturizing ingredients) and have some moisturizing function.

Liposomes
Some products contain structural substances encased in molecules called liposomes that are supposed to enable them to penetrate the skin. It is unlikely that liposomes actually allow large enclosed substances to penetrate to the deeper layers of the skin. However, there is evidence that liposomes can help moisturizing ingredients to penetrate the skin surface more effectively and that they may make some moisturizers more effective.

Aloe Vera
Aloe vera is often added to moisturizers as a humectant because of its ability to retain water. Tests done by Consumers Union showed that products with aloe vera were often rated subjectively more pleasant than other moisturizers. Many other healing properties have also been ascribed to aloe vera; however, these are less well proven. Chemical analysis of the aloe vera plant does reveal several ingredients that individually have anti-inflammatory effects, lending plausibility to the claim that the substance has healing properties. Whether commercially available aloe vera has healing properties is difficult to determine conclusively because aloe extracts vary depending on the particular crop of aloe plant used, and the time of year and method of extraction.

Vitamins
Although often added to moisturizers, the fat-soluble vitamins A, D, and E will not penetrate the skin and therefore will not "nourish" the skin in any manner. Vita-mins A and D may be mild emollients but probably have no other significant moisturizing effects. Vitamin E may have some ability to cross the epithelial barrier, but more studies are needed to establish this point.

Vitamins C and E are antioxidants, and it has been suggested that they may act as scavengers to destroy harmful substances called free radicals, which are created when sunlight strikes the skin. Products containing vitamins C or E may claim to give "environmental protection or defense." Again, it has not been established that this actually occurs in the concentrations used in these products. On the contrary, vitamin E has caused occasional allergic reactions (as has vitamin B_1).

OILS AND MOISTURIZERS

Natural Oils
Natural oils, including vegetable oils of all types and mink oil, have sometimes been purported to have special benefits when added to moisturizers. Some of these oils are thicker than others, but none of them has been shown to have any major advantage over the others, except possibly aroma.

On the contrary, some natural oils such as linseed oil, peanut oil, sesame oil, olive oil, grape seed oil, and cocoa butter appear to be comedogenic (able to induce blackheads and whiteheads in some individuals). Some studies have shown the same to be true of mineral oil and petrolatum, two of the most common ingredients found in moisturizers. Oil-containing moisturizers are probably not the best choice for anyone prone to acne. Oil-free moisturizers are preferred (if a moisturizer is needed at all by acne-prone women).

Natural Moisturizing Factor and NaPCA
Two patented ingredients called natural moisturizing factor (NMF) and sodium PCA (NaPCA) are found in some moisturizers. Although these ingredients are very good humectants, there is no convincing evidence that they are superior to other humectant ingredients or have any additional special properties.

*Moisturizers for Specific Uses
or Areas of the Body*
Some moisturizers claim to be of special benefit to specific areas of the body, but there is seldom any obvious difference in these products that would make them more suitable for a given region of the body. However, some are less suitable for certain areas. For example, cosmetics with color ingredients made from coal tar are unsuitable for use around the eyes or on the lips. There is also nothing that clearly makes moisturizers that claim to be useful for certain specific purposes (such as "after-sun" moisturizers) more suitable for that purpose than other moisturizers.

CLEANSERS

Abrasive Scrubs and Exfoliants
These products sometimes extol the benefits of removing dead surface skin cells; however, it is debatable whether these benefits are significant or whether the appearance of the skin is improved. Dead skin cells are shed naturally when they reach the skin surface, and it is doubtful whether accelerating this process can improve appearance or "replenish" or "rejuvenate" the skin in any meaningful way.

Mask Cleansers
Masks are products designed to be applied to your face, left on the skin for 20 to 30 minutes, then washed off. Claims for these products vary, but there is no convincing evidence that they have substantially different effects from other cleansers that are washed off immediately.

*Toners, Astringents, Skin Fresheners,
and Clarifiers*
Toners, astringents, skin fresheners, and clarifiers are useful to decrease oil on the skin; however, they do not tighten the skin (except by drying it), decrease oil production, or shrink oil glands.

Refiners
Refiners are usually solutions containing water and humectants that often promise to deliver major benefits. These products are essentially very light oil-free moisturizers that usually do not have any obvious further useful properties. A few refiners do not have humectant ingredients; these products are probably merely pleasant-smelling rinses.

TAN ACCELERATORS

It has not been shown that these products are capable of speeding up the tanning process. In general, these are oils or oil-containing products designed to be used instead of sunscreens. (These products do not contain sunscreen ingredients or dihydroxyacetone, the active ingredient in self-tanners.) It can be argued that since these products do not provide any significant sun protection, they therefore offer an accelerated tan compared to products containing sunscreen. However, they have not been shown to offer an accelerated tan when compared to applying nothing at all! By eliminating sunscreen protection, they can actually accelerate sun damage to the skin.

FIRMING AND ANTICELLULITE CREAMS

Although these products may dry on the skin to produce a firm-feeling film that can perhaps help slightly to hide loose hanging skin and cellulite briefly, it has not been shown that these products produce any lasting shrinkage of the skin or reduction in cellulite. Furthermore, the implication that they can lead to firmer skin or less cellulite when used regularly is very unlikely to be true.

HORMONE CREAMS

Hormone-containing moisturizer creams are an example of how an ingredient in cosmetics may be found to be dangerous only after years on the market. In the past, certain cosmetics contained high enough levels of added hormones to cause side effects when absorbed through the skin. Only after consumers and the medical community noted the occurrence of the side effects were limits placed on the amount of estrogen in skin-care products.

Hormone-containing creams have now been classified by the FDA as drugs because manufacturers claimed these products reversed some signs of skin aging.

An FDA advisory panel reviewed cosmetics containing hormones and concluded that there was no evidence that moisturizing products with hormones added in the amounts allowed without prescription are more effective than the same products without hormones. The FDA has recommended that these products no longer be sold; however, some manufacturers ignore these recommendations and continue to sell products containing hormones.

PLANT AND ANIMAL EXTRACTS

A current trend in many cosmetic products is the inclusion of multiple extracts from plants and animals. Companies that market these products often make substantial claims for these ingredients. These extracts are complex mixtures of natural organic substances rather than single ingredients; furthermore, the actual composition of different batches of these substances may vary significantly. For these reasons, it is difficult to prove exactly what benefits, if any, these substances deliver. Perhaps more important, it is equally difficult to *disprove* claims about benefits these substances purportedly deliver. The consumer

> Consumers are advised to avoid over-the-counter products that contain hormones.

is well advised to view product claims of these substances with "informed skepticism." In addition, it is important to realize that plant extracts can cause allergic reactions in some individuals.

A review of currently available cosmetics reveals that a number of companies use animal extracts in their products. These extracts are usually derived from cows (bovine extracts) or from horses (equine extracts). Some examples are spleen extract, brain extract, placenta extract, horse serum, spinal cord extract, serum albumin, aorta extract, calf skin extract, bovine embryo lipid fraction, and bovine thymus extract. Although these ingredients may not be dangerous, their presence may offend the sensibilities of some consumers. Women are advised to read the labels of the cosmetics they purchase very carefully.

"NATURAL" COSMETICS

Cosmetics claiming to be made entirely from "natural" ingredients are not necessarily superior in any way to other similar products. Like many similar products, these also often contain preservatives and other ingredients that can cause allergic reactions.

Choosing Cosmetics Wisely

FIND A KNOWLEDGEABLE SALESPERSON

It's helpful to work with a knowledgeable, objective salesperson. But shopping for a good cosmetics salesperson can be as difficult as shopping for a good doctor. Some cosmetics salespeople are both well informed and dedicated to helping you find the cosmetics that are the very best for your needs. However, most cosmetics salespeople are hired to sell one line of cosmetics and are often paid on commission. This can act as an incentive to sell the most expensive products exclusively from their line even if you would fare better with a less expensive product from a different cosmetics company. The common practice of placing cosmetics behind different counters with separate salespersons makes it difficult to compare specific products, lines of products, and prices.

If you're unable to get help from a knowledgeable salesperson, you are likely to fare poorly. You may not know how to choose the proper cosmetic type and color for the desired effect. Even if you're successful at this, you may not know how to apply the product properly. If you master application, you may not know your skin type and how to choose a product that is right for your skin. Moreover, if you've had a skin irritation from one product, you may be easily convinced you have an allergy and persuaded to abandon one line of products for a so-called hypoallergenic one.

Your most effective first step in finding the right salesperson is to find a store where the atmosphere is friendly and courteous. While department stores are more likely to have knowledgeable salespeople, drugstore and discount store personnel can also be helpful in steering you toward appropriate products. Look for a salesperson who is willing and able to answer questions. Since many of the cosmetics companies carry full lines of products for each type of skin, it is often more important to get the right help than the right manufacturer.

EVALUATE EACH PRODUCT

Although there are differences between comparable products offered by various companies, no company provides products that are uniformly better than the competition. Therefore, each product must be evaluated on its own merits and suitability for your particular skin. It's important to

> It is important to realize that cosmetic products from different brands will work perfectly well together if chosen carefully.

realize that cosmetics from different brands will work perfectly well together if chosen carefully. Don't allow a salesperson to convince you that a particular brand of cosmetics will only work well with other products made by the same company.

COMPARE PRICES

Since many of the attributes of cosmetics are subjective, it is often difficult to determine whether the difference in quality obtained from an expensive product is worth the greater price tag.

More expensive foundations sometimes provide better coverage or can be worn successfully for a longer period of time without loosing their optimal appearance. The colors found in more costly cosmetics may sometimes be more stylish. The texture of more expensive products may be smoother and may apply to the skin more easily, with less dragging or smudging. The more expensive products will sometimes use more expensive ingredients that may or may not be better for your needs.

Many inexpensive cosmetics have performed extremely well and are equal or superior to more expensive products. Often, much of the extra price you pay for an expensive cosmetic is for the brand name or fancy packaging. In most cases, the difference in ingredients between an expensive and inexpensive product is minor. The charts in this book will enable you to identify cosmetics with similar attributes but very different price categories.

COMPARE COSMETICS PACKAGING

Before the "throwaway" era, many cosmetics were sold in durable containers that the consumer could refill when the product was depleted. Metal lipstick tubes for which refills could be purchased and durable rouge and powder compacts were available. The container would last for months or even years. The initial cost of the durable container and the product was relatively high, but the cost of the refills was very low. The overall result: very little generation of solid waste and very little environmental impact.

Today, most lipsticks, rouges, powders, and other cosmetics are sold in disposable containers. Once the product is used up or found to be stale, the whole package must be thrown out. Lately, some consumers have expressed a need for a return to the refillable, durable containers. Body Shop, Origins, and some other companies have already responded.

The quantity and design features of cosmetics packaging have also become controversial. A tiny amount of eye shadow is often sold in a large, intricately designed plastic case inside a cardboard and film plastic blister pack. In fact, the package is often larger in weight and volume than the cosmetic it contains. Besides generating unnecessary solid waste, the large, intricate containers often cost more. Packaging trade journals talk about the importance of *ambiance*—the role of cosmetics packaging in glamorizing the product and, by extension, the buyer. But such a "total package" generally costs much more than a similar product that is minimally packaged. Consumers should consider whether they are willing to pay for the ambiance as well as the product.

Consumer Reports suggests considering the following package-savvy points before purchasing cosmetics:

• Do not choose a product that is packaged with extras, such as a mirror or compact, that you might not need or want.
• When choosing between cosmetics of equal quality, choose the brand/model with the least amount of packaging.
• When the quantity of packaging is similar, choose the product packaged in recyclable materials, such as cardboard, in favor of nonrecyclable plastic or mixed materials.
• Look for refillable cosmetics containers, which should be entering the market in increasing frequency.

FIND PRODUCTS THAT ARE RIGHT FOR YOUR SKIN

A knowledgeable salesperson can give you some suggestions and introduce you to various colors and lines. Use this book to double-check your information and provide additional facts.

Learn Your Skin Type
The charts in this book group together the products appropriate for each skin type. Determining your skin type is the key to using this book. Chapter 5 tells you how.

The appropriate chart shows many products from the inexpensive to the deluxe brands that are suitable for your type of skin. You should be able to find a "best value" by trying several products from the appropriate chart and zeroing in on the cheapest one that meets your needs.

Find Problem-free Cosmetics
This book contains specific strategies on how to choose products if you tend to get allergic reactions, irritations, or acne. It provides information on how to prevent infections and guard against problems that might occur if certain cosmetic products are used on areas of the body for which they were not formulated.

THE PRODUCT CHARTS

The products chosen to appear on the charts in this book include the nationally advertised and distributed brands that have the largest market share of cosmetic sales as well as many lesser-known brands. Since the market is constantly changing and some brands are only distributed locally, not every product or every brand will be found on these lists.

The charts should provide enough guidance to help you make informed choices about products that do not appear in this book. Read the labels of all products carefully. Any product whose label lists ingredients designated as "Possible Comedogenic Ingredients" (may cause pimples) or "Other Possible Sensitizers" (can cause local irritation or allergic reaction) may cause reactions similar to those caused by products listed in this book.

> Ingredients and brand names change constantly. Be sure to review carefully the package information provided by the manufacturer before using any product.

PRICE CODES

While it is impossible to include specific pricing information for the hundreds of products included in the charts, many of which can be found at discount stores for less than the suggested retail price, the charts do provide price codes. As you look for certain attributes and ingredients, the price codes enable you to compare at a glance the inexpensive, moderately priced, and expensive brands.

Finding safe, appropriate, affordable cosmetics requires knowledge and care. The charts in the following chapters will help you make informed choices.

Price codes are based on a sampling of products from each brand found in a shopping survey done in retail stores in the New York City area.

BRANDS AND PRICE CODES

KEY

A—Inexpensive ($5.00 and under)
B—Moderate ($5.01 to $11.99)
C—Expensive ($12.00 to $19.99)
D—Deluxe ($20.00 and up)

Brand	Code
Adrien Arpel	C
Alexandra de Markoff	D
Allercreme	A
Almay	A, B
Alo Sun	A

Brand	Code
Andrew Jergens	A
Avon	B
Aziza	A
Banana Boat	A
Beecham	A
Beiersdorf (Nivea)	A
Biotherm	C, D
Black Radiance	A
Bonne Bell	A
Chanel	D
Charles of the Ritz	C
Chattem (Bullfrog)	A
Chesebrough Ponds	A
Christian Dior	C, D
Clairol	A
Clarins	C, D
Clarion	A, B
Clinique	C
Colgate Palmolive	A
Color Style (Revlon)	A
Commerce	A
Corn Silk	A
Cosmyl	B
Coty	A
Cover Girl	A
Cutex	A
Dep	A
Dial	A
Doak (Formula 405)	B
Dr. Scholl	A
Dubarry	B
Eboné	A
E. E. Dickinson	A
Elancyl	C, D
Elizabeth Arden	C, D
Erno Laszlo	D
Estee Lauder	C, D
Fashion Fair	C
Finger Mates (Formula 10)	A, B
Flame Glo	A
Flori Roberts	C

Brand	Code
Frances Denney	C
Germaine Monteil	D
Giorgio of Beverly Hills	D
Helene Curtis (Suave)	A
Johnson & Johnson	A, B
Kelmata (Orlane)	C, D
Lancôme	C, D
La Prairie	D
Lever Brothers	A
L'Oreal	B
Mary Kay	B, C
Max Factor	A, B
Maybelline	A
Mennen	A
Merle Norman	B, C, D
Moon Drops (Revlon)	B
Naomi Sims	C, D
Natural Wonder (Revlon)	A
Neutrogena	A, B
Norcliff Thayer	A, B
Noxell	A
Nu Skin	C, D
Oil of Olay	A, B
Orlane	D
Pfeiffer	A
Plough	B
Posner	A
Prescriptives	D

Brand	Code
Princess Marcella Borghese	D
Procter & Gamble	A
Quencher (Sally Hansen)	A
Rachel Perry	C
Revlon	A, B
Richardson Vicks	
(Bain de Soleil)	B
(Clearasil, Wondra Lotion)	A
Ron Ric Hawaiian Tropic	B
Rydell (Aveeno)	A
Sally Hansen	A
S. C. Johnson	A
Shades of You (Maybelline)	A
Shiseido	D
Simply Satin	A
Soft Soap	A
St. Ives	A
Stendhal	D
3-M (Buf)	A
Ultima II	C, D
Warner Lambert	A
West Cabot	A
Westwood (Keri)	A
Wet 'N' Wild	A
Winthrop	A
Yardley	A
Yves Saint Laurent	D

PART TWO

SKIN:
THE FACE

CHAPTER 4

The Skin: Structure, Growth, and Development

In order to discuss how cosmetics and beauty products work, it is helpful to understand the structure of the skin and how it changes at different stages of life.

The skin is the largest organ of the body. In addition to affecting appearance, it serves as an important window on internal disease. Major layers of the skin include the epidermis, the dermis, and the subcutaneous fat layer.

THE EPIDERMIS

The epidermis, the outermost layer of the skin, is a constantly changing blanket of millions of individual skin cells. New cells are continually being formed deep within the epidermis. These cells migrate to the surface as they grow and develop. When skin cells reach the surface, they die and are shed and are replaced by the cells growing in the deeper layers of the epidermis. Products such as abrasive masks and exfoliants are designed to remove dead surface skin cells, which in large numbers can make the skin appear cosmetically dull and lifeless. Since normal skin does not usually retain an excess amount of dead surface skin cells, it is questionable whether abrasive products are successful at giving the skin a more vibrant sheen.

As epidermal skin cells mature and migrate to the skin surface, they produce a material called keratin. Keratin, skin oils, and phospholipids in the epidermis form a barrier to outside substances. The epidermal barrier also helps keep the skin moist by preventing evaporation of water in the skin. When the moisture content in the skin drops below 5 to 10 percent water, the skin becomes dry.

Cosmetically, dry skin will look dull and lifeless. In this state, the skin is prone to becoming itchy, red, and scaly, creating a condition called eczema or dermatitis. Women with dry skin will look their best and have healthier skin when using cosmetics that are moisturizing. Some cosmetics companies have added phospholipids to moisturizing products. However, it has not been shown that these products are better than any other moisturizers.

Melanin

At the deepest layer of the epidermis are cells called melanocytes that produce the

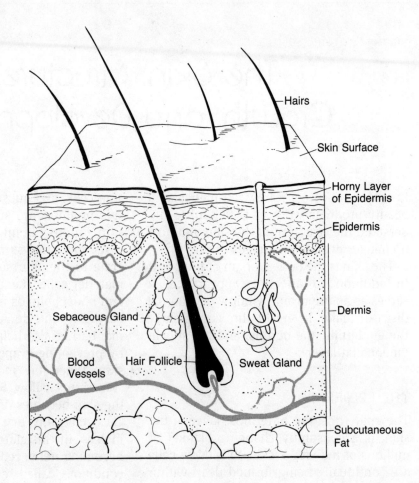

Structure of the skin

melanin responsible for the pigmentation of the skin. Melanocytes are uniformly spaced among the deep epidermal skin cells. Interestingly, black and Caucasian individuals have the same number of melanocytes in the skin. However, in Caucasians the individual granules of melanin are smaller and packaged in bundles rather than dispersed individually.

Moles and Liver Spots

An area of skin that is abnormal is referred to as a skin lesion. Two common examples of pigmented skin lesions are moles and liver spots.

Pigmented nevi is the medical term for moles, collections of pigment-containing cells related to melanocytes. They can be skin colored, reddish, brownish, or black and can be either raised or flat depending on the depth and size of the collection of pigmented cells. Solar lentigo is the medical term for liver spot, a flat, light brown patch on sun-exposed skin. Years of cumulative sun exposure lead to an increased number of melanocytes deep in the epidermis creating a solar lentigo.

THE DERMIS

The dermis is the layer of skin beneath the epidermis that is responsible for providing structural support and elasticity to the skin.

Collagen and Elastin

Collagen is the major structural component of the dermis. In addition to collagen, the dermis contains elastin that gives the skin the ability to stretch and then to return to its original shape. The dermis also is rich in mucopolysaccharides, such as hyaluronic acid. Some cosmetics companies make products that contain hyaluronic acid or other mucopolysaccharides. Although these ingredients may be useful as humectants (water-retaining ingredients) when applied to the skin surface, they consist of molecules that are too large to penetrate down to the dermis to "replenish the skin." These ingredients may be more costly but are probably no better than other humectant ingredients.

> Claims that the addition of collagen or elastin to cosmetics will reverse sun-induced aging of the skin should be met with great skepticism.

As the total amount of sun exposure increases during a lifetime, there is increasing damage to the collagen and elastin of the dermis, and the skin sags and develops wrinkles. Although skin does change with age, much of the sagging and wrinkling that is observed in older people is due to the cumulative effects of the sun. The addition of collagen or elastin to cosmetics to reverse these changes has the same limitations as mucopolysaccharides. These molecules are effective as humectants when deposited on the skin but are too large to penetrate the skin and replenish the dermis. Claims that these ingredients will help reverse sun-induced aging of the skin should be met with great skepticism.

Skin Pores, Sweat Glands, Oil Glands, and Other Structures

The dermis also contains blood vessels, nerves, hair follicles (skin pores), sweat glands, and sebaceous glands (oil glands). In addition, when the skin is irritated or inflamed there may be inflammatory cells present as part of the body's response to the problem.

Sebaceous glands produce skin oils and related substances that prevent drying of the skin caused by evaporation of water. The areas of the body that have the most sebaceous glands have the oiliest skin. Two of the oiliest areas of the body, the scalp and the T-zone of the face (i.e., the forehead and middle of the face), have approximately 400 to 900 sebaceous glands per square centimeter of skin. Oily skin has a greasy and shiny appearance. Many people with oily skin develop plugged skin pores that develop into acne pimples. Therefore, women with oily skin will look their best and have healthier skin when using cosmetics that help to dry out or absorb excess oil.

THE SUBCUTANEOUS FAT

The deepest layer of the skin is the subcutaneous fat layer. It is here that fat is stored. It also contains blood vessels, nerves, deep hair follicles, sweat glands, and sebaceous glands. This layer of the skin is too deep to be affected by the use of existing cosmetics. It is highly unlikely that firming or anticellulite skin-care products can penetrate deep enough to affect the fat layer in any way.

HOW SKIN AGES

Changes occur in the skin as we age. During childhood, the hair follicles and sebaceous glands are small; oily skin and acne are uncommon. During puberty, hormones are produced that cause the sebaceous glands to enlarge and become more active; the skin becomes much oilier and acne becomes more common. As we go through adulthood, the skin becomes a little thinner with each passing year and less effective at holding on to moisture. Thus, the skin becomes drier in most adults after middle age. In addition, women develop much drier skin after menopause since skin oil production drops because of changes in hormone levels. Hormones added to cosmetics are not effective in reversing this problem and may, in fact, have harmful side effects. (See page 13).

PROPER SKIN CARE

It is important to wash your face for cleanliness. However, washing too frequently may irritate your skin. Washing your face twice daily with either warm or cold water and an appropriate cleanser should be sufficient to clean the skin thoroughly so that you can wear makeup every day without clogging the pores.

If you have dry skin, you might want to use a moisturizer after washing. If you have oily skin and want to use a moisturizer, choose an oil-free product.

Skin Care for Older Women

Skin generally becomes less oily with increasing age. Although the same general principles of skin care apply to all age groups, oilier moisturizers and cosmetics are often needed as age increases. However, there are always exceptions. Some women continue to have oily skin well into adulthood. These women may experience adult acne or rosacea and will need to use oil-free cosmetics (usually designed for younger people) on areas of oily skin.

CHAPTER 5

Skin Types

THE IMPORTANCE OF SKIN TYPE

Skin type is the single most important piece of information needed to select cosmetics properly. The major skin types are oily, normal, and dry. When cosmetics manufactured for a specific skin type are used on a different skin type, they can cause irritation and other skin problems, as well as detract from appearance.

DETERMINING SKIN TYPE

It is easy to estimate the oiliness of the skin and determine your skin type. Wash your face with a nonmoisturizing soap (such as Neutrogena or Purpose), wait several hours, then hold a separate small piece of eyeglass lens-cleaning paper to each region of the face (forehead, nose, chin, cheeks, and lower and upper eyelids) for 10 seconds. The paper will show little oil when applied to dry areas and will be oily when applied to oily areas. On normal skin, the pieces of paper held to the T-zone areas (forehead, nose, sides of nose, chin) will be oily, whereas the paper applied to other areas of the face will show less oil. The eyelids will be the least oily. On oily skin, the paper from all areas (except the eyelids) will be oily; on dry skin, the paper from all areas will be dry.

Skin type changes at various stages of life. It is therefore necessary to retest the skin periodically to ensure that changes in skin type have not occurred and that new cosmetics are not needed. Skin type may also change at different seasons of the year—often becoming drier in winter—so you may have to use different skin-care products, depending on the season.

Combination Skin

In a strict sense, all women have combination skin, but the cosmetics industry uses a more narrow definition of the term. The areas in the T-zone (the forehead, on and around the nose, and the mid-chin) are always oilier than the rest of the face, because the T-zone contains the largest concentration of oil glands. The majority of women between puberty and menopause have what is called "normal skin type," in which the skin is slightly oily in the T-zone and slightly dry on the rest of the face. The cosmetics industry calls this type of skin "combination skin" because there are both oily and dry facial areas. Using this defi-

> Skin type changes at various stages of life and even at different seasons of the year.

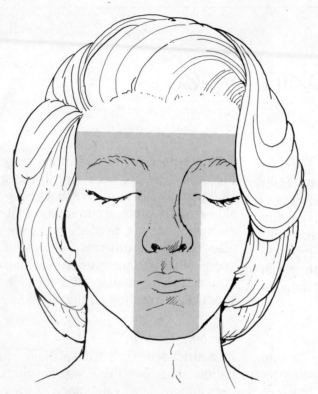

"T-Zone" of the face

nition, "combination skin type" and "normal skin type" are identical and are used interchangeably throughout this book.

Oily or Dry Skin
There are people in whom the entire face is either predominantly oilier or drier than the average face. These people are said to have "oily skin type" or "dry skin type." Although some young women have dry skin, it is much more common in post-menopausal women.

Oily Skin and Acne
Although many young women have "normal" skin, a large number of young women have oilier than average skin. Many, but not all, of these women have problems with acne (pimples). Acne almost always occurs on oily skin, and under most circumstances it is safe to assume the skin is oily in areas where there is acne. It is possible that other areas of the face that do not have acne, such as the region around the eyes, may be much drier. Oil is not the only factor in the development of acne, how-

ever, and not all women with oily skin have acne.

Flaky Facial Skin and Seborrheic Dermatitis

Many women who actually have oily skin believe that they have dry skin that requires a moisturizer. One common cause for this misconception is seborrheic dermatitis, a condition caused by excess oil production and characterized by red scaly skin on the facial T-zone, the scalp, or other oily skin regions of the body. The affected skin will be red, irritated, and scaly and may feel as if it is dry—symptoms that easily lead to an incorrect diagnosis of dry skin. However, since seborrheic dermatitis is an oily condition, oily moisturizers applied to these areas will only aggravate the problem.

CHAPTER 6

Types of Cosmetics and Skin-Care Products

Once you have determined your skin type, you need to find the right cosmetics. The old adage about how dermatologists take care of the skin—"If it's wet, dry it and if it's dry, wet it"—is surprisingly accurate when it comes to choosing cosmetics and skin-care products. Women with oily skin should use products to dry the skin, and women with dry skin should moisturize it. In this way, the skin will be closer to the mean or ideal (neither oily nor dry) and will look its best cosmetically. Four types of products are used to affect the moisture of the skin.

Water-free   Water-in-oil   Oil-in-water   Oil-free
more moisturizing ← → less moisturizing

WATER-FREE PRODUCTS

Water-free products contain oils, fats, and other lipids but no water. They are very moisturizing because they form a thick barrier on the skin that prevents water loss. The lipids in these products also repair faulty skin barrier function and recondition the skin lipids in the epidermis. However, they are very greasy ointments and oils that will usually feel unpleasant except on extremely dry skin. Examples of water-free products include petroleum jelly, water-proof foundations, and many foundations marketed for cover-up.

WATER-IN-OIL PRODUCTS

Water-in-oil products are oil-based creams and lotions that contain some water. They are less moisturizing and less greasy than water-free products but are still very strong moisturizers. Water-in-oil products are designed for moderately dry skin. Most cold creams are water-in-oil products. Another example is oil-based foundation.

OIL-IN-WATER PRODUCTS

Oil-in-water products are the opposite of water-in-oil products. They are water-based creams and lotions that contain some oil. They are less moisturizing and less greasy than water-in-oil products and are mild moisturizers. Oil-in-water products are designed for normal to slightly dry skin. Water-based foundation makeups, regular mascaras, and most light moisturizers are examples.

OIL-FREE PRODUCTS

The term *oil-free* is not as simple as it seems. All oil-free products are free of most ingredients that contain the word *oil* (mineral oil). However, the names of many oils and fats do not contain the word *oil* (glyceryl tribehenate, lard, lanolin). In addition, waxes (carnauba and ozokerite) and oily hydrocarbons (petrolatum and squalene) are similar to oils in many ways. They should probably not be included but are often found in products labeled oil-free. In this book, only products devoid of all the above-mentioned ingredients are classified as oil-free.

This book further subdivides oil-free products into two groups. The first group includes strictly oil-free products. The second group includes borderline oil-free products that contain lipid ingredients called *emollient esters;* these products contain ingredients that act somewhat like oils.

Fragrance ingredients called essential oils (clove oil, lemon oil) do not behave like other oils and are included in products designated as oil-free. Lipids that do not appear to aggravate acne (fatty acids, fatty alcohols, and sterols) and occlusive silicone derivatives are also included in oil-free products. Occlusive silicone derivatives act as moisturizing ingredients by preventing evaporation of water and are unlikely to aggravate acne since they are not lipids.

Solutions and Gels

Strictly oil-free products are usually solutions or gels. They are designed primarily for oily skin but can sometimes be used on other skin types.

A solution consists of a substance dissolved in a large amount of liquid (usually alcohol, water, propylene glycol, and/or glycerin). Alcohol solutions are very drying because they evaporate rapidly, whereas water solutions are only mildly drying because water evaporates more slowly. Alcohol solutions are most useful for oily skin and may be quite irritating to dry skin. Water solutions are best used on oily or normal skin. Skin toners are solutions that contain large quantities of alcohol, whereas skin refiners are predominantly water solutions.

Gels are clear, non-oily, semiviscous solid products usually consisting of cellulose or substances called carbomers dissolved in a small amount of solvent (water, alcohol, or acetone). They are usually mildly drying because the solvent evaporates and are most useful for oily and normal skin.

On the other hand, alcohol-free solutions and gels that contain a large amount of propylene glycol or glycerin are mildly moisturizing because these ingredients behave as humectants (non-oily moisturizing ingredients). These products are usable on all types of skin.

THE EFFECTS OF ALCOHOLS ON DRY SKIN

Many women with dry skin know that simple alcohols (ethanol, methanol, isopropyl) are drying; these women usually read product ingredient labels to avoid purchasing or using one that contains alcohol. However, the fatty alcohols used in cosmetic products are moisturizing, not drying, and do not need to be avoided by women with dry skin. Fatty alcohols include caprylic, cetearyl, cetyl, decyl, isocetyl, isostearyl, lauryl, myristyl, oleyl, and stearyl alcohols.

THE EFFECTS OF HUMECTANTS

A humectant is a non-oily ingredient that helps the skin hold on to water. A humectant will make a product more moisturizing than it would otherwise be. Humectants can be added to oil-free gels and solutions to increase their moisturizing ability to the extent that they behave as mild moisturizers. In fact, this is how oil-free moisturizers are made. Humectants added to relatively mildly moisturizing oil-in-water products make their moisturizing ability equal to that of much greasier products. A few of the most effective humectants for this purpose currently on the market are lactic acid, glycolic acid, and urea. Because they are effective and pleasant to use, moisturizers with significant amounts of these humectants are often recommended by dermatologists for patients with dry skin. However, products containing these ingredients may sting when applied to cracks or fissures that often accompany dry skin.

THE EFFECTS OF POWDERS

Powders are ingredients that make a product more drying than it would otherwise be, because the powder will absorb water and oil. A plain loose powder is a drying product useful for people with oily skin. Oil-containing lotions, creams, or sticks that have powder added are less moistur-

> A humectant is a non-oily ingredient that helps the skin hold on to water. The addition of a humectant will make a product more moisturizing.

izing than those that do not contain powder. If enough powder is added to an otherwise moisturizing product, it can behave like a mildly drying product. For example, certain cakes of pressed powder containing oil may behave as mildly drying products.

Talc

Talc is widely used in compact makeups because it can easily be compressed into a pressed powder cake, it spreads easily, feels smooth, has a bright white color, and can easily be converted into products in a variety of colors.

Concerns were voiced in the early 1970s that talc usage might be associated with an increased risk of cancer. Talc used prior to 1972 was often contaminated with asbestos, but recent regulations require that products contain no detectable asbestos fibers. Nevertheless, there is circumstantial evidence that talc itself may, under certain circumstances, be associated with an increased risk of cancer. Women's use of talcum powder as a dusting powder on the genital area, for example, has been suspected of being associated with an increased risk of ovarian cancer. However, there are almost no reports of adverse effects from the use of talc-containing cosmetics, and the current belief is that these products are completely safe.

COSMETICS FOR WOMEN OF COLOR

Women of color need to use bright colors of blusher, eye makeup, lipstick, and nail polish to achieve a noticeable effect. Moreover, dark skin introduces color shades into the makeup equation that are rarely factors in the tonal variations of light skin. Cosmetics companies must therefore make a wider variety of products to match the subtle skin shades of women of color properly.

Color is the only difference in cosmetics designed for dark skin. All other aspects of composition and proper use of cosmetics apply equally to products for dark or light skin.

Several companies specialize in cosmetics for African-American women and other women of color. Products made by Color Magic, Eboné, Fashion Fair, Flori Roberts, Honey and Spice, Mahogany Image, Montaj, Naomi Sims, Posner, and Simply Satin are evaluated in each section of this book. Some of the larger cosmetics companies are now expanding to provide cosmetics suitable for women with dark skin. In some cases, these cosmetics will be designated with a separate line such as Color Style (Revlon), Black Radiance (Pavion), and Shades of You (Maybelline). When not certain, a salesperson can probably tell you

> Color is the only difference in cosmetics designed for dark skin. All other aspects of composition and proper use of cosmetics apply equally to products for dark or light skin.

whether a particular company produces dark makeup colors.

Special Concerns for African-American Women

Dry dark skin may have a grayish appearance because of the dull effect created by light reflecting off dry scale. This problem can be corrected by using a proper moisturizer.

Women with dark skin are much less likely to develop sunburn, sun-related skin damage (such as wrinkles or discoloration), and skin cancer than are women who have light skin. Most women of color will not need to be concerned with sunscreen products unless they have relatively light skin.

However, women with dark skin can occasionally develop skin cancers. The most serious of the common skin cancers is melanoma, which may be very aggressive. Melanoma is most apt to appear on the lighter pigmented skin of the palms, soles, and nailbeds of African-Americans.

Cosmetics for
Skin with Acne

The medical name for pimples is *acne*. Viewed most simply, acne pimples occur when plugs form in the pores (follicles) of the skin. Shallow pimples such as blackheads and whiteheads are called *comedones;* deeper pimples are referred to as *papules, pustules,* and *cysts.* Deep, inflamed pimples can leave permanent scars; however, a discussion of the causes of acne is beyond the scope of this book.

ACNE AND SKIN TYPE

Acne occurs predominantly on oily skin. Oil is an important factor in the development of pimples. Women with acne-prone skin should choose oil-free products that decrease oil or help dry out the skin. Acne is often aggravated by oily products that make the skin even more oily.

NONCOMEDOGENIC PRODUCTS

Many products and product ingredients have been tested by the manufacturers to determine if they are noncomedogenic. Comedogenic refers to the ability of a product or ingredient to create comedones (blackhead or whitehead pimples) either on normal rabbit ears in the laboratory or in actual use on people without acne. The term *comedogenic* is starting to be replaced by *acnegenic,* which refers to the ability of a product to cause any type of pimple, not just comedones.

Unfortunately, the fact that a product does not create acne on normal rabbit ears or skin free of acne does not mean that it will not aggravate skin with acne. A product labeled noncomedogenic does not mean it is necessarily desirable to use when acne is already present. Studies are needed that test products in actual use on persons with acne to determine whether or not the products aggravate the condition. This has not yet been done for most products.

CHOOSING COSMETICS FOR
USE WITH ACNE

Because of the wide variety of available cosmetics, there is almost always a choice among a number of products. A woman with acne should not choose products that contain oils or ingredients that have been found to be comedogenic. Products with these ingredients *are certainly more likely* to be aggravating to acne than products

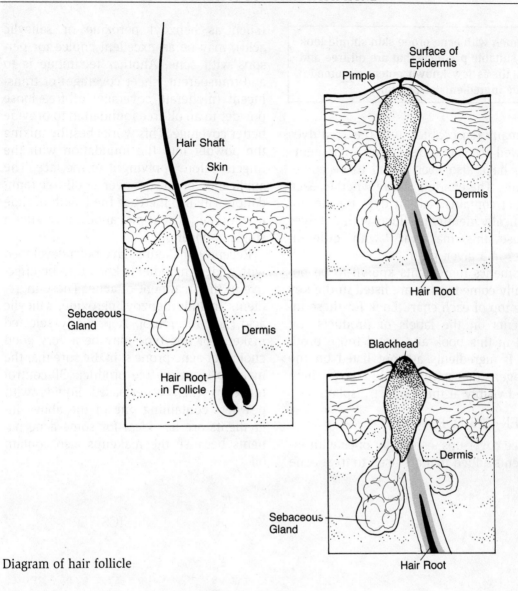

Diagram of hair follicle

without these ingredients. It is recommended that women with acne-prone skin look for suitable products that are oil-free and contain as few known potentially co-medogenic ingredients as possible. The charts in this book include information on whether products contain oil or possible comedogenic ingredients. Keep in mind

> Women with acne-prone skin should look for suitable products that are oil-free and contain as few known potential comedogenic ingredients as possible.

that many red coal tar dyes (i.e., red dyes followed by a number on an ingredients label) have also been found to be comedogenic. The charts indicate whether each product contains coal tar dyes but do not specifically identify products with red dyes because this may vary with different shades in a given product.

Cosmetics ingredients known to be potentially comedogenic are listed in the key at the top of each chart. Look for these ingredients on the labels of products not listed in this book and avoid those products. If ingredients are not listed on the package, the store should have them posted visibly at the product display.

COVER-UPS FOR ACNE

Oil-free cover-ups, especially ones with ingredients added that are used to treat acne (such as benzoyl peroxide or salicylic acid), may be an excellent choice for persons with acne. Another technique is to add transparent (sheer coverage) or translucent (moderate coverage) oil-free loose powder to an oil-free foundation to provide better coverage. This works best by mixing the powder into the foundation with the fingers before applying it to the face. The application of powder over an oil-free foundation will also increase the length of time it will retain its optimal appearance after a single application.

Recently, makeups have been developed with added ingredients known to be effective in the treatment of acne. These ingredients include benzoyl peroxide, salicylic acid, and resorcinol. A properly selected makeup of this type may be a very good choice for acne-prone skin. Be sure that the makeup is an oil-free product. Oil-control makeups (i.e., water-based liquids with powder) containing one of the above ingredients are not ideal for some acne patients because the makeups also contain oil.

Cosmetics for
Sensitive or Allergic Skin

Many women are unable to tolerate certain cosmetics. Reactions usually take the form of red, swollen, itchy skin with or without small blisters. Not all of these reactions, however, are allergic reactions. Many adverse reactions are caused by irritation rather than allergy. A true allergy, called *allergic contact dermatitis,* occurs when sensitivity develops to a specific ingredient that does not cause a reaction in most other people. If this ingredient can be identified, the problem can be solved by using alternative products that do not contain the offending ingredient.

IRRITANT REACTIONS
TO COSMETICS

An irritant reaction may look almost identical to an allergic reaction but has very different implications. An irritant is an ingredient that will cause a reaction on the skin of most people if they are exposed to enough of the substance. Some individuals have very sensitive skin that becomes irritated by relatively small amounts of a variety of irritating substances. In addition, inflamed skin such as occurs with eczema will be much more prone to irritant reactions. These reactions are much more difficult to avoid than allergic reactions because no single substance causes the problem. Finding a usable product is a trial-and-error proposition and sometimes there may not be an acceptable alternative product.

Products Likely to Cause Irritant Reactions
Irritant reactions are more common to soaps, detergents, shampoos, deodorants, antiperspirants, eye makeups, and bubble baths than are allergic reactions to the same products. Allergic and irritant reactions are both fairly common to moisturizers, permanent hair dyes, and hair permanent-wave products.

Products containing possible allergenic ingredients need to be avoided only if you are experiencing allergic reactions to cosmetics. A potential allergenic ingredient is harmless to a person not allergic to that ingredient.

ALLERGIC REACTIONS TO COSMETICS

Allergic contact dermatitis, a common problem seen by dermatologists, occurs when sensitivity develops to a specific ingredient that does not cause a reaction in most other people. The exact incidence of contact allergy to cosmetics is difficult to determine because many cases are never reported.

A group of dermatologists studied 13,216 people with suspected contact dermatitis and determined the percentage of these cases caused by cosmetics. When these people were tested, 713 allergic reactions to cosmetics were discovered. That is, approximately 5.4 percent of patients seen with contact dermatitis were found to be allergic to cosmetics (Adams and Maibach).

Cosmetics Ingredients Most Likely to Cause Allergic Reactions

Of the 713 allergic reactions in the Adams and Maibach study, 538 were analyzed according to causative agent. The results are listed in the following table. The ingredients listed in the table are labeled "possible sensitizers" in the charts contained in this book.

ANALYSIS OF 538 COSMETIC ALLERGIC REACTIONS BY CAUSATIVE AGENT

Agent	Reactions
fragrance	161
quaternium-15	65
paraphenylenediamine	41
lanolin derivatives, wool wax, or wool alcohol	29
propylene glycol	25
glyceryl thioglycolate (in permanent-wave products)	25
toluene sulfonamide/ formaldehyde resin	23
imidazolidinyl urea	21
sunscreens	20
parabens	19
formaldehyde	19
bronopol (2-bromo-2- nitropropane-1,3 diol)	16
sorbic acid	6
other substances with <3 reactions	62

Fragrance and Fragrance-Free Products

Fragrance is found in a wide variety of cosmetic products. It is obvious from the table above that fragrance is responsible for relatively large numbers of allergic reactions to cosmetics. This is partially because fragrance is not a single ingredient but a generic name given to a large number of individual fragrance ingredients. Individual ingredients in fragrance are usually not listed on ingredients labels. However, products without fragrance will often be labeled "fragrance-free." Products labeled "unscented" are not the same as fragrance-free, because they may contain masking fragrance designed to eliminate odors from ingredients used to make the product.

Essential Oils

Ingredients called essential oils are derived from plants and used to add scent to cosmetics. Oils, as well as parts, extracts, and resins of these plants, may cause allergic reactions in anyone allergic to fragrance. These ingredients are often listed by name on the product ingredient list. The presence of essential oils in cosmetic products is indicated in the charts in this book.

The following is a partial list of commonly used essential-oil plants.

anise	lime
balm mint	lovage
bay	mandarin
bergamot	matricaria
bitter almond	nutmeg
calendula	*Ocotea cymbarum*
camellia	orange
caraway	parsley seed
cardamom	peppermint
carrot	pine
chamomile	pine tar
cinnamon	primrose
clove	rose
cloveleaf	rosemary
coriander	rue
eucalyptus	sage
geranium	sambucus
ginger	sandalwood
grapefruit	sassafras
henna	spearmint
hops	sweet marjoram
ivy	tar
lavender	tea tree
lemon	vanilla
lemon grass	yarrow
lily	

Preservatives

Quaternium-15 is a preservative found in many cosmetics. People may be allergic to the substance itself, and those who are allergic to formaldehyde can potentially have problems with this ingredient.

Recently, it has been found that quaternium-15 can react in the body with other chemicals to produce nitrosamines, known carcinogens (substances able to cause cancer). However, it is not clear whether or not enough quaternium-15 can be absorbed through the skin for the carcinogen-producing reaction to occur.

At the present time, parabens (methylparaben, ethylparaben, butylparaben, etc.) are the most common cosmetics preservatives, currently found in the vast majority of cosmetic products. Given the prevalence of parabens, there are relatively few allergic reactions to these substances and almost all occur on inflamed or cracked skin. This has been called the "paraben paradox."

Formaldehyde is a preservative in some cosmetics and is often present in shampoos. Persons who are allergic to formaldehyde may also have problems with quaternium-15, imidazolidinyl urea, diazolidinyl urea, 2-bromo-2-nitropropane-1,3 diol (bronopol), DMDM hydantoin, 5-bromo-5-nitro-1,3 dioxane (bromidox), or tris (hydromethyl) nitromethane.

Imidazolidinyl urea and the related substance diazolidinyl urea are preservatives found in many cosmetics and can cause allergic reactions. These substances can also release formaldehyde, creating potential problems for people allergic to formaldehyde.

Bronopol, or 2-bromo-2-nitropropane-1,3 diol, is a less common preservative used in some cosmetic products. People who are allergic to formaldehyde can potentially have problems with this ingredient.

Sorbic acid is a common cosmetics preservative that occasionally causes allergic reactions. People allergic to sorbic acid may also react to a related ingredient called potassium sorbate. Sorbic acid is also frequently used as a preservative in contact lens solutions.

Two newer cosmetics preservatives that have been used in Europe for some time but have only recently been introduced into products in this country are methylchloroisothiazolinone and methylisothiazolinone (collectively referred to as Kathon CG). These ingredients have been responsible for numerous allergic reactions in Europe. However, in this country, they have been used in lower concentrations and have not yet been found to be a major cause of contact allergy. The newest preservative system found in cosmetics, euxyl K 400, is a combination of phenoxyethanol and methyldibromoglutaronitrile. Although the latter ingredient has caused documented cases of allergic contact dermatitis, it is still too soon to tell if allergy to this preservative will turn out to be a significant problem.

OTHER POSSIBLE ALLERGENIC INGREDIENTS

Paraphenylenediamine (ppd) is found in permanent hair dyes. Approximately 25 percent of people who are allergic to ppd will also be unable to tolerate semipermanent hair dyes since these products may contain some closely related ingredients. Reactions to ppd can usually be avoided by the use of temporary hair dyes. However, anyone allergic to ppd may also react to similar chemicals such as PABA and its derivatives (found in sunscreens) or benzocaine (found in skin anesthetics such as sunburn medications).

Lanolin and wool wax are complex substances found in moisturizers and other moisturizing cosmetics. Most allergic reactions are to the alcohol fraction of these substances. Therefore, anyone allergic to lanolin should avoid products with any of the following ingredients: lanolin, wool wax, lanolin alcohol, or wool wax alcohol.

Propylene glycol is a versatile ingredient that is both a solvent and a humectant. It can occasionally be an irritant that stings when applied to inflamed or cracked skin. Irritant and allergic reactions to propylene glycol occur more frequently on skin with eczema. It can occasionally cause true allergic reactions.

Glyceryl thioglycolate is found in hair permanent-wave or "perming" products and can cause allergic reactions.

Toluene sulfonamide/formaldehyde resin is found in nail polish. Some polishes use polyester resin instead of formaldehyde resin; these polishes can be used by people who are allergic.

Sunscreen ingredients that can cause allergic contact dermatitis include PABA, PABA derivatives, benzophenone, cinnamates, and avobenzone (butylmethoxydibenzoylmethane). Many people are allergic to PABA (para-aminobenzoic acid) and its derivatives, glyceryl PABA and octyl dimethyl PABA (also called Padimate O). People allergic to PABA should avoid products containing all these ingredients. Unfortunately, there are products on the market that claim to be PABA-free but contain PABA derivatives. Read the label carefully.

The benzophenones, which include oxybenzone and dioxybenzone, have also caused allergic reactions. In fact, allergic reactions to benzophenones are now more common than allergic reactions to PABA. There are numerous cases of people allergic to benzophenones who assumed they were allergic to PABA. They switched to another PABA-free sunscreen only to experience an allergic reaction from benzophenones contained in the substitute product.

Cinnamates (including cinoxate) are occasional photosensitizers. This means that they can cause allergic reactions when the product is worn in the sun. Since sunscreens are designed to be worn in the sun, allergic reactions caused by cinnamates will appear identical to the types seen with PABA, PABA derivatives, and benzophenones. People allergic to cinnamates will often react to some perfumes, flavorings, and toothpastes.

Sunscreen ingredients are also found in many other cosmetic products, including foundations, pressed powders, anti-aging products, lip and nail products, moisturizers, and toners. If you are allergic or sensitive to any of the ingredients mentioned, avoid them in all cosmetic products.

Some other ingredients that sporadically cause allergic reactions are PEG 200-400, butylated hydroxyanisole or hydroxytoluene (BHA or BHT), vitamin E (tocopherol or tocopherol acetate), captan, rosin (colophony), thimerosol, propyl gallate, di-tert-butyl hydroquinone, dihydroabietyl alcohol, bismuth oxychloride, benzalkonium chloride, chlorhexidine, benzoin, chloroxylenol, phenylmercuric acetate, trietha-nolamine, cetyl alcohol, urea-formaldehyde resin, and stearyl alcohol.

Coal tar colors in cosmetics (especially reds and yellows) can occasionally cause allergic reactions; however, the specific dyes used often vary from shade to shade in a given product. Therefore, the charts in this book contain a column that indicates products containing coal tar dyes but not which specific dyes are present.

FINDING YOUR OWN SAFE PRODUCTS

Hypoallergenic Products

Hypoallergenic products do not cause allergic reactions in a large percentage of the population. However, cosmetics companies generally do not use chemicals that are likely to cause allergic reactions. Therefore, by this definition, all cosmetics are hypoallergenic. It is possible to have an allergic reaction to a hypoallergenic product. Also, it is possible to become allergic to a product used safely for many years in the past. Hypoallergenic does not mean *non*allergenic! In fact, products that claim to be hypoallergenic may or may not be less allergenic than ones that do not make this claim. Hypoallergenic products are usually, but not always, fragrance-free, because fragrance is the most frequent cause of allergic reaction to cosmetics.

"Allergy-Tested" and "Dermatologist-Tested" Products

Testing of products by cosmetics companies is to be commended because it is voluntary. However, adjectives such as "allergy-tested" and "dermatologist-tested" are meaningless because they do not indicate how well a product fared when it was tested! Furthermore, the testing may range from sophisticated laboratory tests to merely mailing product samples to dermatologists and then asking their opinions.

While cosmetics chemists are very sophisticated and nearly all marketed cosmetics are unlikely to cause large numbers of bad reactions, almost all cosmetics require preservatives and other ingredients that will cause allergic reactions in a small number of individuals.

Switching Cosmetics Brands
It is important to realize that different products produced by the same company usually have very different ingredients. Women experiencing allergic reactions will often be confronted by cosmetics salespeople who will claim that the problem can best be solved by switching brands of cosmetics. This approach is not likely to be helpful. There may very well be alternative products made by the same company that do not contain the ingredient responsible for the allergic reaction. Alternatively, it is quite possible to choose products made by

a new company that contain the ingredient responsible for the allergic reaction.

Choosing Cosmetics When
Allergy Is Suspected
See the charts in this book for possible allergenic ingredients in the product (or products) suspected of causing an allergic reaction. Next, look for alternative products that do not contain any of the same potentially allergenic ingredients. If the suspect product was causing an allergic reaction, an alternative product chosen in this manner will often be tolerated well.

Obtaining Help from a Dermatologist
A dermatologist can often help identify the cause of a reaction to cosmetics and can provide suggestions to help solve the problem. The dermatologist may suggest a procedure called patch testing, which can often identify the offending substance. Cosmetics patch testing involves placing small amounts of suspected cosmetics or cosmetic ingredients onto metal or plastic chambers that are attached with tape to the patient's back. After 48 to 72 hours, the dermatologist removes the test materials and examines the sites. A positive reaction shows redness and sometimes swelling or blisters.

Dermatologists are the doctors most likely to have specific expertise in patch testing for allergic contact dermatitis. Allergists specialize in identifying allergic reactions to inhaled substances. Most nondermatologists who offer patch testing usually offer only the most rudimentary type.

> Testing of products by cosmetics companies is commendable because it is voluntary. However, adjectives such as "allergy-tested" and "dermatologist-tested" are meaningless because they do not indicate how well a product fared when it was tested.

Avoiding Products that List
"and Other Ingredients"
The expression "and other ingredients" means that the ingredients list does not include all ingredients contained in the product. Since it is not clear what these products contain, they are best avoided by anyone who has had an adverse reaction to a cosmetic product.

CHAPTER 9

Foundation Makeups, Powders, Bronzers, Self-Tanners, and Makeup Removers

HOW TO USE FOUNDATION

Foundation is the base makeup used to improve the appearance of facial skin. The color of the makeup should match skin color as closely as possible when viewed in natural sunlight. Most experts suggest matching makeup color to the skin color at the jawline or throat. For oily skin, it may be necessary to choose makeup one shade lighter than the skin color, because makeup (especially oil-free products) may turn darker when applied to the skin as it mixes with skin oils. However, a makeup one shade darker than the skin color will provide superior cover-up.

Foundation should be applied to the face with the fingers and then smoothed with a sponge. To avoid the possibility of infec-

> To avoid the possibility of infection, never use a friend's sponge to apply makeup. When testing makeup in a store, be sure to use a new applicator/sponge.

tion, never use a friend's sponge to apply makeup. When testing makeup in a store, be sure to use a new applicator/sponge. If there is none available, try the product on your arm or wrist, but be aware the match may not be as accurate as if it had been tried on the face.

Using Regular Foundation and Concealer near the Eyes or on the Lips

Some women use regular foundation makeup near the eyes or on the lips instead of products specifically designed for use in these areas, such as eye shadow setting creams or lip sealants. It is important to know that some foundations contain coal tar colors and are not safe for use near the eyes because they contain carcinogens or can cause blindness. Also, some coal tar colors cannot be used on the lips. The charts in this book indicate which products contain coal tar colors.

Concealers do not usually contain coal tar colors and can be used anywhere

> Some foundations contain coal tar colors and are not safe for use near the eyes or on the lips.

needed for cover-up. However, it is still wise to examine the ingredients list before purchasing a concealer to make sure it does not contain coal tar colors.

*Coal Tar Colors and Where
They Can Be Used Safely*
Coal tar colors will be found on the ingredients label and will begin with the abbreviation FD&C (e.g., FD&C Red #3) or D&C (e.g., D&C Red #7). Never use products containing coal tar colors near the eyes— such usage may be potentially carcinogenic (may lead to development of cancer) or even cause blindness.

Although some coal tar colors are safe to use on the lips, products with ingredients containing the abbreviations D&C and Ext. (e.g., Ext. D&C Violet #2) should not be used there. Also, products stating "external use only" should not be used on the lips.

Other ingredients use a color as part of the ingredient name, such as ultramarine blue, manganese violet, and carmine. If these color ingredients do not contain a number in their name, they are not coal tar colors and are probably safe for use on the eyelids or lips.

TYPES OF FOUNDATION MAKEUPS

It is important to know your skin type (see Chapter 5) to choose optimal makeup products. The chart below will help you quickly locate the type of foundation that is best for your skin type.

Type of Foundation	Skin Type	Class of Product	Moisturization	Usual Duration	Finish
water-free	very dry	water-free	extremely high	usually full day	shiny
oil-based	dry	water-in-oil	high	half to full day	shiny
water-based or oil control	slightly dry to normal	oil-in-water	moderate	up to half day	semimatte
oil-free	slightly dry to oily	oil-free	slight to drying	couple of hours to half day	matte, semimatte
pressed or loose powder (with oil)	dry to normal	powder plus oil	moderate to none	usually full day	matte
pressed or loose powder (oil-free)	normal to oily	powder	slight to drying	up to full day	matte

Water-free Foundations

Water-free foundations contain predominantly oils but no water. These products are very oily or waxy, are extremely moisturizing, and are designed for the very dry skin that is common in older women. Water-free products are not usually the first choice for normal skin because they will feel too oily. They are not advised for oily skin and may aggravate acne. Nevertheless, these products do have several desirable characteristics that can be successfully used for moderately dry or normal skin. First, they are often called "waterproof makeup" or "workout makeup" because they usually will not smear when a user perspires during exercise. In addition, they are very thick (and often opaque) and will hide skin color irregularities and flat scars. However, they should not be used on depressed scars or deep wrinkles because their shininess will draw attention to such defects.

Water-free makeups are usually creams or sticks. Sticks are simply creams made more solid by adding wax to the product. Water-free foundations are very stable and will usually last all day with one application. They are also slow drying and usually have a shiny finish caused by their large oil content.

Oil-based Foundations

Oil-based foundations are water-in-oil products that contain predominantly oil but also some water. These products are somewhat less oily than water-free foundations. They are not quite as moisturizing as water-free foundations but are still strongly moisturizing and are usually best for dry skin. They can be used on normal skin but are not advised for oily skin or acne.

Oil-based foundations may be creams, liquids, or soufflés (i.e., whipped creams). They are fairly stable and will usually last from about half a day to all day with one application. These products are slow drying and therefore easy to apply. Oil-based foundations usually have a shiny finish. A duller finish can be achieved by using powder over these foundations.

Water-based Foundations

Water-based foundations are oil-in-water products that contain mostly water but also some oil. These products are mildly oily, moderately moisturizing, and are usually best for normal or slightly dry skin. They can be used on other types of skin but are not usually the first choice. That is, for dry skin, oilier makeups moisturize better, are easier to apply, and wear longer than water-based foundations. Similarly, for oily skin, oil-free foundations are less likely to aggravate acne and will wear longer without showing saturation from facial oils. Color drift sometimes occurs with these products. If this happens, an oil-free foundation primer can be used to minimize this problem.

Water-based foundations may be creams, liquids, soufflés, or mousses (aerosol liquid). Mousse is very sheer, provides less coverage, and requires more frequent application; only a thin layer of makeup is sprayed onto the palm of the hand and then applied to the face. Usually, water-

Although some products clearly contain more water than oil, this cannot always be determined accurately from the ingredients label. The total amount of several oily ingredients may exceed the amount of water present even if water is listed as the primary ingredient.

based foundations will only last up to about half a day at optimal appearance with one application. These products dry more quickly than oilier foundations and must be applied with more skill to avoid uneven coverage as the product dries. They usually have a semimatte (medium) finish. Women with normal to slightly dry skin can use oilier products for a shinier look or oil-free products for a duller look.

Keep in mind that although some products on the market clearly contain more water than oil, this cannot always be determined accurately from the ingredients label. This is because the total amount of several oily ingredients may exceed the amount of water present in a product even if water is listed as the primary ingredient. Therefore, it is possible that some of the makeups listed as water-based may actually be oil-based products. For most people, this should not present problems. How-

ever, women with oilier skin are better off using oil-free products.

Oil-free Foundations

Oil-free foundations may be slightly moisturizing to drying. Some oil-free products contain emollient esters and are best for slightly dry to slightly oily skin. Other products are strictly oil-free and are the best choice for very oily skin or acne.

Oil-free foundations are liquids. Some require shaking to disperse the powder in the product evenly and are referred to as *shake lotions*. These products tend to cover the skin less evenly than the oil-free products that require less shaking. Oil-free foundations generally last from a couple of hours to about half a day at optimal appearance with one application. They may become significantly darker in color when applied to the face as they combine with skin oils; consequently, oil-free foundations should be one shade lighter than actual skin color. These products dry quickly and should be applied on one area of the face at a time so that they do not dry before properly applied. Oil-free products have a dull matte or semimatte (medium) finish. There is really no appropriate foundation with a shiny finish for oily skin.

Chart 9–1
FOUNDATION MAKEUPS

The charts are designed to help you minimize adverse reactions and choose products with the proper oil content for your skin type. If you have cosmetics-related acne, you should also choose products with the least amounts of potentially comedogenic ingredients.

Although most cosmetics contain potentially sensitizing ingredients, there is no reason to avoid any ingredient unless you are experiencing adverse reactions to cosmetic products. If you know you are allergic to certain ingredients, the charts will show you which products to avoid. If you are experiencing reactions to a certain cosmetic product, the charts can help you select alternative products that do not contain the same potentially sensitizing ingredients. To choose new products that are least likely to cause allergic reactions, keep in mind that fragrance is by far the most frequent cause of allergic reactions to cosmetics, followed by ingredients listed as "possible sensitizers." The ingredients listed as "other possible sensitizers" cause allergic reactions less frequently. Using these charts should help solve many cosmetics-related skin problems; however, if a problem persists, consult a dermatologist for advice and possible patch testing.

The products listed in these charts include many of the nationally advertised and distributed brands that have the largest market share of cosmetics sales; an extensive sampling of other brands available in the Chicago area is also included.

After locating several suitable products, use the pricing information on pages 18–19 for comparison shopping.

KEY

Possible Comedogenic Ingredients

BS—butyl stearate
CB—cocoa butter
DO—decyl oleate and derivatives
II—isopropyl isostearate
IM—isopropyl myristate
IN—isostearyl neopentanoate
IP—isopropyl palmitate
IS—isocetyl stearate and derivatives
LA—lanolin, acetylated
LO—linseed oil/extract
L4—laureth-4
M—mineral oil
ML—myristyl lactate
MM—myristyl myristate
O—oleic acid
OA—oleyl alcohol
OO—olive oil

OP—octyl palmitate
OS—octyl stearate and derivatives
PGS—propylene glycol stearate
PPG, PPG-2, PPG-4—myristyl ether propionate
PT—petrolatum
S—sesame oil/extract
SLS—sodium lauryl sulfate

Possible Sensitizers

B—benzophenones
BP—bronopol (2-bromo-2-nitropropane-1,3-diol)‡
C—cinnamates
D—diazolidinyl urea‡
DM—DMDM hydantoin‡
E—essential oils and biological additives
F—fragrances
I—imidazolidinyl urea‡
L—lanolin and derivatives that may cross-react with lanolin
P—parabens
PB—PABA and PABA derivatives
PG—propylene glycol
PS—potassium sorbate
Q—quaternium-15‡
SA—sorbic acid

Other Possible Sensitizers

BHA—butylated hydroxyanisole
BHT—butylated hydroxytoluene
BO—bismuth oxychloride
CA—captan
CH—chlorhexidine and derivatives
CX—chloroxylenol
HQ—hydroquinone and derivatives
HS—horse serum
MCZ—methylchloroisothiazolinone
MD6—methyldibromoglutaronitrile
MO—mink oil
MZ—methylisothiazolinone
PGL—propyl gallate
R—rosin (colophony) and derivatives
T—triethanolamine and derivatives that may cross-react
VE—vitamin E (tocopherol and derivatives)

*may contain [see column head]
†does contain (coal tar colors)
‡formaldehyde-releasing ingredients

Names of products and product lines, and ingredients, are continually changing. Read the labels carefully before purchasing any beauty or skin-care product.

WATER-FREE FOUNDATIONS

Product name	Form	Possible comedogenic ingredients	Possible sensitizers	Other possible sensitizers	Coal tar colors
Adrien Arpel					
(Two-in-One) Powdery Cream Makeup	Cream	OP	P		
Alexandra de Markoff					
Countess Isserlyn Makeup	Liquid	M	F,P		
Powder Finish Creme Makeup	Cream	II,M	F,P	BHA,MO	
Allercreme					
Satin Finish Make-Up for Dry Skin	Cream	BS,IM,M	F,L	PGL	
Almay					
Cream Makeup	Cream		P	VE	
Avon					
Advanced (Moisture) Foundation Natural Finish Creme Powder	Cream	M,OS,PPG	C,F,L,Q	BHT,VE	
Black Radiance					
Maximum Coverage Cream Foundation	Cream	IM,M,MM	P,SA	VE	
Coty					
Airspun Powderessence Foundation Creme	Cream	IM,IN	D,E,P		
Dubarry					
Sophisti-Creme Makeup	Cream	IM,M	F,L,P		
Eboné					
Maximum Coverage Creme Foundation	Cream	M	L	R,VE	
Elizabeth Arden					
Flawless Finish Sponge-On Cream Makeup	Cream	IM,M,PT	F,L,P	BHA,BHT	*
Fashion Fair					
Perfect Finish Creme Makeup	Cream	M	F,L,P,PG	BHA,PGL,R	
Flori Roberts					
Touche Satin Finish Creme Cake Makeup	Cream	M,PT	P		
Frances Denney					
Incandescent Makeup	Lotion	IM,M	F,L,P,SA		
Lancôme					
Teint Majeur Creme Compact Makeup	Cream	OP	F,P		

Product name	Form	Possible comedogenic ingredients	Possible sensitizers	Other possible sensitizers	Coal tar colors
Mary Kay					
Day Radiance Cream Foundation	Cream		F,P	BHA	
Max Factor					
Pan-Stik Ultra-Creamy Makeup	Stick	M	F,P,SA		
Satin Splendor Flawless Complexion Makeup SPF 15	Cream	II,M	P,PB	BHA	
Waterproof Cream Makeup	Cream	IM,M	F,L,P	BHA,BO*	
Waterproof Protection Makeup SPF 6	Cream	IM,IP,M	C,F,L,P	BO*	
Naomi Sims					
Skin Enhancer Cream Foundation	Cream	M,MM,OP	P,SA	VE	
Orlane					
Powder Creme Foundation	Cream		C,E,F	VE	
Physician's Formula					
Le Velvet Film Makeup SPF 15 (compact)	Cream	IN	P		
Posner					
Cream Compact Makeup	Cream	O,OS	P,PG	BHA,PGL	
Princess Marcella Borghese					
Molto Bella Liquid Powder Makeup with Sunscreen	Lotion	OP	C,E,P	BHA,BO*	
Pupa					
Compact Makeup	Cream	IM,LA,PT	F,P	R,VE	
Creamy Makeup	Cream	LA,M,PT	F,P	BHA	
Shiseido					
Stick Foundation	Stick		F	VE	*
Simply Satin					
Creme Foundation (pressed)	Cream	M,PT	L,P	BHA	
Ultima II					
Beautiful Creme Makeup	Cream	IN,M	F,L,P,PB	BHA	

OIL-BASED FOUNDATIONS

Product name	Form	Possible comedogenic ingredients	Possible sensitizers	Other possible sensitizers	Coal tar colors
Clarion					
Protection 15 Makeup	Liquid	IP,M	B,C,D,P,PG	BHA,BHT,VE	
Cover Girl					
Replenishing Ultra-Finish Cream Makeup	Cream	II	B,C,D,F,P,PG	T	

Product name	Form	Possible comedogenic ingredients	Possible sensitizers	Other possible sensitizers	Coal tar colors
Merle Norman					
Powder Base Makeup Cream	Cream	CB,MM	F		

WATER-BASED AND OIL-CONTROL FOUNDATIONS

Product name	Form	Possible comedogenic ingredients	Possible sensitizers	Other possible sensitizers	Coal tar colors
Adrien Arpel					
Sheer Souffle	Cream	IP,M	P,PG,PS		
Alexandra de Markoff					
Countess Isserlyn:					
Cream Makeup	Cream	DO,LA	F,I,L,P,PG	T	
Luminous Finish	Liquid	II,IM,M,OP	B,L,P,PB,PG	VE	
New Perfection Makeup	Cream	IS,M	P,PG,Q	T,VE	
Premiere Protection					
Makeup SPF 15	Liquid	IP	B,C,E,P,PG,Q	T,VE	
Allercreme					
Velvet Finish Make-up	Cream	IM,M,SLS	P	PGL	
Almay					
Cream Makeup	Cream	IS,M	I,P	VE	
Extra Protection Liquid					
Makeup SPF 8	Liquid		B,C,I,P		
Just Enough Light Finish					
Makeup	Liquid	M	I,P	T	
Liquid Makeup	Liquid	M	I,P	VE	
Light Makeup	Liquid	M	I,P		
Luxury Performance Makeup	Liquid	M	C,I,P	T	
Moisture Balance Makeup for					
Normal Skin	Liquid	M	I,P,PG		
Moisture Renew Makeup	Liquid	M,OS	I,P,PG		
Artmatic					
Liquid Makeup	Liquid	M	F,I,L,P,PG	T	
Avon					
Advanced Foundation					
Perfecting Creme	Cream	M,OP,OS	F,I,P,PB	T,VE	
Color Active Casual Makeup	Liquid		F,I,L,P,PB	T	
Color-Free Liquid Foundation	Liquid	IS,M	C,F,I,L,P	T	
Biotherm					
BioClimat 12 Hour					
Weatherproof Face Tint					
SPF 8	Cream		B,C,D,F,P,PG	T	
Bioperfection Liposome				BHA,BHT,MCZ,	
Treatment Makeup	Cream	LO,OO	B,C,D,E,F,P,PG	MZ,PGL,T,VE	
Black Radiance					
Oil-Free Liquid Foundation	Liquid	II,IN,OP,OS	C,I,L,P,PB,PG	T	

Product name	Form	Possible comedogenic ingredients	Possible sensitizers	Other possible sensitizers	Coal tar colors
Body Shop					
Colourings Foundation	Cream	M,MM	B,P,PG	T,VE	
Bonne Bell					
Color Care Makeup SPF 4	Liquid	DO,M	D,P,PB,PG,Q		
Medicated Makeup with SPF 4	Liquid	DO,M	I,L,P,PB,PG	T	
White White Creme Makeup	Cream	IP,M	I,L,P,PG	T	
Chanel					
Blanc de Chanel Perfecting Colour	Liquid	IN,M,OP,PGS	BP,F,L,P,PG	T	
Luxury Cream Makeup	Cream		C,F,P,PG	BHT,PGL	
Tient Naturel Liquid Makeup SPF 8	Liquid	IN,M,OP	BP,F,L,P,PB,PG	T	
CHR					
Anti-Aging Firming Foundation	Cream	M	C,E,P,PG		
Extraordinary Creme Makeup	Cream	M,LA,PGS	F,L,P,PG	VE	
Extraordinary Face Makeup	Liquid	M,LA,PGS	F,L,P,PG	T,VE	
Charles of the Ritz					
Perfect Finish Makeup Natural Finish SPF 6	Liquid		E,P,PG		
Revenescence: Moisture Reservoir Cream Makeup	Cream	DO	L,P,PG	T,VE	
Moisture Reservoir Liquid Makeup	Liquid	II,IM,M,OP	L,P,PG	T,VE	
Superior Moisture Makeup	Liquid	IP,M,O	I,L,P,PB,PG	BHA,T,VE	
Christian Dior					
Line Softening Makeup	Liquid	IM,LA,M,OP	C,F,P,PG	T	
Moisturizing Makeup	Liquid	IP,M,O,SLS	C,F,L,P,PG	BHT,T	
Clarion					
Face Protection-15	Liquid	IM,M	B,C,D,P	BHA,BHT,VE	
Moisturizing Makeup	Liquid	II,IP,M	D,P,PG		
Natural Finish Makeup	Liquid	II,IP,M	D,P,PG		
Clientele					
Moisturizing Skin-Tone Balancer	Liquid	IP,M,OA	L	MCZ,MZ	
Clinique					
Balanced Makeup Base	Liquid	M,PGS	I,L,P,PG		
Continuous Coverage SPF 11	Cream	M	P,PG	BO*,T	
Extra-Help Makeup	Liquid	M,OS,PGS	I,L,P,PG	BO*,HQ,VE	
Workout Makeup	Cream	M,PT	C,L,P,PG	BO*,CA	
Color Me Beautiful					
Color Adjuster	Liquid	DO,IP,S	F,I,L,P,PG	T	
Liquid Foundation	Liquid	DO,IM,IP,S	F,L,P,PB,PG,Q	T	

Product name	Form	Possible comedogenic ingredients	Possible sensitizers	Other possible sensitizers	Coal tar colors
Corn Silk					
Oil-Absorbent Liquid Makeup	Liquid		F,P,PG,Q	BHA,PGL,T	
Cosmyl					
Hydra-Cell Maximum Moisture Foundation	Liquid	M,O,OS	I,P,PG	BHA,T,VE	
Coty					
All-in-One Makeup	Liquid	M,PGS,PT,SLS	F,I,L,P,PB,PG	BHA,PGL,T	
Cover Girl					
Clean Makeup	Liquid	IM,M	E,F,I,P,PG	T	
Extremely Gentle Fragrance-Free Liquid Makeup	Liquid	IP,M	D,P,PG		
Moisture Wear Moisturizing Cream Makeup	Liquid	DO,M,MM,SLS	F,P,PG	T	
Moisture Wear Moisturizing Liquid Makeup	Liquid	IP,M,PGS,PT	F,L,P,PG	BHA,BHT,T	
Oil Control Makeup	Liquid	DO,ML,SLS	E,F,P,PG	T	
Perfecting Makeup	Liquid	IP,M	D,E,F,P,PG	T	
Replenishing Liquid Makeup	Liquid	IP,M,PGS,PT	F,I,L,P,PG	BHA,BHT,T	
Dubarry					
Flatter-Glo Fluid Makeup	Liquid	IM,M,SLS	F,P,THN		
Ebené					
Oil-Free Liquid Foundation	Liquid	IM,O,PGS,PT	I,L,P,PG	T,VE	
Elizabeth Arden					
Flawless Finish:					
Liquid Makeup Dewy Finish SPF 4	Liquid	II,IS,M,PT	C,L,P,PG	T,VE	
Liquid Makeup Matte/SPF 4	Liquid		C,L,P,PG	VE	
Liquid Perfection Makeup	Liquid	M,OS	F,I,L,P,PG	PGL,T	
Simply Perfect Mousse Makeup	Mousse	II,IM,IP,M, OP,OS,PT	F,L,P,PG	T	
Erno Laszlo					
pHelitone Fluid Makeup	Liquid	M,PGS	B,C,DM,F,P	MO	
Estee Lauder					
Fresh Air Makeup Base	Liquid	O,PGS,PT	F,L,P,PB,PG	VE	
Country Mist Liquid Makeup	Liquid	II,IM,IP,M,OP,OS	F,L,PB		
Polished Performance Liquid Makeup	Liquid	M,OP,OS,PGS	F,I,L,P,PB,PG	VE	
Re-Nutriv Souffle Makeup	Souffle	BS,II,IP,M,OP	D,F,L,P,PB,PG	VE	
Fashion Fair					
Fragrance-Free Oil-Free "Perfect Finish" Souffle Makeup	Souffle		I,P,PB,PG	T	
Sheer Foundation	Liquid	IM,M,SLS	F,I,P,PG	T	

Product name	Form	Possible comedogenic ingredients	Possible sensitizers	Other possible sensitizers	Coal tar colors
Fernand Aubry					
Gel Foundation	Liquid	M	F,I,L,P,PG	T	
Satin Foundation Aubryissmes	Cream	M	C,F,I,L,P,PG	T	
Frances Denney					
Moisture Silk Liquid Makeup (Normal/Dry)	Cream	IM,PGS,SLS	C,I,P,PG	T	
Moisture Silk Liquid Makeup (Normal/Oily)	Cream	IM,PGS,SLS	C,I,P,PG	T	
Germaine Monteil					
Antidote des Rides Daily Resistant Color Tint with Sunscreen SPF 25	Liquid	IN,PGS,PT	B,C,E,I,P		
Soft Cover Creme Makeup SPF 8	Cream	IM,M,MM,PGS	B,C,D,E,L,P, PG,Q	T,VE	
Soft Cover Liquid Makeup SPF 6	Liquid	IP,M,PGS	B,F,I,L,P,PB,PG	VE	
Supplegen Lasting Makeup	Liquid	IM,M,PGS,PT	E,F,I,L,P,PG	BHA,BO*,PGL	
L'Oreal					
Visuelle Invisible Coverage Liquid Makeup	Liquid	IP,M,OP	B,I,L,P,PB,PG	T	
Lancôme					
Maqui-Eclat Natural Finish Treatment Foundation	Liquid		B,D,F,P,PB,PG	VE	
Maquimat Fluid Foundation	Liquid		I,P,PB,PG	T	
Maquivelours Liquid Makeup	Liquid	IP,M,OP	B,F,I,P,PB,PG	T	
La Prairie					
Cellular Treatment Foundation	Liquid	IN,S	B,C,F,I,L,P,PG	T,VE	
Mahogany Image					
Creme Foundation	Cream	IP,ML,PGS	F,I,L,P,PG,Q	T	
Matte Tint Foundation	Liquid	IM,PGS	F,L,P,PG,Q	T	
Mary Kay					
Day Radiance Liquid Foundation	Liquid	M	I,P,PG	T,VE	
Max Factor					
Active Protection Makeup with Sunscreen SPF 6	Liquid	PT	I,L,P,PB	BHA,BO*	
Invisible Makeup Foundation	Liquid	LA	B,D,E,L,P,PB,PG		
Light and Natural Mousse Makeup	Mousse	PGS	F,I,L,P,PG	BHA,BO*	
Light and Natural Water-Based Liquid Makeup	Liquid	IM,M,PGS	F,I,L,P,PG	BHA,BO*,T	
Maxi-Fresh Moisturizing Makeup	Liquid	IM,M,PGS	F,P,PG,Q	T	

Product name	Form	Possible comedogenic ingredients	Possible sensitizers	Other possible sensitizers	Coal tar colors
Sun Smart Sheer Makeup & Suntan Lotion:					
For Cheeks SPF 6	Liquid	M	P,PB,PG		*
For Eyes SPF 6	Liquid		L,P,PB	BHA,BO*	
For Faces SPF 6	Liquid	M	P,PB,PG		
Whipped Creme Makeup	Souffle	IM,M,PGS,S	F,P,PG,Q	PGL	
Whipped Creme Cream Makeup (Light)	Souffle	IM,M,PGS,S	F,P,PG,Q		
Whipped Creme Makeup (Sheer to Light)	Souffle	IM,PGS,S	F,P,PG,Q		
Whipped Creme Shimmering Fluid Makeup	Liquid	IM,M,PGS,S	F,P,PG,Q		
Maybelline					
Active Wear Makeup with Sunscreen SPF 8	Liquid	M	E,I,P,PG	VE	
Moisture Whip Liquid Makeup	Liquid		F,I,L,P,PG	T,VE	
Moisture Whip Liquid Makeup with Sunscreen	Liquid		F,I,L,P,PG	T,VE	
Sheer Essentials Makeup	Liquid		I,L,P,PG	T,VE	
Sheer Essentials Makeup with Sunscreen	Liquid		I,L,P,PG	T,VE	
Ultra Performance Pure Makeup	Liquid	M	I,P,PG		
Merle Norman					
Aquabase Cream Base	Cream	IP,PGS	F,I,P,PG		
Aquabase Water-Base Protective Makeup	Cream	IP,PGS	F,I,P,PG		
Liquid Makeup	Liquid	M	F,P,PG	T.	
Luxiva Creme Foundation	Cream	DO,MM,PT	DM,F,L,P,PG	BHA	
Luxiva Liquid Creme Foundation	Liquid	IP,M	DM,F,L,P,PG	BHA	
Sheer Tint SPF 4 Natural Tint Foundation	Cream	ML,OP,OS	B,C,DM,P,PG		
Natural Wonder					
Equalizing Makeup	Liquid	M,PGS,PT	C,L,P,PG	T,VE	
Keep Moisturizing Makeup	Liquid	IS	P,PG,Q	BHA,T	
New Essentials					
Skin Balancing Foundation SPF 8	Liquid	M	C,I,P	VE	
Orlane					
Water-Based Special Effects Creme Makeup	Cream	IS,M,MM,S	E,F,I,L,P	T	
Physician's Formula					
Oil-Control Matte Makeup	Liquid		D,P,PG,Q	BHA,PGL	

Product name	Form	Possible comedogenic ingredients	Possible sensitizers	Other possible sensitizers	Coal tar colors
Sheer Protection Moisture Makeup	Liquid	M	D,L,P	BHA,BHT,MO	
Sun Shield Liquid Makeup SPF 15	Liquid	M	B,D,L,P,PB		
Posner					
Souffle Makeup	Souffle	PGS	C,I,P,PG	T,VE	
Prescriptives					
Exact Color Makeup #1	Liquid	M,OS,PGS	F,I,L,P,PB,PG	VE	
Princess Marcella Borghese					
Effetto Bellizza Targeted Treatment Makeup	Liquid	IS	E,P,PG,Q		
Hydro-Minerali Natural Finish Makeup	Liquid		F,P,PG		
Lumina Creme Foundation	Cream	LA,M,PGS,S	F,L,P,PB,PG	VE	
Lumina Liquid Foundation	Liquid	LA,M,PGS	F,L,P,PB,PG	T,VE	
Velluto Liquid Foundation	Liquid	LA,M,PGS,S	F,L,P,PG,Q	VE	
Velluto II Liquid Foundation	Liquid	M,PGS,PT	F,L,P,PG		
Pupa					
Natural Base	Liquid	LA,M,PT	E,I,P,PG	T	
Revlon					
Touch and Glow Moisturizing Liquid Makeup	Liquid	M,PGS,PT	F,L,P,PG		
Touch and Glow Moisturizing Makeup	Liquid	M,PGS,PT	F,L,P,PG		
Shades of You (Maybelline)					
100% Oil-Free Souffle Water-Based Make Up	Souffle	SLS	I,L,P,PG	BHA,T	
Liquid Water-Based Make Up	Liquid	PGS	I,L,P,PG	T	
Shiseido					
Fluid Foundation	Liquid	PT	B,F,P	T,VE	†
Simply Satin					
Liquid Foundation	Liquid	M,OP	P,PG,L	T	
Sisley					
Botanical Makeup	Cream	IM,M,OA	F,P,PG	HS,MCZ,MZ	
Stagelight					
Hydro Face Tint	Liquid	IM,M,PGS	F,L,P,PG,Q	T	
Stendhal					
Hydro-Matte Fluid Foundation	Liquid	M,PGS	F,I,L,P,PG		
Moisturizing Foundation	Cream	M,PPG	C,F,I,L,P,PG	BHT,VE	
Recette Marvelleuse Protective Firming Base	Cream	IP,M	C,F,I,L,P	MCZ,MZ,VE	
Ultima II					
A Better Makeup	Liquid	M,PT	F,L,P,PG		

Product name	Form	Possible comedogenic ingredients	Possible sensitizers	Other possible sensitizers	Coal tar colors
Advanced Formula Makeup	Liquid	L4	DM,F,P,PG	T	
Beautiful Nutrient Makeup	Liquid	M,PGS,S	F,L,P,PG,Q	VE	
Nearest to Natural Makeup	Liquid	M,PGS,PT	E,L,P,PG	T	
Yves Saint Laurent					
Line Smoothing Foundation	Liquid	IP,M,O	F,L,P,PG,SA	T,VE	
Liquid Creme Foundation	Cream	IM	F,P,PB,PG	BO*,T,VE	
Velvet Complexion Hydro-Protective Makeup	Cream	IP,M,O,PGS	F,L,P,PB,PG	T,VE	

OIL-FREE LIQUID FOUNDATIONS CONTAINING EMOLLIENT ESTERS

Product name	Possible comedogenic ingredients	Possible sensitizers	Other possible sensitizers	Coal tar colors
Alexandra de Markoff				
Countess Isserlyn Soft Velvet Makeup	O,PGS	B,L,P,PB,PG	VE	
Allercreme				
Oil-Free Matte Finish Make-Up	IM,SLS	P,PG		
Almay				
Matte Finish Makeup	PGS	I,P	VE	
Avon				
Advanced (Moisture) Foundation Enhancing Liquid	IS	C,F,I,P,Q	T,VE	
Pure Care Foundation	PPG	C,I,P		
Bonne Bell				
Medicated Makeup for Normal/Oily Skin	DO	C,D,L,P,PG	T	
Chanel				
Oil-Free Makeup	PGS	BP,E,P	T	
Tient Pur Satin Makeup SPF 8	PGS	B,BP,E,P,PB,PG	T,VE	
Charles of the Ritz				
Superior Makeup	O,PGS	L,P,PB,PG	T,VE	
Christian Dior				
Reflet du Tient Emulsion Teintee Unifiante (Light Reflecting Moisturizing Makeup)	IP,OP,OS	C,E,F,P,PG	T	
Clarion				
Individual Beauty: Oil-Free Liquid Makeup		D,P,PG	BHA	
Oil-Free Makeup		D,P,PG	BHA	
Clinique				
Stay-True Makeup		I,P,PG	BO*,T	
Color Style (Revlon)				
Natural Color Oil-Free Makeup	IS	P,PG,Q	T	

Product name	Form	Possible comedogenic ingredients	Possible sensitizers	Other possible sensitizers	Coal tar colors
Cosmyl					
Perfection Liquid Makeup		II,IN,OP,OS	F,I,L,P,PG	T	
Coty					
Airspun Powderessence Foundation Liquid		IM,PGS	D,E,F,P,PG	BHA,T	
Oil-Free Makeup with Astringent		IN	D,F,P,PB,PG	T	
Cover Girl					
Clarifying Anti-Acne Formula Makeup			D,F,P,PG		
Fresh Complexion Oil Control Makeup		IP	D,F,P,PG	T	
Elizabeth Arden					
Gentle Makeup		LA	E,P,PB,PG,Q		
Extra Control Oil-Free Makeup			P,PG	CH	
Soothing Care Gentle Makeup SPF 4			E,P,PB,PG,Q		
Erno Laszlo					
Oil-Free Normalizer Base			B,C,DM,F,P		
Estee Lauder					
Demi-Matte Makeup		PGS	I,P,PG,T		
Lucidity Light-Diffusing Makeup SPF 8			C,E,I,P,PG	BHT,T,VE	
Fashion Fair					
Fragrance-Free Oil-Free Liquid Makeup		II,IN,OP,OS	C,I,L,P,PG	T	
Fernand Aubry					
Foundation Aubryissmes		IM	B,C,F,P,PG	VE	
Flame Glo					
Natural Glow Sheer Liquid Powder Makeup		IP,PGS	C,E,I,P,PG	T,VE	
Flori Roberts					
Gold/Hydrophylic Foundation		DO,MM	I,P,Q	T	
Frances Denney					
FD-29 Foundation Formula SPF 15			B,C,D,P,PG		
Sensitive Soft Matte Makeup		PGS	B,C,D,P,PG	T	
Sensitive Soft Moisture Makeup		PGS	B,C,I,P	T,VE	
Velvet Fresh Foundation			C,DM,P,PG	BO*	
Germaine Monteil					
Duplex Foundation			E,P,PG,Q	T,VE	
Foundation		IS	C,E,P,PG,Q	T,VE	
Oil-Free Foundation		PGS	D,P	CX,T	
L'Oreal					
Mattique Illuminating Matte Makeup			P,PG	T,VE	

Product name	Form	Possible comedogenic ingredients	Possible sensitizers	Other possible sensitizers	Coal tar colors
Lancôme					
Maquicontrole Oil-Free Liquid Makeup			P,PG	T	
Mary Kay					
Oil-Free Foundation		PGS	I,P,PG	T	
Max Factor					
Color and Light Makeup			P		
Maxi Un-Shine Oil-Free Makeup		IN,PGS	I,P,PG	BHA,T	
Maybelline					
Finished Matte Water-Based Liquid Makeup		PGS	F,I,P,PG	T	
Long Wearing Makeup		PGS	F,I,L,P,PG	T	
Long Wearing Makeup with Sunscreen		PGS	F,I,L,P,PG	T	
Shine Free:					
Normal to Combination Skin Makeup		PGS	F,I,L,P,PG	T	
Oil-Control Liquid Makeup			E,I,P,PG	T	
Merle Norman					
Protection Plus Water-Free Makeup with Sunscreen		IP,ML	DM,P,PB		
Naomi Sims					
Oil-Free Skin Enhancer		II,IN,OP,OS	C,I,L,P,PB,PG	T	
Natural Wonder					
Shine Stopper Makeup		IN,L4	P,PG	T	
New Essentials					
Skin Balancing Foundation (100% oil-free)		PGS	I,P	VE	
Orlane					
Oil-Free Foundation with a Matte Finish		PGS	F,I,P,PB,PG	T,VE	
Posner					
Oil-Free Makeup		II,IN,LA,OP,OS	F,L,P,PG,Q	T	
Prescriptives					
Exact Color Makeup (100% oil-free)		PGS	C,P	BO*,T	
Princess Marcella Borghese					
Milano 2000 Makeup		IS	C,F,P,PG,Q	T	
Revlon					
SpringWater Makeup		PGS	E,I,P,PG	BO*,T	
Ultima II					
Beautiful Nutrient Makeup (matte finish)		IM,L4	F,P,PG,Q	BHA,T	

Product name	Possible comedogenic ingredients	Possible sensitizers	Other possible sensitizers	Coal tar colors
STRICTLY OIL-FREE LIQUID FOUNDATIONS				
Almay				
Oil-Control Makeup for Oily Skin		P		
Oil-Free Makeup		I,P		
Avon				
Advanced Moisture Oil-Free Foundation		F,I,P,PB	T,VE	
Shine Defense		F	T	
Chanel				
Tient Pur Mat Matte Makeup		BP,C,P,PG	PGL	
Clientele				
Oil-Free Skin Tone Balancer				
Clinique				
Pore Minimizer Makeup		PG,PS		
Mary Kay				
Oil-Free Foundation		I,P,PG		
Prescriptives				
Oil-Free Exact Color Makeup		I,P,PB,PG		

THE EFFECTS OF POWDER IN MAKEUP

All foundations contain powders, such as talc and titanium dioxide. Powders are inherently drying and when added to a product will make that product more drying than it would otherwise be. The addition of powders tends to increase the length of time a given foundation can be worn with optimal appearance after a single application. Powders tend to dull the finish when added to a foundation and plain powder when used alone has a dull matte finish. Powder can also be made "opalescent" or shimmery by the addition of bismuth oxychloride, mother of pearl, mica, aluminum, or bronze. Powders such as titanium dioxide and zinc oxide are used to increase foundation coverage. Foundation coverage may be sheer (transparent), moderate (translucent), or heavy (opaque) depending on the amounts of powders added to the product. Foundations designed for cover-up will contain larger than average amounts of added titanium dioxide and zinc oxide.

Powders are used not only for foundations and cover-up but also to provide a matte finish and smooth appearance when used over makeup foundation. Oil-containing powders are best for dry skin, oil-free powders with emollient esters are best for normal skin, and strictly oil-free powders are best for oily skin. Loose powders are more likely to be oil-free than pressed powders but check labels carefully!

Pressed Powder Foundations

Pressed powders contain large amounts of powder compressed with varying amounts of oil or other ingredients. These products generally do not contain water. Some of these products are marketed as powder foundation makeups, while similar products are marketed only as pressed powders (i.e., for use over other foundations). Because of the drying effect of powder, pressed powders with oil are usually less oily than water-free or oil-based foundations, but are still not the best choice for oily or acne-prone skin. They are best suited to women with drier skin. All of the oil-free pressed powder foundations examined to date contain emollient esters and are best for normal to slightly oily skin. Pressed powder foundations can often last all day with one application. Apply a light coat using downward strokes; then blend with a cosmetic sponge, cotton, or blending brush.

Oil-control Foundations

Some water-based foundations with added absorptive powders have been marketed as oil-control foundations, claiming they will make combination skin more uniform by absorbing oil in oily areas of the face despite the presence of oil in the product. These products are often excellent foundations that are less oily and longer wearing than other water-based foundations. However, it is probably more effective to make combination skin more uniform by applying a moisturizer to the drier areas of the face if needed and by using a drying toner on the oilier T-zone prior to applying foundation. Oil-control makeups are used like other water-based foundations.

Many companies promote oil-control foundations for persons with acne, and these products are often suitable for use on mildly oily skin. However, oil-free foundation is still better for persons with very oily skin or acne.

MAKEUPS WITH SUNSCREEN

Several newer makeups are available with added sunscreens. With the current concern about skin cancer and sun-related skin damage (e.g., wrinkles and discoloration), it has become very important to develop the habit of using sunscreen. Since most women wear makeup, this type of combination product makes it easy to achieve sun protection for facial skin without any change in skin-care habits. Users who have allergies or are sensitive to certain sunscreen ingredients should check labels.

Chart 9–2

POWDER FOUNDATIONS, PRESSED POWDERS, AND LOOSE POWDERS

The charts are designed to help you minimize adverse reactions and choose products with the proper oil content for your skin type. If you have cosmetics-related acne, you should also choose products with the least amounts of potentially comedogenic ingredients.

Although most cosmetics contain potentially sensitizing ingredients, there is no reason to avoid any ingredient unless you are experiencing adverse reactions to cosmetic products. If you know you are allergic to certain ingredients, the charts will show you which products to avoid. If you are experiencing reactions to a certain cosmetic product, the charts can help you select alternative products that do not contain the same potentially sensitizing ingredients. To choose new products that are least likely to cause allergic reactions, keep in mind that fragrance is by far the most frequent cause of allergic reactions to cosmetics, followed by ingredients listed as "possible sensitizers." The ingredients listed as "other possible sensitizers" cause allergic reactions less frequently. Using these charts should help solve many cosmetics-related skin problems; however, if a problem persists, consult a dermatologist for advice and possible patch testing.

The products listed in these charts include many of the nationally advertised and distributed brands that have the largest market share of cosmetics sales; an extensive sampling of other brands available in the Chicago area is also included.

After locating several suitable products, use the pricing information on pages 18–19 for comparison shopping.

KEY

Possible Comedogenic Ingredients

BS—butyl stearate
DO—decyl oleate and derivatives
II—isopropyl isostearate
IM—isopropyl myristate
IN—isostearyl neopentanoate
IP—isopropyl palmitate
IS—isocetyl stearate and derivatives
LA—lanolin, acetylated
L4—laureth-4
M—mineral oil
MM—myristyl myristate
OA—oleyl alcohol
OP—octyl palmitate
OS—octyl stearate and derivatives
PT—petrolatum
S—sesame oil/extract

> Names of products and product lines, and ingredients, are continually changing. Read the labels carefully before purchasing any beauty or skin-care product.

Possible Sensitizers

A—and other ingredients
B—benzophenones
BP—bronopol (2-bromo-2-nitropropane-1,3-diol)‡
C—cinnamates
D—diazolidinyl urea‡
E—essential oils and biological additives
F—fragrances
I—imidazolidinyl urea‡
L—lanolin and derivatives that may cross-react with lanolin
P—parabens
PB—PABA
PG—propylene glycol
PS—potassium sorbate
Q—quaternium-15‡
SA—sorbic acid

Other Possible Sensitizers

BHA—butylated hydroxyanisole
BHT—butylated hydroxytoluene
BO—bismuth oxychloride
CA—captan
CX—chloroxylenol
MCZ—methylchloroisothiazolinone
MZ—methylisothiazolinone
PGL—propyl gallate
T—triethanolamine and derivatives that may cross-react
UFR—urea/formaldehyde resin
VE—vitamin E (tocopherol and derivatives)
Z—zinc pyrithione

*may contain [see column head]
†does contain (coal tar colors)
‡formaldehyde-releasing ingredients

OIL-CONTAINING PRESSED POWDER FOUNDATIONS

Product name	Possible comedogenic ingredients	Possible sensitizers	Other possible sensitizers	Coal tar colors
Almay				
SPF 15 Cream Powder Makeup		B,C,I,P	BHA,BO	
Avon				
Advanced Foundation Oil-Control Pressed Powder		C,F,I,P,Q	BHT,BO*,VE	
3 in Wonder Makeup	M	P	BO*	*
Body Shop				
Colourings All-in-One Face Base	M,OP,OS	B,C,P	BO	
Charles of the Ritz				
Perfect Finish Solid Powder Foundation	M	I,L,P		
Christian Dior				
Tient Poudre Dual Powder Foundation		P,SA		
Color Style (Revlon)				
Cremepowder Make Up	II,IS,M	P	BHA	
Coty				
Chronologix Line Minimizing Make Up	M	D,F,P		*
Cover Girl				
Clean Makeup	M	E,F,P,Q	BHA	
Extremely Gentle Makeup	M	P,Q	BHA	
Oil-Control Makeup	M	E,F,P,Q	BHA	
Damascar				
Compact Pressed Powder Foundation	IM,M	F,I,L	BHA	
Fernand Aubry				
Powder Foundation	LA	BP,SA	BO	
Germaine Monteil				
Couvrage-Complete Cream Compact Makeup with Sunscreen	BS,II,M,S	L,P	BHA,VE	
Lancôme				
Dual Finish Creme/Powder Makeup	M,PT	F,L,P	T	
Max Factor				
Creme Puff Pressed Powder Makeup	IS,M,OS	F,I,P		*
Pan-Cake Water-Activated Makeup	M	F,L,P,SA	T	
Merle Norman				
Total Finish Compact Makeup	IS,M	F,P	BHA,BHT	
Princess Marcella Borghese				
Lumina Compact Makeup	M,OP	F,P	BHA,BO*	*
Revlon				
Powder Creme Makeup	II,IS,M	P	BHA	

Product name	Possible comedogenic ingredients	Possible sensitizers	Other possible sensitizers	Coal tar colors
Shiseido Compact Foundation (Pressed Powder)	M,PT	F,P	VE	*
Stendhal Radiantly Smooth Compact Powder		F,P	BHA	
Ultima II Advanced Formula Compact "Liquid" Makeup	M,OP	F,P	BHA	
Yves Saint Laurent Powder Foundation		B,F,P,PB	VE	

OIL-FREE PRESSED POWDER FOUNDATIONS CONTAINING EMOLLIENT ESTERS

Product name	Possible comedogenic ingredients	Possible sensitizers	Other possible sensitizers	Coal tar colors
Estee Lauder Simply Sheer Creme-to-Powder Makeup SPF 4	OA	P	BHT,BO*,VE	
Ultima II The Nakeds Brush-On Foundation	II,IN,OS	E,P	BHA	

OIL-CONTAINING LOOSE POWDER

Product name	Possible comedogenic ingredients	Possible sensitizers	Other possible sensitizers	Coal tar colors
Alexandra de Markoff Lasting Luxury Finishing Powder	IM	F,I,P	BO*,VE	*
Almay Loose Finishing Powder Luxury Finish Loose Powder				*
Avon Advanced Foundation Translucent Loose Face Powder		C,F,P	BHT,BO*,VE	
Black Radiance Loose Finishing Powder		I,P		
Chanel Luxury Powder		F,P		*
Charles of the Ritz Ready-Blended Powder	M	F,I,L,P		*
Clinique Blended Face Powder	IM	PS	BO*,Z	*
Cosmyl Perfection Translucent Face Powder	M	I,P		
Coty Airspun Face Powder	M	F,I,L,P		*
Airspun Natural Finish Loose Face Powder	M	F,I,L,P		*
Totally Transparent: Shine-Control Loose Powder	M,OS	F,I,P		
T-Zone Control Loose Powder	M,OS	F,I,P		

Product name	Possible comedogenic ingredients	Possible sensitizers	Other possible sensitizers	Coal tar colors
Cover Girl				
Oil-Control Colorless Finishing Powder	IM,M	E,F,P,Q	BHA	
Professional Finishing Powder	IM,M	E,F,P,Q	BHA	*
Replenishing Finishing Powder	M	F,P,Q	BHA	
Elizabeth Arden				
Flawless Finish Loose Powder		P	BO*,VE	
Erno Laszlo				
Controlling Face Powder	MO	F		
Estee Lauder				
Moisture-Balance Translucent Face Powder	II,IP,M	F,I,L,P	BO*	*
Signature Face Powder	M	I,P	BHT,BO*,VE	*
Fashion Fair				
Trans-Glow Face Powder	M	F,I,P	BHA	
Fernand Aubry				
Translucent Loose Powder		BP,F,SA		
Flame Glo				
Natural Glow Natural Finish Loose Powder	M	L,P,Q	BO*	
Flori Roberts				
Gold/Chromatic Loose Powder with Silk	IP	P		
Melanin Face Powder		F,I,P		
Germaine Monteil				
Perfect Texture Loose Powder		D,F,P,PB,PG	BHA,BO*,PGL,VE	*
Lancôme				
Poudre Majeur Loose Powder with Micro Bubbles	M	F		*
La Prairie				
Foundation Finish Loose Powder	M	F,I,P	BHA	
Max Factor				
Powder Pure Translucent Loose Powder		I,P	BHA,BO*	†
Maybelline				
Moisture Whip Loose Powder	M	F,I,P		
Merle Norman				
Matte Finish Face Powder	M	F		
New Essentials				
Pure Finish Loose Powder				*
Physician's Formula				
Oil-Control Blotting Face Powder	M	I,P		
Oil-Control Blotting Powder	M	I,P		
Princess Marcella Borghese				
Translucent Loose Powder	IM,M	F,L,P	BHA,BO*,T	

Product name	Possible comedogenic ingredients	Possible sensitizers	Other possible sensitizers	Coal tar colors
Revlon Touch & Glow Loose Face Powder	IM,M	L,P	T	
Stendhal Silk Finish Loose Powder	IM	F,P	VE	
Ultima II Translucent Brush-On Face Powder	M	F,L,P	BO*	

OIL-FREE LOOSE POWDER CONTAINING EMOLLIENT ESTERS

Product name	Possible comedogenic ingredients	Possible sensitizers	Other possible sensitizers	Coal tar colors
Charles of the Ritz Blemish Control Powder	IN	F,I,P,PG	BHA,BO*,PGL	
Christian Dior Loose Powder		F,P,SA		*
Cover Girl Professional Finishing Powder Translucent Loose Powder	IM	F,P,Q	BHT	
Eboné Loose Setting Face Powder	OP	I,P	VE	
Estee Lauder Lucidity Translucent Loose Powder		F,P,PS	BHT,BO*,VE	
Frances Denney Moisture Silk Finishing Powder	DO	F,I,P	BO*	
Mahogany Image Translucent Face Powder	IM	I,P		*
Maybelline Shine-Free Oil-Control Loose Powder		I,P		*
Merle Norman Oil-Control Loose Powder	OP	P	BHT	
Posner Oil-Absorbing Loose Powder	OP	I,P		
Revlon Pure Radiance Sunglow Effects Loose Powder	II,OS	C,P	BO*	
Yves Saint Laurent Silk Finish Loose Powder	II,LA	F,P		*

STRICTLY OIL-FREE LOOSE POWDER

Product name	Possible comedogenic ingredients	Possible sensitizers	Other possible sensitizers	Coal tar colors
Adrien Arpel Transparent Face Powder		I,P	BO*	†
Allercreme Translucent Loose Powder		P		
Bonne Bell Translucent Face Powder		F,I,P		

Product name	Possible comedogenic ingredients	Possible sensitizers	Other possible sensitizers	Coal tar colors
Chanel				
Translucent Loose Powder		F,P		
Clientele				
Oil-Control Powder		P		
Color Me Beautiful				
Translucent Loose Powder		P		
Corn Silk				
Oil-Absorbent Loose Powder		F,I,P		
Coty				
Correctives Loose Face Powder		D,E,F,P,PG		
Dermablend				
Setting Powder		P		
Dubarry				
Face Powder		F,P		†
Elizabeth Arden				
Illusion Translucent Face Powder		F,I,P,PG	BHA,PGL	
Estee Lauder				
Demi-Matte Loose Powder		I,P		*
Mary Kay				
Exquisite Dusting Powder		F,P		
Loose Face Powder		I,P		
Powder Perfect Loose Powder		I,P	BO*	
Max Factor				
Face Powder		F,I,P		†
Powder Bar Solid Loose Powder		D,P		
Ultra-Sheer Face Powder (loose)		F,I,P		
Merle Norman				
Plush Powder		F		*
Sheer Face Powder		F		*
Naomi Sims				
Skin Enhancer Translucent Loose Powder		I,P		
Orlane				
Translucent Loose Powder		F,P		
Physician's Formula				
Translucent Face Powder				*
Princess Marcella Borghese				
Powder Milano		F,P	BO*	*
Pupa				
Face Powder		F,P		
Sisley				
Botanical Translucent Free Powder		E,F,P,Q		

Product name	Possible comedogenic ingredients	Possible sensitizers	Other possible sensitizers	Coal tar colors
Stagelight				
Highlighting Powder				
Translucent Loose Powder		F,P		*
Ultima II				
The Nakeds Face Powder		D,P	BO*	*

OIL-CONTAINING PRESSED POWDER

Product name	Possible comedogenic ingredients	Possible sensitizers	Other possible sensitizers	Coal tar colors
Adrien Arpel				
Real Silk Kaleidoscope Brightening Finish	M	I,P	BO*	
Real Silk Powder	IM,IP,M	I,L,P	BHA,BO*	
Mix and Match Translucent Finishing Powder	IP,M	F,P,Q		
Alexandra de Markoff				
Lasting Luxury Pressed Powder	II	F,I,L,P	BO*	*
Powder-Finish Creme (Soft Matte)	II,M	F,P		
Allercreme				
Translucent Pressed Face Powder	IM,M	I,P	BHA	
Almay				
Matte Finish Pressed Powder				
Pressed Powder				
Avon				
Advanced Foundation Translucent Pressed Powder		C,F,P	BHT,BO*,VE	
Black Radiance				
Matched Pressed Powder	L4,M	I,P		
Chanel				
Poudre Facettes Perfecting Powder		P,PG,PS	VE	*
Poudre Lumiere Perfecting Powder		BP,P	BO*	*
Sheer Pressed Powder		BP,F,P	BO*,VE	*
Christian Dior				
Pressed Powder	M,OP	F,P,SA	BHT,PGL	*
Terra Bella Poudre de Soleil Sun Powder	II	F,P	VE	
Clarion				
Natural Finish Powder	II,M	P,Q	BHA	
Translucent Finishing Powder	II,M	P,Q	BHA	
Clinique				
Super Powder Double Face Powder	M,OS	I,L,P	BO*,CX,VE	*
Transparent Blended Pressed Powder	II,M	PS	Z	*
Color Me Beautiful				
Translucent Pressed Powder	IP	I,L,P	BHA	*
Color Style (Revlon)				
Color Balancing Pressed Powder	M	P	BO*	
Cosmyl				
Perfection Compact Powder	IP	I,L,P	BO*,VE	

Product name	Possible comedogenic ingredients	Possible sensitizers	Other possible sensitizers	Coal tar colors
Coty				
Airspun Pressed Moisturizing Powder	IP,LA,M	F,I,P		*
Totally Transparent Shine Control Pressed Powder	M,OS	F,I,P		
Cover Girl				
Extremely Gentle Pressed Powder	M	P,Q	BHA	
Moisture Wear Perfecting Pressed Powder	II,M	F,P,Q	BHA	
Replenishing Pressed Powder	II,M	F,P,Q	BHA	
Eboné				
Oil-Free Pressed Translucent Powder	OP	I,P	VE	
Erno Laszlo				
Duo-pHase Pressed Powder Compact (transparent)	OP	F	BO	
Estee Lauder				
Moisture-Balance Translucent Face Powder	II,IP,M	F,I,L,P	BO*	*
More Than Powder	M,OA	A,I,P	BO,CX,VE	*
Signature Face Powder	M	I,P	BHT,VE	
Fashion Fair				
Fragrance-Free Trans-Glow Pressed Powder	IP	I,L,P	BHA,BO*	*
Trans-Glow Pressed Powder	IP	F,I,L,P	BHA,BO*	*
Fernand Aubry				
Compact Powder		BP,F,L,SA		
Sun Compact (+ sunscreen)	LA	BP,C,SA		
Flame Glo				
Natural Glow Natural Finish Pressed Powder	M	L,P,Q	BO*	
Flori Roberts				
Gold/Pressed Powder	M	P		
Pressed Powder	M	I,L,P*		
Frances Denney				
Moisture Silk Pressed Powder	IM,IP	F,I,L,P		
Sensitive Pressed Powder		I,P		
Germaine Monteil				
Perfect Texture Pressed Powder		D,F,P,PB,PG	BHA,BO*,CA,PGL,VE	*
L'Oreal				
Visuelle Pressed Powder	IM,M	F,I,L,P	BO*	
Mahogany Image				
Translucent Pressed Powder	IM,IP,M	I,L,P	BHA	
Mary Kay				
Translucent Pressed Powder	M,OS	I,P		

Product name	Possible comedogenic ingredients	Possible sensitizers	Other possible sensitizers	Coal tar colors
Maybelline				
Moisture Whip Translucent Pressed Powder	M	I,P,PB		
Shine-Free Oil-Control Dual Powder Base	M	I,P		
Merle Norman				
Matte Finish Pressed Powder	M	F,L		
Sheer Pressed Powder Compact	M	F		
Natural Wonder				
Keep Moisturizing Pressed Powder	MM,OS	P,PB,Q	BHA,BO*	
New Essentials				
Pure Finish Pressed Powder				
Orlane				
Transparent Pressed Powder	LA,M	F,L,P,Q		
Prescriptives				
A Better Powder	M,OP,OS	A,C,P,PG	BO*	*
Princess Marcella Borghese				
Lumina Radiant Finish Moisturizing Pressed Powder	IM,M	F,L,P	BHA,T	
Translucent Pressed Powder Compact	IM,M	F,L,P	BHA,BO*,T	
Revlon				
Love Pat Moisturizing Pressed Powder	IM,M,OP	F,L,P	BO*	*
New Complexion Powder (Normal/Dry)		P,PB	BO*,T	
New Complexion Powder (Normal/Oily)		P,PB	BO*	
Pure Radiance Sunglow Effects Powder	M	C,L,P	BO*	
Touch and Glow Pressed Powder	IM,M	L,P	T	
Touch and Glow Translucent Pressed Powder	IM,M	L,P	T	
Stagelight				
Clown White	M	P		
Ultima II				
Pressed Face Powder	IM,M	F,L,P	BHA,BO*,T	†
Translucent Face Powder	IM,M	F,L,P	BHA,BO*,T	
Wet 'N' Wild				
Silk Finish Translucent Pressed Powder	II,M	D,F,L,P	BO*	
Yves Saint Laurent				
Pressed Powder	II	F,L,P,PG	BHA,PGL	*

OIL-FREE PRESSED POWDER CONTAINING EMOLLIENT ESTERS

Product name	Possible comedogenic ingredients	Possible sensitizers	Other possible sensitizers	Coal tar colors
Black Radiance				
Translucent Pressed Powder	OP	I,P		
Bonne Bell				
Translucent Pressed Powder	OP	F,I,P		

Product name	Possible comedogenic ingredients	Possible sensitizers	Other possible sensitizers	Coal tar colors
Clarion				
Individual Beauty: Silk Perfection Pressed Powder	M,OS	P	BHT	
Oil-Free Translucent Powder	II	P,Q	BHA	
Cover Girl				
Fresh Complexion Oil Control Translucent Pressed Powder	IM	F,P,Q	BHT	
Estee Lauder				
Lucidity Translucent Pressed Powder	OS	F,L,P,PS	BHT,BO*	
Flori Roberts				
Gold/Compact Face Powder		I,P		
Lancôme				
Poudre Majeur Pressed Powder with Micro-Bubbles	OS	A,F,P	BO*,MDG	
Max Factor				
New Definition Perfecting Pressed Powder	OS	I,P	BO*	†
Maybelline				
Satin Complexion Pressed Powder		I,P		
Shine-Free Oil-Blotting Translucent Pressed Powder		I,P		
Merle Norman				
Oil-Control Powder	IN,OP	P	BHT	
Physician's Formula				
Translucent Pressed Powder	OP	I,P,PG	BHA,BO*	*
Posner				
Custom Cover Powder	OP	I,P	BHA,BO*	
Oil-Absorbing Pressed Powder	OP	I,P		
Revlon				
Clean Pressed Powder	OS	E,F,P,Q	BHT	
SpringWater Powder	OS	D,E,P	BO*	
Simply Satin				
Pressed Translucent Powder	OS	I,P	BO*	
Ultima II				
The Nakeds Pressed Powder		D,P	BO*	

STRICTLY OIL-FREE PRESSED POWDER

Alexandra de Markoff				
Professional Accent Powder		D,E,P	BO	
Almay				
Oil-Blotting Pressed Powder				
Artmatic				
Pressed Powder		F,I,P,PG		

Product name	Possible comedogenic ingredients	Possible sensitizers	Other possible sensitizers	Coal tar colors
Corn Silk Oil-Absorbent Pressed Powder		F,I,P		
Coty Correctives Pressed Face Powder		D,E,F,P,PG		
Estee Lauder Demi-Matte Face Powder		I,P		*
Mary Kay Powder Perfect Pressed Powder		I,P		
Natural Wonder Shine Stopper Pressed Powder		C,P	BHA	
Princess Marcella Borghese Powder Milano Pressed Powder		D,F,P	BO*	
Sisley Botanical Pressed Powder with Hawthorne		F,P	MCZ,MZ	
Stagelight Translucent Pressed Powder/Face Powder				*
Ultima II The Nakeds Rice Powder		D,P	BO*	

COVER-UP MAKEUPS AND CONCEALERS

Concealers are makeup products used to cover up minor irregularities of facial color or texture. A green-hued color-correcting cream can be used under foundation to hide facial ruddiness (see color-correcting creams on page 79).

The most effective cover-ups are usually water-free and designed for use on dry skin predominantly. Although they may feel rather greasy, water-free cover-ups and concealers can also be used on normal skin but should be avoided by people with oily skin or acne. These products will hide skin color irregularities and flat scars, but the shininess of the products will draw attention to defects such as depressed scars or deep wrinkles. Water-free cover-ups are available as creams or sticks.

In addition, there are water-based cover-ups for people with normal skin and oil-free cover-ups and concealers for those with oily skin. These products are less shiny than water-free products and may work well on depressed skin defects.

Choose cover-ups one shade darker than skin color since darker colors provide superior cover-up. Cover-ups must usually be covered with loose powder and/or powder blush to keep them from looking too unnatural. Cover-ups for the body are similar to those for the face but less thick because they are designed to cover larger areas of skin. If the coverage with a body cover-up cream proves insufficient, a facial cover-up cream may give better results.

Techniques for Hiding Minor Blemishes
Many minor blemishes can be adequately covered with the sheer-to-moderate coverage obtained with regular foundations. A foundation that is slightly darker than skin color will maximize the coverage obtained. For more coverage, add transparent (sheer coverage) or translucent (moderate coverage) loose powder to regular foundation.

Chart 9–3
CONCEALERS AND COVER STICKS

The charts are designed to help you minimize adverse reactions and choose products with the proper oil content for your skin type. If you have cosmetics-related acne, you should also choose products with the least amount of potentially comedogenic ingredients.

Although most cosmetics contain potentially sensitizing ingredients, there is no reason to avoid any ingredient unless you are experiencing adverse reactions to cosmetic products. If you know you are allergic to certain ingredients, the charts will show you which products to avoid. If you are experiencing reactions to a certain cosmetic product, these charts can help you select alternative products that do not contain the same potentially sensitizing ingredients. To choose new products that are least likely to cause allergic reactions, keep in mind that fragrance is by far the most frequent cause of allergic reactions to cosmetics, followed by ingredients listed as "possible sensitizers." The ingredients listed as "other possible sensitizers" cause allergic reactions less frequently. Using these charts should help solve many cosmetics-related skin problems; however, if a problem persists, consult a dermatologist for advice and possible patch testing.

The products listed in these charts include many of the nationally advertised and distributed brands that have the largest market share of cosmetics sales; an extensive sampling of other brands available in the Chicago area is also included.

After locating several suitable products, use the pricing information on pages 18–19 for comparison shopping.

> Names of products and product lines, and ingredients, are continually changing. Read the labels carefully before purchasing any beauty or skin-care product.

KEY

Possible Comedogenic Ingredients

DO—decyl oleate and derivatives
IM—isopropyl myristate
IN—isostearyl neopentanoate
IP—isopropyl palmitate
IS—isocetyl stearate and derivatives
LA—lanolin, acetylated
M—mineral oil
ML—myristyl lactate
MM—myristyl myristate
OA—oleyl alcohol
OP—octyl palmitate
OS—octyl stearate and derivatives
PGS—propylene glycol stearate
PT—petrolatum
SLS—sodium lauryl sulfate

Possible Sensitizers

B—benzophenones
C—cinnamates
D—diazolidinyl urea‡
DM—DMDM hydantoin‡
E—essential oils and biological additives
F—fragrances
I—imidazolidinyl urea‡
L—lanolin and derivatives that may cross-react with lanolin
P—parabens
PB—PABA
PG—propylene glycol
PS—potassium sorbate
Q—quaternium-15‡
SA—sorbic acid

Other Possible Sensitizers

BHA—butylated hydroxyanisole
BHT—butylated hydroxytoluene

BO—bismuth oxychloride
CH—chlorhexidine and derivatives
MCZ—methylchloroisothiazolinone
MO—mink oil
MZ—methylisothiazolinone
PGL—propyl gallate
R—rosin (colophony) and derivatives

T—triethanolamine and derivatives that may cross-react
VE—vitamin E (tocopherol and derivatives)

*may contain [see column head]
†does contain (coal tar colors)
‡formaldehyde-releasing ingredients

WATER-FREE CONCEALERS				
Product name	Form	Possible comedogenic ingredients	Possible sensitizers	Other possible sensitizers
Alexandra de Markoff				
Countess Isserlyn Secret Cover	Cream	IN,M,OP	I,P	BHA
Almay				
Complexion Perfector	Cream		P	BHA
Concealing Coverup	Cream	M	P	VE
Black Radiance				
Concealer Stick	Stick	M,ML	L,P	VE
Body Shop				
Colourings Concealer	Stick	IM	P	BHT
Bonne Bell				
Cover Cream	Cream	M,PT	P,SA	
Clientele				
Treatment Conceal	Pressed powder	IP,M,PT	L,P	
Clinique				
Advanced Concealer	Cream		P	BHT,BO*
Cover Girl				
Moisture Wear Moisturizing Concealer	Cream	IP,LA,M	L,P	BHA,BHT
Replenishing Concealer Pen SPF 8	Cream	PT	P	VE
Dermablend				
Cover Cream	Cream	M	P	
Elizabeth Arden				
Concealing Cream	Cream	IM,M,PT	F,L,P	BHA,BHT
Estee Lauder				
Cream Concealer	Cream		C,L,P,PB	BHT,BO*,VE
Fashion Fair				
Fragrance-Free Covertone Concealing Creme	Cream	M	P	
Frances Denney				
Concealer Base Cream	Cream	M	L,P,PG,SA	
Mary Kay				
Cream Concealer	Cream		P	

Product name	Form	Possible comedogenic ingredients	Possible sensitizers	Other possible sensitizers
Max Factor				
Erace Extra Cover	Cream	M	F,L	BHA,BHT,PGL
Merle Norman				
Oil-Free Concealing Creme	Cream		I,P	
Retouch Cover Creme	Cream	M,PT	F,P	BHA,BHT
Pupa				
Cover Cream[1]	Cream	LA,M,PT	F,P	BHA
Ultima II				
Moisturizing Cream-On Concealer	Cream	M,OP	L,P	BHA,BO

WATER-BASED CONCEALERS

Product name	Form	Possible comedogenic ingredients	Possible sensitizers	Other possible sensitizers
Adrien Arpel				
Porcelain Cover Base	Cream	M	L,P,PG,PS	T
Almay				
SPF 8 Extra Protection Concealer (automatic)	Liquid		I,P	
Avon				
Advanced Foundation:				
Concealer Plus	Liquid	M,OP	C,E,F,I,P	T,VE
Hide 'N' Blend Body Cover	Liquid		C,D,F,L,P,Q	BHT,R,VE
Hide 'N' Perfect Correcting Cream	Cream	M	C,F,I,P,Q	VE
Pure Care Concealer	Liquid	IM,M	I,P	T
Aziza				
Flawless Finish Retouch Cream Concealer	Cream	IP,M	I,P,PG	T
Retouch Cream Concealer SPF 2	Cream	IP,M	I,P,PG	T
Biotherm				
Ecran Naturel Eye Block Concealer	Cream	OP	E,I,P,PG	T,VE
Bonne Bell				
Cream Concealer	Cream	IM,M,OP	I,P,PG	T
Charles of the Ritz				
Hide and Chic Cream Concealer	Cream	M,OP,PGS	D,L,P,PG	
Perfect Instant Concealer	Cream	M,PGS	I,L,P,PG	T
Clarion				
Flawless Concealer	Liquid	IP,M	D,P,PG	
Individual Beauty:				
Flawless Concealer	Liquid	IP,M	D,P,PG	
Protection-15 Concealer	Liquid	IP,M,PT	B,C,D,P,PG	BHA,BHT,VE
Color Style (Revlon)				
Natural Blend Concealer	Liquid	M,PGS	D,I,L,P,PG	
Cosmyl				
Concealing Cream	Cream	II,M,OP,OS	I,P,PB,PG	T,VE

[1]This product contained coal tar colors in one of its formulations.

Product name	Form	Possible comedogenic ingredients	Possible sensitizers	Other possible sensitizers
Cover Girl				
Clarifying Anti-Acne Blemish Concealer	Liquid	OS	DM,P	
Invisible Concealer	Liquid	IP,M	F,I,P,PG	T
Dermablend				
Leg and Body Cover	Cream		P	
Elizabeth Arden				
Flawless Finish Cream-On Concealer	Cream	M	L,P,PG	
Simply Perfect Mousse Concealer	Mousse	M,PGS	PG	BO*
Estee Lauder				
Automatic Creme Concealer	Cream	M,PGS	L,P,PG	
Germaine Monteil				
Duplex Concealer (creamy)	Liquid	M,PGS	I,L,P,PG	
Hides Anything Moisturizing Concealer	Cream	M,OP,PGS	D,I,L,P,PG	T
Mary Kay				
Touch-On Concealer	Liquid	M	I,P,PG	T,VE
Maybelline				
Liquid Cover (+ sunscreen)	Liquid		E,I,P,PG	
Shine Free Blemish Concealer	Cream	DO,OP,SLS	I,L,P,PG	T
Undetectable Cream Concealer	Liquid	DO,M,OP,SLS	I,L,P,PG	T
Orlane				
Creme Cover-Up	Cream	M,PT	F,I,L,P,PG	MCZ,MZ
Prescriptives				
Camouflage Cream	Cream	M,PGS	L,P,PG	BO*
Princess Marcella Borghese				
Impeccable Absolute Concealer	Liquid	IP,M,PGS	I,L,P,PG	
Revlon				
Line Concealer (liquid)	Liquid	IN,OS,PT	E,L,P,PG	BHA,T
New Complexion Concealer	Liquid	M,PGS	I,L,P,PG	
SpringWater Oil-Free Concealer	Liquid	IS,PGS	E,I,P,PG	
OIL-FREE CONCEALERS CONTAINING EMOLLIENT ESTERS				
Almay				
Touch-On Blemish Treatment (automatic)[2]	Liquid		I,P,PG	
Clinique				
Anti-Acne Control Formula	Liquid			
Corn Silk				
Oil Absorbent Concealer	Liquid	OS	F,P,PG,Q	
Estee Lauder				
Signature Cream Concealer	Compact		C,I,L,P	BHT,BO*,VE
Mary Kay				
Liquid Concealer	Liquid	IS	I,P,PG	T,VE

[2]Contains sulfur.

Product name	Form	Possible comedogenic ingredients	Possible sensitizers	Other possible sensitizers
New Essentials				
SPF 8 Concealer	Liquid		I,P	

STRICTLY OIL-FREE CONCEALERS

Charles of the Ritz				
Disaster Cream	Cream		P	
Flori Roberts				
Blemish Touch (oil-free)	Liquid		P,PG	
Max Factor				
Erace Line Filler	Liquid		I,P	

WATER-FREE UNDER-EYE CONCEALERS

Adrien Arpel				
Cover Away	Cream	M,PGS,PT	L	
Under-Eye Concealer	Cream	M,PT	F,L,P	
Almay				
Extra Moisturizing Under-Eye Cover Cream	Cream	M,PT	P	BHA,BHT
Avon				
Next Generation Concealer	Cream	M,OS	F,Q	VE
Clarion				
Protection 15 Concealer (SPF 15) (automatic)	Cream	IP,M,PT	B,C,D,P,PG	BHA,BHT,VE
Erno Laszlo				
pHelitone Emollient with Duo-pHase Concealer (neutral pressed powder)	Cream		P	BHA,MO
Fernand Aubry				
Under-Eye Concealer	Stick	M	P	
Flame Glo				
Undercover Cover Stick	Stick	M	L,P	BHA
Princess Marcella Borghese				
Eye Duetta Under-Eye Concealer	Cream	M	L,P	BHA
Under Cover Concealer	Cream	DO,M,PT	L,P	BHA
Stendhal				
Under-Eye Concealer	Stick	LA,M,OA,PT	L,P	BHT

WATER-BASED UNDER-EYE CONCEALERS

Allercreme				
Cream Concealer	Cream	M	D,P,PG	T
Avon				
Camouflage Eye Disguise	Cream	OP	C,L,P,Q	VE
Pure Care Under-Eye Concealer	Cream	M	C,I,P	

Product name	Form	Possible comedogenic ingredients	Possible sensitizers	Other possible sensitizers
Clinique Quick Corrector	Cream	M,PGS	L,P,PG	
Lancôme Anti-Cernes Waterproof Under-Eye Concealer	Cream	IP,PT	D,P,PB,PG	BHA

WATER-FREE COVER-UP STICKS

Product name	Possible comedogenic ingredients	Possible sensitizers	Other possible sensitizers
Allercreme Concealer Stick	IP	P,PG	BHA,PGL
Almay Natural Look Cover-Up Stick	IM	L,P,PG	BHA,PGL
Avon Advanced Foundation Concealing Stick	M,OP	C,F,I,P,Q	T,VE
Perfect Point Concealer Pencil		C,F,Q	BHT,VE
Wrinkle Control Stick	IM,M,PT	B,C,P	BHT,VE
Aziza Retouch Cover Stick SPF 4	M	F,L,PG	BHA,BO,PGL
Chanel Estompe de Chanel Corrective Concealer	M,OP	P,PG	PGL,VE
Clinique Concealing Stick	M		
Color Me Beautiful Cover Stick		P	BHA
Dermablend Quick Fix Concealer with Sunscreen	M	C,P	
Fashion Fair Cover Stick	IM,M,PT	F,L	BHA
Fragrance-Free Cover Stick	IM,M,PT	L	BHA
Flame Glo Natural Glow Natural Cover Concealer	M	E,L,P	BHT
Undercover Cover Stick	M	L,P	BHA
Flori Roberts Vanish Stick	M	P	VE
Max Factor Erace Plus Cover-Up	M	F,L	
Erace Secret Cover-Up	IM,OP	F,P	BHA,BO*
Maxi Waterproof Cover-Up Stick	M,MM	P	
Maybelline Shine Free Oil-Control Cover Stick	M	L,P	BHA
Waterproof Cover Stick	M	L,P	BHA

Product name	Possible comedogenic ingredients	Possible sensitizers	Other possible sensitizers
Princess Marcella Borghese Cama Flura Cover Stick	IS,OP	E,F,P	BHA
Revlon Vanishing Stick	IM,M	F,L,P	BHA
Shades of You (Maybelline) 100% Oil-Free Coverstick		P	BHA,BO*
Wet 'N' Wild Silk Finish Cover All Cover Stick	M	F,L,P	BHA
Yves Saint Laurent Concealer		F,P	

OIL-FREE COVER-UP STICKS

Product name	Possible comedogenic ingredients	Possible sensitizers	Other possible sensitizers
Artmatic Oil Free Cover Stick (+ emollient esters)	ML,OS	P	BHA
Lancôme Point Correctif Blemish Stick			CH

COLOR-CORRECTING CREAMS

Product name	Form	Base	Possible comedogenic ingredients	Possible sensitizers	Other possible sensitizers	Coal tar colors
Erno Laszlo pHelitone Emollient with Duo-pHase Concealer (Blush)	Cream	Water-free		P		
Estee Lauder Color Primer Skin Tone Perfecting Creme	Cream	Water-free	OS	I,P	B0*,VE	
Merle Norman Color Mist with Sunscreen	Cream	Water-based	IP	DM,F,P, PB,PG		
Stagelight Incandescent Light Balancer	Lotion	Water-based	IM,M,PGS	F,L,P,PG,Q		
Stendhal Les Bio Program Soin Beaux Roses Creme for Redness	Cream	Water-based	M	F,P,PG		†

FOUNDATION PRIMERS						
Product name	Form	Base	Possible comedogenic ingredients	Possible sensitizers	Other possible sensitizers	Coal tar colors
Adrien Arpel Glycerine Liquid Powder	Shake lotion	Oil-free and water-free		PG		
Flori Roberts Oil-Free Melanin Makeup Base	Lotion	Oil-free and water-free		P,PG		
La Prairie Cellular Treatment Foundation Primer	Cream	Water-based		I,F,P,PB,PG	T,VE	
Pupa Makeup Base	Cream	Water-based	LA,M,PT	E,P,PG		
Sisley Creme Lisley Lily Makeup Base	Cream	Oil-based	IM,M,OA	F,P,PG,SA	HS,MCZ, MZ	
Stendhal Recette Marvelleuse Revitalizing Night Care Cream	Cream	Water-based	LA,M,PT	F,I,L,P,PG	T	†
Yves Saint Laurent Makeup Primer	Cream	Oil-free and water-free	IM	F,P	BHA	

COLOR-CORRECTING CREAMS, FOUNDATION PRIMERS, AND BRONZERS

Color-correcting creams are used to mask undesirable color tones. A cream with green tint will tone down a ruddy complexion, and one with purple will tone down yellowish skin. White creams will help disguise wrinkles and other surface imperfections. These products are often water-free and are best used for dry to normal skin types. They are likely to aggravate acne. Color-correcting creams are designed to be worn under other foundations.

Foundation primers are essentially makeup products designed to wear under foundation to obtain a longer optimal wear time. Some are silicone-based products that contain no water or oil and can be used by any skin type. Other products contain oil and are best avoided by women with oily skin or acne.

Bronzers are usually suntan-colored makeup creams, gels, or powders. The creams are water-based oil-containing products that are moisturizing for drier skin. Gels and powders with oil are most suitable for normal skin whereas those with emollient esters are relatively neutral products that can be used on any type of skin.

Some products are misleadingly labeled bronzers when they are in fact sun-free tanning creams containing dihydroxyacetone as a staining agent. Look for this ingredient on the label to be sure which type of product you are buying. There are also bronze-tinted moisturizers on the market.

THE NEWER SELF-TANNING PRODUCTS

It is possible to obtain the appearance of a suntan artificially through the use of sun-free tanning products called self-tanners. These products contain dihydroxyacetone, a staining ingredient designed to stain the outer layer of the skin. The stained surface skin cells are shed in about a week; this looks like a normal fading tan. These products are applied to the skin, then washed off after about three hours. If the skin does not appear tan enough after three hours, the product can be reapplied for an additional period of time. Many people require two to four applications to reach an optimal color and can maintain this color with reapplication every few days. Care must be taken to wash the product off the palms after use or they will develop an unnatural-looking tan.

Dry skin will absorb more color, and best results are obtained by first removing dry skin using a mild abrasive, such as a loofah. A moisturizer can also be used prior to the self-tanner on dry areas of skin. Less of the product should be applied to the elbows and knees, which absorb more color. In order to prevent fabric staining, wait 30 minutes after application before dressing or going to bed; wait at least 2 hours before exercising to prevent streaking. Dihydroxyacetone degrades and should be used within 6 months of opening the container.

Self-tanners are either water-based creams or lotions or oil-free lotions with emollient esters. Most of the currently available self-tanners are water-based products that contain oil and may therefore aggravate acne. An oil-free product is the best choice for people prone to acne.

Chart 9–4
BRONZERS AND SELF-TANNING PRODUCTS

The charts are designed to help you minimize adverse reactions and choose products with the proper oil content for your skin type. If you have cosmetics-related acne, you should also choose products with the least amount of potentially comedogenic ingredients.

Although most cosmetics contain potentially sensitizing ingredients, there is no reason to avoid any ingredient unless you are experiencing adverse reactions to cosmetic products. If you know you are allergic to certain ingredients, the charts will show you which products to avoid. If you are experiencing reactions to a certain cosmetic product, the charts can help you select alternative products that do not contain the same potentially sensitizing ingredients. To choose new products that are least likely to cause

> Names of products and product lines, and ingredients, are continually changing. Read the labels carefully before purchasing any beauty or skin-care product.

allergic reactions, keep in mind that fragrance is by far the most frequent cause of allergic reactions to cosmetics, followed by ingredients listed as "possible sensitizers." The ingredients listed as "other possible sensitizers" cause allergic reactions less frequently. Using these charts should help solve many cosmetics-related skin problems; however, if a problem persists, consult a dermatologist for advice and possible patch testing.

The products listed in these charts include many of the nationally advertised and distributed brands that have the largest market share of cosmetics sales; an extensive sampling of other brands available in the Chicago area is also included.

After locating several suitable products, use the pricing information on pages 18–19 for comparison shopping.

KEY

Possible Comedogenic Ingredients

CB—cocoa butter
II—isopropyl isostearate
IM—isopropyl myristate
IN—isostearyl neopentanoate
IP—isopropyl palmitate
LA—lanolin, acetylated
L4—laureth-4
M—mineral oil
ML—myristyl lactate
MM—miristyl miristate

OA—oleyl alcohol
OO—olive oil
OP—octyl palmitate
OS—octyl stearate and derivatives
PGS—propylene glycol stearate
PT—petrolatum

Possible Sensitizers

B—benzophenones
BP—bronopol (2-bromo-2-nitropropane-1,3-diol)‡
C—cinnamates
D—diazolidinyl urea‡
DM—DMDM hydantoin‡
E—essential oils and biological additives
F—fragrances
I—imidazolidinyl urea‡
L—lanolin and derivatives that may cross-react with lanolin
P—parabens
PB—PABA
PG—propylene glycol
Q—quaternium-15‡
SA—sorbic acid

Other Possible Sensitizers

BHA—butylated hydroxyanisole
BHT—butylated hydroxytoluene
BO—bismuth oxychloride
MCZ—methylchloroisothiazolinone
MZ—methylisothiazolinone
PGL—propyl gallate
T—triethanolamine and derivatives that may cross-react
VE—vitamin E (tocopherol and derivatives)

*may contain [see column head]
†does contain (coal tar colors)
‡formaldehyde-releasing ingredients

BRONZERS					
Product name	Form	Possible comedogenic ingredients	Possible sensitizers	Other possible sensitizers	Coal tar colors
Adrien Arpel Real Silk Bronzing Powder	Powder with oil	IM,IP,M	I,L,P	BHA,BO*	
Almay Bronzing Gel	Oil-free gel		I,P		†

Product name	Form	Possible comedogenic ingredients	Possible sensitizers	Other possible sensitizers	Coal tar colors
Avon					
Advanced Foundation Bronzing Powder	Powder with oil	M	C,F,P,Q	BO*,VE	*
Color Active:					
Bronzing Powder	Powder with oil	M	C,P	BO*	*
Bronze Radiance Sheer Mousse	Powder with oil	M	F,I,P,PB	BO*	*
Biotherm					
Gelee Bronzante Triple Protection Bronzing Gel SPF 4	Gel with oil	M,OO	B,C,F,I,L,P	MCZ,MZ,T,VE	†
Body Shop					
Colourings Translucent Bronzer	Water-based cream	OA,PT	P,PB,PG	T	*
Bonne Bell					
Bronzing Gel	Gel with oil	M	I,L,P,PG	T	†
Waterproof Bronzing Cream SPF 8	Water-based cream	M	B,C,D,P,PG	T	
Chanel					
Bronze de Chanel Perfect Bronze SPF 8	Water-based liquid	IN,M,OP	B,BP,C,F,L, P,PB,PG	BHA,PGL,T	
Bronze de Chanel Poudre Perfect Bronzing Powder SPF 8	Powder with oil		B,BP,C,P,PB		
Clinique					
Bronze Gel	Gel with emollient esters		P,PG		†
Dermablend					
Blush-On Bronzer	Powder with oil	M	C,P		
Body Bronzer	Water-based cream		B,C,D,P,PG		
Elizabeth Arden					
Luxury Bronzing Powder	Powder with emollient esters		P		
Flame Glo					
Natural Glow Radiant Finish Bronzing Powder	Powder with oil	M	C,E,L,P,Q	BO*,VE	
Flori Roberts					
Natural Glow Bronzing Powder	Powder with oil	L4,M	P,Q	BO*	
Giorgio of Beverly Hills					
Extraordinary Bronzing Powder	Powder with oil	M	P,PB		

Product name	Form	Possible comedogenic ingredients	Possible sensitizers	Other possible sensitizers	Coal tar colors
Glamatone					
Brush a Tan Bronzing Powder	Powder with oil	M	C,P		
Lancôme					
Conquête du Soleil Special Bronzing Gel/ Creme SPF 6	Gel with oil		B,C,F,I,P	BHA,BHT,MCZ, MZ,T,VE	†
Max Factor					
California Bronze Face Gel	Oil-free gel		D,P,PG		*
Merle Norman					
Sheer Bronzing Powder	Powder with emollient esters	II	F,I,P		
Pupa					
Bronze Makeup	Powder with emollient esters	PGS	F,I,L,P,PG,SA	BHT,T	
Revlon					
Microgems Solid Bronzing Powder	Powder with oil	M	L,P	BHA,BO*	*
Stagelight					
Bronze Toner	Water-based cream		F,I,P,PG	T	†

WATER-BASED SELF-TANNERS

Product name	Form	Possible comedogenic ingredients	Possible sensitizers	Other possible sensitizers	Coal tar colors
Bain de Soleil					
Sunless Tanning Creme for Fair Skin	Cream	CB,OP	DM,E,F,I,L,P		
Sunless Tanning Creme for Medium to Dark Skin	Cream	CB,OP	DM,E,F,I,L,P		
Biotherm					
Lait Bronzeur In-Sun Self-Tanning Milk SPF 8	Lotion	IP,M,OO	B,C,F,I,P	MCZ,MZ,T,VE	
Protecteur Bronzeur Gentle Face Self-Tanner SPF 12	Cream	OO	B,C,F,I,P	VE	
Self-Tanning Lotion	Lotion	IM,M,OO	F,I,P		
Chanel					
Perfect Color Self-Tanning Lotion SPF 8	Lotion	IM,OP	B,C,E,F,P	VE	
Clientele					
Solar Free Tanning System Face Gel	Gel		D,E,P	VE	

Product name	Form	Possible comedogenic ingredients	Possible sensitizers	Other possible sensitizers	Coal tar colors
Clinique					
Self-Tanning Formula	Cream	ML,OP,OS	E,I,P,PG		
Coppertone					
Q.T. Lotion SPF 2	Lotion		C,D,F,P	VE	
Tan Extender	Lotion	IP	D,E,F,P,PG	VE	†
Elizabeth Arden					
Spa for the Sun Sunshine Self-Tanner for the Body	Lotion	OS	C,DM,E,F,P	VE	
SunScience Self-Tanning Lotion	Lotion	LA	F,I,P,PG		
Erno Laszlo					
Self-Tanning Lotion SPF 8	Lotion	MM	B,C,DM,E,F,P	BHA,BHT,VE	
Estee Lauder					
Self-Action Tanning Creme	Cream	ML	F,P,PG,SA		
Frances Denney					
Sun Care Self-Tanner	Lotion	M	L,P,PG		
Germaine Monteil					
Soleil Self-Tanning Creme	Cream	M	D,E,F,P,PG,SA		
Lancome					
Effet du Soleil Self-Tanning Moisture	Lotion	M	B,C,F,I,P		
Lait Auto-Bronzant Self-Tanning Lotion	Lotion	IM,M	F,I,P		
La Prairie					
Sun Care Self-Tanning Cream	Cream	IM	F,P		
Mary Kay					
Sunless Tanning Lotion	Lotion		P		
Max Factor					
California Bronze Sunless Tanning Lotion SPF 6	Lotion	IP,M	B,C,F,P,SA	VE	
Merle Norman					
Light Self-Tanning Moisturizer	Lotion		F,I,P		*
Prescriptives					
Sun-Free Tanner	Lotion	ML	E,P,PG		
Princess Marcella Borghese					
Termi di Montecatini Spa Solare Continuous Tan for Face and Body	Cream	M	D,E,P,PG,SA	VE	

OIL-FREE SELF-TANNERS CONTAINING EMOLLIENT ESTERS					
Product name	Form	Possible comedogenic ingredients	Possible sensitizers	Other possible sensitizers	Coal tar colors
Almay					
Sunless Tanning Lotion	Lotion		I,P	VE	
Sunless Tanning Lotion with SPF 6	Lotion		B,C,I,P	VE	

TYPES OF MAKEUP REMOVERS

Oil-free and water-based facial and eye makeups will wash off easily with soap and water; oilier makeups will not wash off easily. There are three basic kinds of removers especially designed to remove oily makeup: lipid, detergent, and solvent.

Most women who use oily makeup products have dry skin and can therefore use the oilier lipid makeup removers. These products use oils to dissolve and remove oily makeup. They are usually nonirritating and leave a moisturizing film of oil on the skin. Lipid cleansers, cleansing creams, and oil-based moisturizers are products with similar compositions that will serve the same purpose.

Although lipid makeup removers are the least irritating, the detergent and solvent products are usually fairly nonirritating. These products tend to remove skin oils and usually have a drying effect. Oil-free makeup removers are especially useful for eye makeup removal when wearing contact lenses since the oilier products can get onto the lenses and cause cloudy vision. Ideally, you should remove lenses from the eyes before you remove makeup, and thus avoid getting smeary, dissolved makeup on lenses.

Chart 9–5
MAKEUP REMOVERS

The charts are designed to help you minimize adverse reactions and choose products with the proper oil content for your skin type. If you have cosmetics-related acne, you should also choose products with the least amounts of potentially comedogenic ingredients.

Although most cosmetics contain potentially sensitizing ingredients, there is no reason to avoid any ingredient unless you are experiencing adverse reactions to cosmetic products. If you know you are allergic to certain ingredients, the charts will show you which products to avoid. If you are experiencing adverse reactions to a certain cosmetic product, the charts can help you select alternative products that do not contain the same potentially sensitizing ingredients. To choose new products that are least likely to cause allergic reactions, keep in mind that fragrance is by far the most frequent cause of allergic reactions to cosmetics, followed by ingredients listed as "possible sensitizers." The ingredients listed as "other possible sensitizers" cause allergic reactions less frequently. Using these charts should help solve

> Names of products and product lines, and ingredients, are continually changing. Read the labels carefully before purchasing any beauty or skin-care product.

many cosmetics-related skin problems; however, if a problem persists, consult a dermatologist for advice and possible patch testing.

The products listed in these charts include many of the nationally advertised and distributed brands that have the largest market share of cosmetics sales; an extensive sampling of other brands available in the Chicago area is also included.

After locating several suitable products, use the pricing information on pages 18–19 for comparison shopping.

KEY

Possible Comedogenic Ingredients

DO—decyl oleate and derivatives
IP—isopropyl palmitate
M—mineral oil
ML—myristyl lactate
OA—oleyl alcohol
OP—octyl palmitate
OS—octyl stearate and derivatives
PT—petrolatum
SLS—sodium lauryl sulfate

Possible sensitizers

BP—bronopol (2-bromo-2-nitropropane-1,3-diol)‡
D—diazolidinyl urea‡
DM—DMDM hydantoin‡
E—essential oils and biological additives
F—fragrances
I—imidazolidinyl urea‡
L—lanolin and derivatives that may cross-react with lanolin
P—parabens
PG—propylene glycol
Q—quaternium-15‡
SA—sorbic acid

Other Possible Sensitizers

BC—benzalkonium chloride
BHA—butylated hydroxyanisole
BHT—butylated hydroxytoluene
CH—chlorhexidine and derivatives
MCZ—methylchloroisothiazolinone
MZ—methylisothiazolinone
PGL—propyl gallate
PMA—phenylmercuric acetate
T—triethanolamine and derivatives that may cross-react
TH—thimerosal
VE—vitamin E (tocopherol and derivatives)

†does contain (coal tar colors)
‡formaldehyde-releasing ingredients

LIPID MAKEUP REMOVERS

Product name	Possible comedogenic ingredients	Possible sensitizers	Other possible sensitizers	Coal tar colors
Allercreme				
Eye Makeup Remover Pads	M			
Almay				
Gentle Gel Eye Makeup Remover	M	I,P	BHA,BHT,VE	
Moisturizing Eye Makeup Remover Lotion	M	P		
Moisturizing Eye Makeup Remover Pads	M	P		
Avon				
Effective Eye Makeup Remover	DO,M,PT	P	T	
Body Shop				
Orchid Oil Cleansing Milk		E,F,P	T	
Christian Dior				
Equite Demaquillant Integral Visage et Yeux Face and Eye Makeup Remover	M	BP,F,P		

Product name	Possible comedogenic ingredients	Possible sensitizers	Other possible sensitizers	Coal tar colors
Gel Demaquillant Pour les Yeux Fards Waterproof Eye Makeup Remover	M	F		
Huile Douce Demaquillant Pour Mascara Resistant a L'eau Waterproof Makeup Remover	M	F		
Clarion				
Ultra-Pure Eye Makeup Remover	M,OP	P		
Clinique				
Quick Dissolve Makeup Solvent	IP,M	E,I,P,PG		†
Cover Girl				
Clean Eyes Conditioning Makeup Remover	IP,M	E,P,SA	BHA	
Extremely Gentle Cream Rinsable Eye Makeup Remover	DO,IP,M,SLS	F,I,P		
Estee Lauder				
Completely Clear Waterproof Eye Makeup Remover	IP,M	P		
Fernand Aubry				
Makeup Remover for Sensitive and Mixed Skins	M	F,L,P,PG	T	
Johnson & Johnson				
Take-Off Makeup Remover Cloths	M	F,I,SA		
Take-Off Makeup Remover Cloths (fragrance-free)	M	I,SA		
Lancôme				
Effacil Gel Gentle Eye Makeup Remover	IP,M,OS	P	BC,BHT	
Mary Kay				
Eye Makeup Remover	M,PT			
Max Factor				
Hypo-Allergenic Eye Makeup Remover Pads	M	P		
Instant Eye Makeup Remover Stick	IP,M	P,PG	PGL	
Professional Makeup Remover (cream)	M,OA	B,P		
Maybelline				
Mascara Remover	M	L,P		
Mavala				
Gentle Eye Makeup Remover Gel	IP,M	P		
Merle Norman				
Very Gentle Eye Makeup Remover (gel)	IP,M	L,P	BHA,BHT	
New Essentials				
Extra Gentle Moisturizing Eye Makeup Remover	M	P		
Noxell				
Noxzema Dif-Rinse Water Rinsable Cold Cream	DO,IP,M,SLS	F,I,P		

Product name	Possible comedogenic ingredients	Possible sensitizers	Other possible sensitizers	Coal tar colors
Orlane				
Lacta-Creme Cleanser/Makeup Remover	M,ML,OS	F,L,P,PG	T	
Physician's Formula				
Eye Makeup Remover Lotion	M,PT	L,P	BC	†
Eye Makeup Remover Pads	M	L,P	BHA,BHT	
Princess Marcella Borghese				
Waterproof Eye Makeup Remover	IP,M,PT	P,SA	BHA	
St. Ives				
Facial Cleanser and Makeup Remover	M	D,E,F,L,P,PG		†
Stagelight				
Abschminke Makeup Remover		E,L,P		†
Eye Makeup Remover	PT	P,SA		
Stendhal				
Les Bio Program Gentle Eye Cleanser/Eye Makeup Remover	M,OP			

DETERGENT MAKEUP REMOVERS

Product name	Possible comedogenic ingredients	Possible sensitizers	Other possible sensitizers	Coal tar colors
Adrien Arpel				
Gentle Rinse Eye Makeup Remover		P,PG	MCZ,MZ	†
Alexandra de Markoff				
Eye Makeup Remover		I,P		
Triple Effect Gentle Eye Makeup Remover		E,P,PG		
Almay				
Non-Oily Eye Makeup Remover Lotion				
Non-Oily Eye Makeup Remover Pads				
Avon				
Eye Makeup Remover Gel		I		
Pure Care Eye Makeup Remover for Contact Lens Wearers		I		
Aziza				
Contact Lens Eye Makeup Remover		DM		
Body Shop				
Chamomile Eye Make-Up Remover		E,P		
Charles of the Ritz				
Gentle Eye Makeup Remover		P,PG		
Clientele				
Eye Makeup Remover		D,PG,SA	BC	
Clinique				
Rinse-Off Eye Makeup Solvent		P		
Color Me Beautiful				
Eye Makeup Remover		E,I,P,PG		

Product name	Possible comedogenic ingredients	Possible sensitizers	Other possible sensitizers	Coal tar colors
Cosmyl				
Delicate Eye Makeup Remover		I,P		
Estee Lauder				
Gentle Eye Makeup Remover		P		
Frances Denney				
Fast and Gentle Eye Makeup Remover		I,P,PG		
Germaine Monteil				
Gentle Lift Professional Eye Makeup Remover		P,PG		
L'Oreal				
Eye Makeup Remover		F,P	TH	
Plenitude Tender Eye Makeup Remover	OP	P,Q	T	
Lancôme				
Effacil Gentle Eye Makeup Remover		F,P	TH	
La Prairie				
Eye Makeup Remover		E,P,PG	MCZ,MZ	†
Max Factor				
Gentle Eye Makeup Remover		I,P	T	
Merle Norman				
Instant Eye Makeup Remover		E,I		
New Essentials				
Extra Gentle Oil Free Eye Makeup Remover				
Physician's Formula				
Vital Lash Oil-Free Eye Makeup Remover		PQ		†
Prescriptives				
Eye Makeup Remover		P		
Princess Marcella Borghese				
Gel Delicato Gentle Makeup Remover		E,P,PG		
Instant Eye Makeup Remover		P,PG	PMA	
Revlon				
30 Second Eye Makeup Remover		P,PG		
Stagelight				
Amazing Aloe Makeup Remover		D,P,PG		
Ultima II				
Eye Makeup Remover for Sensitive Eyes		P,PG		

Product name	Possible comedogenic ingredients	Possible sensitizers	Other possible sensitizers	Coal tar colors
SOLVENT MAKEUP REMOVERS				
Almay				
Non-Oily Makeup Remover Gel		D		
Chanel				
Demaquillant Douceur Formule Biphase Pour les Yeux Dual Phase Eye Makeup Remover		E,P,Q	CH	
Christian Dior				
Gel Demaquillant Pour les Yeux Eye Makeup Remover Gel		BP,F,P		
Clarins				
Lotion Demaquillant Pour les Yeux Eye Makeup Remover Lotion		E	BC,CH,MCZ,MZ	
Color Me Beautiful				
Skin Care Gentle Eye Makeup Remover Gel		E,I,P,PG	T	
Fashion Fair				
Eye Makeup Remover Dual Purpose		Q		
Fernand Aubry				
Ligne Fondamentale Soft Eye Make-Up Remover	IM	F,P,PG		
Kelemata				
Eye Makeup Remover		E	MCZ	
Eye Makeup Remover Pads		E,I,P,PG		
Lancôme				
Bi-Facil Double Action Eye Makeup Remover		F,Q	BC	
Mary Kay				
Remover Pads	M	F		
Maybelline				
100% Oil-Free Makeup Remover		PG	CH	
Neutrogena				
Eye Makeup Remover Gel	IP	P		
Revlon				
Micropure Eye Makeup Remover for Sensitive Eyes		P,PG		

CHAPTER 10

Blush, Buffers, and Highlighters

HOW TO CHOOSE AND USE BLUSH

Blush or rouge products are designed to add color and give a healthy appearance to the cheeks. They can be used over foundation or without foundation. Most cosmetologists think that blush looks best when color-coordinated with lipstick. In general, the more intense shades usually look best with dark skin (less intense shades are often not noticeable), whereas less intense colors look better with lighter skin. Lighter shades will also highlight an area whereas darker shades will make an area appear to recede. Therefore, a lighter blusher can be used to accentuate the cheekbone and a darker shade can be applied below for further emphasis.

In order to achieve a natural look, it is necessary to choose the proper blusher for your skin type (see Chapter 5). The chart below will help you quickly locate the types of blushers that are best for your skin type.

Cream or Stick Blush

Cream blushers are usually water-free products that leave a shiny finish and are most useful for dry skin. There are also some oil-based and water-based cream (or creamy liquid) blushers that will leave a less shiny finish. Stick blushers, also called facial gleamers, are water-free products with wax added to make a solid product.

Cream or stick blush (especially the water-based products) can be used on normal skin, but should be avoided by people with oily skin or acne. Older women with drier skin who might be tempted to use these products because they are moisturizing should be aware that these products

Type of Blusher	Skin Type	Moisturization	Finish
Cream or stick (water-free)	dry	high	shiny
Cream or creamy liquid (water-based)	dry to normal	moderate	semimatte
Powder (with oil)	dry to normal	moderate to none	matte
Powder (oil-free)	normal to oily	slight to drying	matte
Gel	oily	drying	sheer
Oil-free liquid or mousse	oily	drying	sheer

often accentuate wrinkles and lead to a less than desirable overall result. Water-free cream or stick blusher will smear less oily foundation and will therefore not work over water-based or oil-free makeups. Cream and stick blushers are more difficult to apply correctly than powder blush because they are difficult to blend properly.

Powder Blush
The most widely used blusher is powder blush, essentially pressed or loose powder with added rosy color. Although these are seldom oil-free products, the large amounts of powder make even the oil-containing powder blushers less oily than cream blushers. For dry skin, choose a powder blusher with oil. For oily skin or acne, oil-free powder blushers should be used. Oil-free powder blushers with emollient esters are most suitable for slightly oily skin; strictly oil-free products are best for people with very oily skin or acne. Powder blusher can be used over any foundation and will produce a matte finish.

Gel Rouge and Facial Gloss
Gel rouge contains a moderately drying gel base that is designed for women with oily

skin or acne. However, these products provide little coverage (particularly for acne) and are somewhat more difficult to apply than powder blush. Gels with emollient esters are most suitable for slightly oily skin; strictly oil-free products are best for people with very oily skin or acne.

Oil-free Liquid and Mousse Blushers
Oil-free liquid and mousse blushers are similar to gel blushers. They provide minimal coverage and are more difficult to apply than powder blush.

Buffers and Highlighters
Buffer is powder blush that is less intense in color, and highlighter is powder blush that is more intense in color than typical blush. Buffer is used to blend makeup into the surrounding skin. Highlighters are used to accent facial features a woman wishes to emphasize. Sometimes these products have a shimmery finish to accentuate the skin to which they are applied. Like other powders, products with oil are best for drier skin, oil-free products with esters are good for slightly oily skin, and strictly oil-free products are best for very oily skin or acne.

Chart 10-1
BLUSH, BUFFERS, AND HIGHLIGHTERS

The charts are designed to help you minimize adverse reactions and choose products with the proper oil content for your skin type. If you have cosmetics-related acne, you should also choose products with the least amounts of potentially comedogenic ingredients.

Although most cosmetics contain potentially sensitizing ingredients, there is no reason to avoid any ingredient unless you are experiencing adverse reactions to cosmetic products. If you know you are allergic to certain ingredients, the charts will show you which products to avoid. If you are experiencing reactions to a certain cosmetic product, the charts can help you select alternative products that do not contain the same potentially sensitizing ingredients. To choose new products that are least likely to cause allergic reactions, keep in mind that fragrance is by far the most frequent cause of allergic reactions to cosmetics, followed by ingredients listed as "possible sensitizers." The ingredients listed as "other possible sensitizers" cause allergic reactions less frequently. Using these charts should help solve many cosmetics-related skin problems; however, if a problem persists, consult a dermatologist for advice and possible patch testing.

The products listed in these charts include many of the nationally advertised and distributed brands that have the largest market share of cosmetics sales; an extensive sampling of other brands available in the Chicago area is also included.

After locating several suitable products, use the pricing information on pages 18–19 for comparison shopping.

KEY

Possible Comedogenic Ingredients

BS—butyl stearate
CB—cocoa butter
DO—decyl oleate and derivatives
II—isopropyl isostearate
IM—isopropyl myristate
IN—isostearyl neopentanoate
IP—isopropyl palmitate
IS—isocetyl stearate and derivatives
LA—lanolin, acetylated
L4—laureth-4
M—mineral oil
O—oleic acid
OA—oleyl alcohol
OO—olive oil
OP—octyl palmitate
OS—octyl stearate and derivatives
PGS—propylene glycol stearate
PPG—myristyl ether propionate
PT—petrolatum
S—sesame oil/extract

> **Names of products and product lines, and ingredients, are continually changing. Read the labels carefully before purchasing any beauty or skin-care products.**

Possible Sensitizers

A—and other ingredients
B—benzophenones
BP—bronopol (2-bromo-2-nitropropane-1,3-diol)‡
C—cinnamates
D—diazolidinyl urea‡
DM—DMDM hydantoin‡
E—essential oils and biological additives
F—fragrances
I—imidazolidinyl urea‡
L—lanolin and derivatives that may cross-react with lanolin
P—parabens
PG—propylene glycol
PS—potassium sorbate
Q—quaternium-15‡
SA—sorbic acid

Other Possible Sensitizers

BHA—butylated hydroxyanisole
BHT—butylated hydroxytoluene
BO—bismuth oxychloride
CA—captan
CH—chlorhexidine and derivatives
CX—chloroxylenol
MDG—methyldibromoglutaronitrile
MO—mink oil
PGL—propyl gallate
T—triethanolamine and derivatives that may cross-react
UFR—urea/formaldehyde resin
VE—vitamin E (tocopherol and derivatives)
Z—zinc pyrithione

*may contain [see column head]
†does contain (coal tar colors)
‡formaldehyde-releasing ingredients

WATER-FREE CREAM OR STICK BLUSH

Product name	Possible comedogenic ingredients	Possible sensitizers	Other possible sensitizers	Coal tar colors
Adrien Arpel				
Brush-On Powdery Cream Blush	BS,IN,M,OP,OS,PT	L,P	BO*	*
Almay				
Powder Finish Cream Blush		P	BHA,BO*	*
Artmatic				
Blush/Brush	M	F,I,P	T	*
Avon				
Color Natural Radiance:				
Creme Powder	M,OS,PPG	C,F,L	BHT,BO*	*
Stick	M,OP		BHT,BO*,UFR	*
Colortwists	M	F	BHT,BO*,UFR	*
Ultra Wear Stick Blush	OP		BHT,BO*	*
Bonne Bell				
Veri-Hue Cream Blusher	M,PT	L	BHA	*
Clarion				
Individual Beauty Sheer Illusion Cream				
Powder Blush	OP	P	BHA	*
Clinique				
Cheek Base	OP,OS		BHT,BO*	*
Young Face Creamy Blusher	M	P	BO*,VE	*
Coty				
Nature's Blush (stick)	IM,OA		BHA	†
Dubarry				
Bloom Cheek Tint	IM,M	F,L,P		†
Elizabeth Arden				
Luxury Creme-to-Powder Blush	II,PT	P	VE	*
Estee Lauder				
Signature Soft Color Blush	OP,OS,PT	F,P	BHT,BO*,T,VE	*
Germaine Monteil				
Creme Blush	IP,M,OA,OP	E,P,PG	BHA,BO*,PGL	*
Lancôme				
Blush Majeur				
Brush-On Creme Cheek Colour	IN,OS,PT	F,L,P	BHT,BO*	*
Mary Kay				
Blush Rouge	M,PT	L	BHA	†
Cream Blush	IN,IP,M	F,P	BO*	*
Princess Marcella Borghese				
Lumina Radiante:				
Creme Rouge (new formulation)	IN,M	P	BHA,BO*	*
Creme Rouge (old formulation)	OP	P	BHA	*

Product name	Possible comedogenic ingredients	Possible sensitizers	Other possible sensitizers	Coal tar colors
Pupa				
Creamy Blush	LA,M,PT	F,P	BHA	*
Revlon				
Powder Cream Blush	II,IS,M	P	BHA,BO*	*
Ultima II				
Blushing Cream	IM,M,O	F	BHA,BO*	*

OIL-BASED CREAM BLUSH

Product name	Possible comedogenic ingredients	Possible sensitizers	Other possible sensitizers	Coal tar colors
Merle Norman				
Blush Rouge	CB,M	F		†
Warm Blush	CB,M	F		

WATER-BASED CREAM BLUSH

Product name	Possible comedogenic ingredients	Possible sensitizers	Other possible sensitizers	Coal tar colors
Avon				
Velvet Feel Creme Blush	IS,M,PPG	C,I,P	BO*,T	*
Clinique				
Colour Rub Allover Lustre	M,O,OS,PGS	P,PG	VE	
Max Factor				
Whipped Creme Cream Blush	IM,M,PGS,S	F,P,PG,Q		*
Whipped Creme Fluid Blush	IS,PGS	F,I	BHA,BO*	*

OIL-FREE GEL BLUSH AND FACIAL GLOSS CONTAINING EMOLLIENT ESTERS

Product name	Possible comedogenic ingredients	Possible sensitizers	Other possible sensitizers	Coal tar colors
Bonne Bell				
Bright & Shining Face Gloss		F,I,P	BO,T	†
Good Nature Glo (for entire face)		I,P,PG	BO,T	†
Clinique				
Gel Rouge		B,P,PG		*

STRICTLY OIL-FREE GEL BLUSH AND FACIAL GLOSS

Product name	Possible comedogenic ingredients	Possible sensitizers	Other possible sensitizers	Coal tar colors
Avon				
See-Through Color Portables		I,P,PG	T	*
Bonne Bell				
Blushing Gel		F,I,P	T	*
Flame Glo				
Natural Glow See-Through Blushing Gel		E,I,P	T	*

OIL-FREE LIQUID AND MOUSSE BLUSHERS

Product name	Possible comedogenic ingredients	Possible sensitizers	Other possible sensitizers	Coal tar colors
Elizabeth Arden				
Simply Perfect Mousse Blusher		F,I,P,PG	BHA,BO*	*
Max Factor				
Rosewater Blush		D,P,PG	T	†
Rosewater Blush (automatic)		D,P,PG	T	†

Product name	Possible comedogenic ingredients	Possible sensitizers	Other possible sensitizers	Coal tar colors
Stagelight				
Rose Blush		E,P		†

OIL-CONTAINING POWDER BLUSH

Product name	Possible comedogenic ingredients	Possible sensitizers	Other possible sensitizers	Coal tar colors
Adrien Arpel				
Mix and Match: Cheek Colour/Contour Powder	M	I,L,P		*
Alexandra de Markoff				
Lasting Luxury Cheek Colour Powder	II	B,F,I,L,P,PG	BHA,BO*,PGL	*
Allercreme				
Color Sheers Blush	M	I,P	BO*	*
Almay				
Blush	M	I,P	BO*	*
Brush-On Blush	M	I,P	BO*	*
Cheek Color Blush	M	I,P	BO*	*
Avon				
Advanced Foundation Twist 'n' Powder	M	F,I,P,Q	BO*,VE	*
Color Natural Radiance Powder	M	L,P	BO*,UFR	*
Color Release Long Wearing Blush	M	I,L,P	BO*,UFR	*
Coordinates Powder Blush	M	L,P	BO*	*
Pure Care Powder	M	P	BO*	*
Ultra Wear Powder Blush	M	P	BO*	*
Ultra Wear Powder Restage Blush	DO,M,OS	P	BHT,BO*	*
Aziza				
Sheer Blush Colorations Cheek Color	OP,PT	I,P	BHA,BO	*
Black Radiance				
Sheer Finish Blush	M	I,P		*
Body Shop				
Colourings Cream Blush	OP	P,PB		*
Colourings Powder Blusher	OP,OS	P		*
Colourings Tinted Cheek Color	II,M,PT	C,F,P	VE	*
Bonne Bell				
Blush-Lites Cream Powder Blush	IM,M,PT	P,SA	BHA,BO*	*
Blushettes	M	I,P		*
Chanel				
Powder Blush	M	BP,F,L,P	BO*	
Charles of the Ritz				
Powders à la Carte	OP,OS,PT	P	BO*,VE	
Christian Dior				
Blush Plume	M,OP,OS	C,L,P	BHT,PGL	*
Clarion				
Enhancing Blush	II,M	P,Q	BHA	*

Product name	Possible comedogenic ingredients	Possible sensitizers	Other possible sensitizers	Coal tar colors
Clinique				
Beyond Blusher Oil-Free Everywhere Colour		I,P	BO*,CX	
Young Face Powder Blusher	M	PS	BO*,Z	*
Color Me Beautiful				
Powder Blush	L4,M	I,L,P	BHA,BHT,BO*	*
Color Style (Revlon)				
Soft Color Powder Blush	M	D,P	BO*	*
Cosmyl				
Perfection Powder Blush	IM,M	I,L,P	BHA,BO*	*
Coty				
Dual Pan Bare Blusher	M,OS	F,I,P	BO*	*
Cover Girl				
Cheekers Powder Blush	M	E,F,Q		*
Classic-Color Blush	M	E,F,P,Q	BHA	*
Clean Makeup Blush Mates	M	E,F,P,Q	BHA	*
Continuous Color Moisture-Enriched Blush	M,OS	F,P,Q	BHT	*
Moisture Wear Nourishing All-Day Blush	M	F,P,Q	BHA	*
Oil-Control Fresh Blush	M	E,F,P,Q	BHA	*
Professional Color Match Blush Duet	M	E,F,P,Q	BHT	*
Professional Contouring Blush	M	E,F,P,Q	BHA	*
Replenishing Blush	M	F,P,Q	BHA	*
Shape 'N Blush (Blush and Contour Kit)	M	E,F,P,Q	BHA	*
Soft Radiants Sheer Color Blush	M	E,F,P,Q	BHA	*
Damascar				
Compact Blush-On	IM,M	L,P	BO*	*
Terra-cotta Compact Blush	IM	F,I,L	BHA	
Dermablend				
Soft Color	L4,M	I,L,P	BHA,BHT	†
Dubarry				
Bloom Powder Cheek Tint	M	P		†
Eboné				
Soft Blend Powder Blush	OP	I,P	VE	*
Elizabeth Arden				
Powder Perfection for Cheeks	M	F,P	BO*	*
Erno Laszlo				
Luxurious Blushing Powder		P,PS	BHA,BO*,MO	*
Estee Lauder				
Just Blush! Eye and Cheek Powder	II,M,PT	P	BHT,BO*,VE	
Signature Powder Blush	II,M		BHA,BO*,Z	*

Product name	Possible comedogenic ingredients	Possible sensitizers	Other possible sensitizers	Coal tar colors
Fernand Aubry				
Blush-On Aubrylights/Aubryssimes	LA	B,L,SA		*
Flame Glo				
Natural Glow Sheer Cheek Color Powder				
Blush	M	L,P,Q	BO*,VE	
Radiant Blush	M	F,L,P,Q	BO*	*
Shine Control Powder Blush	M	F,L,Q	BO*,VE	*
Flori Roberts				
Radiance Pressed Powder Blush	L4	P,Q	BHA,BO*	*
Frances Denney				
Moisture Silk Powder Blush	IM,IP	F,I,L,P	BO*	*
Germaine Monteil			BHA, BO*,	
Silk Powder Blush	IM,LA,M	F,I,L,P,PG	CA,PGL,VE	*
L'Oreal				
Microblush	OP,PT,S	F,L,P	BHT,BO*	*
Visuelle Powder Blush	M,ML,OO	F,I,L,P	BO*	*
Lancôme				
Maquiriche Blushing Powder	IM,M	F,I,L,P	BHA,BO*,T	*
Mahogany Image				
Pressed Powder Blush	L4,M	I,L,P	BHA,BHT,BO*	*
Mary Kay				
Blusher	M	I,P		*
Creamy Cheek Color	IN,IP,M	L	BHA	†
Max Factor				
Maxi-Fresh Blush	M	I,P		*
New Definition Perfecting Blush	IN,OS,PT	C,D,L,P,PG	BO*	*
Maybelline				
Brush/Blush		I,L,P	BHA,BO*	*
Brush/Blush II		I,L,P	BHA	†
Brush/Blush III	M	I,P	BO*	*
Shine Free Blush-A-Little Oil-Control				
Brush		I,L,P	BHA,BO	†
Sleek Cheeks Powder Blush	M	I,P	BO*	*
Merle Norman				
Powdery Creme Cheek Color		P	BHA,BHT	*
Sheer Powder Blusher	M	I,P	BO	*
Naomi Sims				
Pressed Powder Blush Cheek Enhancer				
Blusher	M	I,P	BHA,BO*	*
New Essentials				
Cheek Color	M	I,P	BO*	*

Product name	Possible comedogenic ingredients	Possible sensitizers	Other possible sensitizers	Coal tar colors
Orlane				
Powder Blush	BS,II	P		*
Physician's Formula				
Gentle Blush	M	P	BHA,BO*	*
Prescriptives				
Powder Cheek Color	IP,M	F,L,PS	BO*,Z	*
Princess Marcella Borghese				
Blush Milano	M	P	BHA,BO*	*
Perlati Colour Brilliance for Eyes, Cheeks and Lips (loose)	II,OS	P	BO*	
Perlati Colour Pastello for Eyes, Cheeks and Lips (pressed)	IM,PT	F,P,Q	BO*,CH,VE	
Pupa				
Blush	IM,IP	BP,SA		*
Revlon				
Naturally Glamorous Blush-On	M	D,P	BO*	*
Powder Creme Blush	II,IS,M	P	BHA,BO*	*
Sheer Face Color	M,OP	D,L,P	BO*	*
Soft Lustre Blush	IM,M	L,P	BHA,T	*
Sisley				
Botanical Powder Blush	M	E,L,P		†
Ultima II				
Advanced Formula Blush	IN,M	P	BHA,BO*	*
Creamy Powder Blush	IM,M	L,P	BHA,BO*,T	*
Wet 'N' Wild				
Silk Finish Blush 'N' Glo	M,OP,OS	D,F,P		*
Yves Saint Laurent				
Blushing Powder	II	F,L,P,PG	BHA,PGL	*
Tender Blusher		P		*

OIL-FREE POWDER BLUSH CONTAINING EMOLLIENT ESTERS

Product name	Possible comedogenic ingredients	Possible sensitizers	Other possible sensitizers	Coal tar colors
Charles of the Ritz				
Perfect Finish Powder Blush	IM,OP	B,P	BO*	*
Christian Dior				
Powder Blush	OP	F,P,SA	BHT,PGL	*
Elizabeth Arden				
Luxury Cheek Color	IM	P	BO*,VE	*
Fashion Fair				
Beauty Blush	IP	I,L,P	BHA,BO*	*
Fragrance-Free Beauty Blush	IP	F,I,L,P	BHA,BO*	
Flori Roberts				
Gold/Chromatic Blush	IM	P		*

Product name	Possible comedogenic ingredients	Possible sensitizers	Other possible sensitizers	Coal tar colors
Mary Kay				
Powder Perfect Cheek Color		I,P		*
Max Factor				
Satin Blush		P	BO*	*
Maybelline				
Shine Free Oil Control Blush		DM,I,P	BO*	*
Natural Wonder				
Keep Blushing Powder Blush	OP	E,P	BO*,T	*
Revlon				
Air Blush	OP	P	BO*	*
SpringWater Blush	OS	D,E,P,PG	BO*	*
Shades of You (Maybelline)				
100% Oil-Free Powder Blush		I,P	BO*	*
Shiseido				
Blusher		F,P	VE	†
Simply Satin				
Powder Blush	OS	I,P		*
Stagelight				
Powder Blush/Cheek Powder	IM	P		†
Stendhal				
Powder Blush	IM	BP,P		*
Ultima II				
Color Shots for Cheeks	IN,OS	F,P	BHA,BO*	*
The Nakeds Cheek Color		D,P	BO*	*
Translucent Blush	OP	P	BO*	*

STRICTLY OIL-FREE POWDER BLUSH

Product name	Possible comedogenic ingredients	Possible sensitizers	Other possible sensitizers	Coal tar colors
Clientele				
Contour Blush		I,P		†
Corn Silk				
Oil-Absorbent Blush and Highlighter		F,I,P,PG	BHA,BO*,PGL	*
Lancôme				
Blush Subtil Delicate Powder Blush		A,F	MDG	*

OIL-CONTAINING POWDER BUFFERS AND HIGHLIGHTERS

Product name	Possible comedogenic ingredients	Possible sensitizers	Other possible sensitizers	Coal tar colors
Clinique				
Transparent Buffer (pressed powder)	II,M	PS	BO*	*
Fashion Fair				
Beauty Highlighter (pressed powder)	IP	F,I,L,P	BHT,BO*	*
Mary Kay				
Facial Highlighter (pressed powder)		P		

OIL-FREE POWDER BUFFERS AND HIGHLIGHTERS CONTAINING EMOLLIENT ESTERS

Product name	Possible comedogenic ingredients	Possible sensitizers	Other possible sensitizers	Coal tar colors
Alexandra de Markoff Lasting Luxury Radiant Colour (highlighter)	II	B,DM,P,PG	BO*	*
Mary Kay Buffing Cream Facial Highlighter	IS	F,P,Q I,P,PG	T,VE	†
Merle Norman Duskglow Highlighting Powder		F		
Ultima II Color Shots for Face (pressed powder beads/highlighter)	IN,OS	F,P	BHA,BO*	*
STRICTLY OIL-FREE POWDER BUFFERS AND HIGHLIGHTERS				
Clientele Contour Blush Highlighter (loose powder)		D,P		*
Corn Silk Oil-Absorbent Blush Duo (blush and highlighter)		F,I,P,PG	BHA,BO*,PGL	*

CHAPTER 11

Moisturizers and Emollient Products

There are more moisturizers on the market by far than any other single cosmetic or skin-care product. You need to know your skin type in order to choose appropriate moisturizers from the vast array of available products (see Chapter 5).

HOW MOISTURIZERS AND EMOLLIENTS WORK

Moisturizers are products designed to increase the water content of the skin. Cosmetics chemists have sometimes used the term *moisturizer* to refer to water-soluble hydrating ingredients and the term *emollient* to refer to occlusive softening ingredients. However, since increasing the water content of the skin tends to soften the skin, both terms tend to be used interchangeably.

Dry skin is caused by decreased water content in the skin. If the outer skin layer contains less than about 5 to 10 percent water, skin will feel dry. Although dry skin is not caused by a decrease in oil, oil plays an important part in preventing dry skin by providing a barrier that prevents evaporation of water. Traditional moisturizing products are oil-containing products. The more oil a moisturizer contains, the better the moisturizer becomes but the greasier it feels.

Experts consider petrolatum (petroleum jelly) to be one of the best moisturizers because it provides such a good barrier against moisture loss from the skin. Recent studies have shown that petrolatum also works by restoring skin barrier function and reconditioning skin lipids.

The best moisturizer will be a product that moisturizes the skin just to the extent needed. Any additional moisturizing is unnecessary and will feel greasy. Use the chart below to find the type of moisturizer that is best for your skin type.

Skin Type	Type of Moisturizer	Net Effect
extremely dry	water-free	extremely moisturizing
very dry	absorption	very moisturizing
dry	water-in-oil	moderately moisturizing
normal to dry	oil-in-water	mildly moisturizing
normal to oily	oil-free	slightly moisturizing

TYPES OF MOISTURIZERS

Water-free Moisturizers

Water-free moisturizers contain predominantly oily ingredients and no water. These products are usually translucent-appearing ointments (if solid) or oils (if liquid). They are very moisturizing because the oily barrier they form on the skin prevents water loss; however, they are very greasy and will feel unpleasant except on extremely dry skin. Examples include petroleum jelly and mineral oil.

Absorption Moisturizers

Absorption moisturizers are also water-free but contain either anhydrous lanolin or cholesterol to absorb water. Although they look very similar to water-free moisturizers, they are slightly less greasy and slightly less moisturizing.

Water-in-Oil Moisturizers

Water-in-oil moisturizers contain predominantly oily ingredients and some water. Since there are both water and oil present, emulsifiers are added so that the oil mixes with the water rather than floating on top of it. In the process, these products become opaque creams (if solid) or lotions (if liquid). They are less moisturizing and less greasy than water-free or absorption products but are still moderately strong moisturizers.

Some products clearly contain more oil than water. However, oil content cannot always be determined accurately from the ingredients label, because the total amount of several oily ingredients may exceed the amount of water, even if water is listed as the primary ingredient. The products listed as water-in-oil on the charts in this book either clearly fall into this category or are marketed as maximum moisturizers or "night creams" that are likely to fall into this category.

Oil-in-Water Moisturizers

Oil-in-water moisturizers contain more water than oil. They are less moisturizing and less greasy than water-in-oil products and are mild moisturizers for normal-to-dry skin. Most moisturizers fall into this category since consumers tend to choose these pleasant light moisturizers over heavier ones.

Oil-free Moisturizers

Humectants, such as glycerin or propylene glycol, are non-oily ingredients that help the skin hold water. Propylene glycol– and glycerin-based solutions are mild, oil-free moisturizing products that can be used on oilier skin. Even gels (which normally have a drying effect) containing large amounts of humectants can have a net moisturizing effect. Thus, there are propylene glycol– and/or glycerin-containing gels that are also mild oil-free moisturizers.

Strictly oil-free moisturizers are usually gels or solutions with large amounts of humectants. A few strictly oil-free moisturizers are emulsions of water and mildly moisturizing fatty acids and alcohols. These ingredients have been allowed in strictly oil-free products using the definition employed in this book. Less strictly oil-free moisturizers can be made by emulsifying water with emollient esters.

Strictly oil-free products are probably the best choice for people with significant acne. Oil-containing foundation makeups are often difficult or impossible to apply over oil-free moisturizers. An oil-free foundation is the best choice to use over oil-free moisturizers.

HUMECTANTS AS ADDITIVES TO OIL-CONTAINING MOISTURIZERS

Although most oil-containing moisturizers also contain some humectant, the addition of large amounts of humectants can make a mildly oily product moisturize as well as a much greasier product. Some of the most effective humectants are lactic acid, glycolic acid, and urea. Moisturizers with significant amounts of these humectants are often recommended by dermatologists for patients with dry skin, because these moisturizers are as effective and more pleasant to use than oilier moisturizers.

Lactic acid and glycolic acid are the first of the alpha-hydroxy acids to appear on the market. These humectants are currently receiving a lot of attention in dermatology because they appear to alter skin fundamentally. Continued use of prescription-strength products containing high concentrations of lactic or glycolic acid will alter dry skin so that it looks like normal skin when viewed under a microscope. These prescription products are considered drugs (rather than cosmetics) because they may actually alter the physiology of skin instead of simply adding moisture. The extent to which similar physiologic effects are produced by products containing nonprescription-strength ingredients is not entirely

clear. It is clear, however, that these products are generally excellent moisturizers.

Unfortunately, products containing high amounts of urea, lactic acid, glycolic acid, or propylene glycol may sting when used on dry skin that has small cracks or fissures.

ALOE VERA IN MOISTURIZERS

Aloe vera is an ingredient that adds a silky feel to a moisturizer. Although it may not have any special moisturizing properties, consumer testing has demonstrated that products with this ingredient are often subjectively rated more pleasant than other products. Aloe vera does not change the oiliness of a moisturizer and can be used by persons with any skin type. However, it is important to make sure that you choose the right type of aloe vera moisturizer for your skin type.

COMEDOGENIC INGREDIENTS IN MOISTURIZERS

Some moisturizers contain individual ingredients that have been found to be comedogenic (i.e., cause acne) in laboratory testing on rabbit ears or normal skin. However, often the product containing these ingredients will not be comedogenic when similarly tested. This has led to controversy about whether these products should be used on skin prone to acne.

The best way to determine if a product aggravates acne is to test it on skin with acne rather than on clear skin. Unfortunately, this type of testing has rarely been done. It is safe to say that when choice is available, the product that contains fewer known comedogenic ingredients is *less likely* to aggravate acne.

NIGHT CREAMS, DAY CREAMS, AND MAXIMUM MOISTURIZERS

Night creams are usually water-in-oil products that are often too oily to use during the daytime. Day creams are light daytime moisturizers and are included with the oil-in-water products in the charts in this chapter. Maximum moisturizers are thick water-in-oil creams designed primarily for older women with dry skin and are essentially the same consistency as night creams.

You will not need a thick night cream or maximum moisturizer unless you have at least moderately dry skin. Because these products are often more expensive, many people assume they are better for the skin. Although they may indeed be more effective for dry skin, these products may lead to problems for people with oily skin or acne.

SPECIAL MOISTURIZERS FOR VARIOUS PARTS OF THE BODY

Various types of moisturizers have been marketed for specific body areas; these products are listed separately in the charts. In most cases, there is no obvious difference in these products that would make them more suitable for a given region of the body. However, the prices of many products would make them prohibitively expensive to use all over the body.

Eye area and lip moisturizers are exceptions. Eye area moisturizers often contain wax to hide wrinkles and are devoid of coal tar colors, which can lead to cancer and even blindness when used near the eyes. Regular moisturizers can also be used near the eyes, but only if they do not contain coal tar colors. Coal tar colors begin with the abbreviation FD&C (e.g., FD&C Red # 3) or D&C (e.g., D&C Red #7) and will be listed on the ingredients label.

Lip moisturizers often have enough added wax to make a stick preparation and will avoid the coal tar colors that are approved only for external use. These color ingredients contain the abbreviations D&C and Ext. (e.g., Ext. D&C Violet #2). Lipsticks usually moisturize quite well so that lip moisturizers are needed only if lipstick is not worn. When using a general moisturizer on the lips, avoid products that contain coal tar colors approved only for external use.

Chart 11–1
MOISTURIZERS AND EMOLLIENT PRODUCTS

The charts are designed to help you minimize adverse reactions and choose products with the proper oil content for your skin type. If you have cosmetics-related acne, you should also choose products with the least amounts of potentially comedogenic ingredients.

Although most cosmetics contain potentially sensitizing ingredients, there is no reason to avoid any ingredient unless you are experiencing adverse reactions to cosmetic products. If you know you are allergic to certain ingredients, the charts will show you which products to avoid. If you are experiencing reactions to a certain cosmetic product, the charts can help you select alternative products that do not contain the same potentially sensitizing ingredients. To choose new products that are least likely to cause allergic reactions, keep in mind that fragrance is by far the most frequent cause of allergic reactions to cosmetics, followed by ingredients listed as "possible sensitizers." The ingredients listed as "other possible sensitizers" cause allergic reactions less frequently. Using these charts should help solve many cosmetics-related skin problems; however, if a problem persists, consult a dermatologist for advice and possible patch testing.

The products listed in these charts include many of the nationally advertised and distributed brands that have the largest market share of cosmetics sales; an extensive sampling of other brands available in the Chicago area is also included.

After locating several suitable products, use the pricing information on pages 18–19 for comparison shopping.

KEY

Possible Comedogenic Ingredients

BS—butyl stearate
CB—cocoa butter
DO—decyl oleate and derivatives
II—isopropyl isostearate
IM—isopropyl myristate
IN—isostearyl neopentanoate
IP—isopropyl palmitate
IS—isocetyl stearate and derivatives
LA—lanolin, acetylated
LO—linseed oil/extract
L4—laureth-4
M—mineral oil
ML—myristyl lactate
MM—myristyl myristate
O—oleic acid
OA—oleyl alcohol
OO—olive oil
OP—octyl palmitate

> Names of products and product lines, and ingredients, are continually changing. Read the labels carefully before purchasing any beauty or skin-care product.

OS—octyl stearate and derivatives
PO—peanut oil
PGS—propylene glycol stearate
PPG—myristyl ether propionate
PT—petrolatum
S—sesame oil/extract
SLS—sodium lauryl sulfate

Possible Sensitizers

A—and other ingredients
B—benzophenones
BP—bronopol (2-bromo-2-nitropropane-1,3-diol)‡
C—cinnamates
D—diazolidinyl urea‡
DM—DMDM hydantoin‡
E—essential oils and biological additives
F—fragrances
I—imidazolidinyl urea‡
L—lanolin and derivatives that may cross-react with lanolin
P—parabens
PB—PABA
PG—propylene glycol
PS—potassium sorbate
Q—quaternium-15‡
SA—sorbic acid

Other Possible Sensitizers

BC—benzalkonium chloride
BHA—butylated hydroxyanisole
BHT—butylated hydroxytoluene
BO—bismuth oxychloride
CH—chlorhexidine and derivatives
CX—chloroxylenol
ED—ethylenediamines
HS—horse serum
MCZ—methylchloroisothiazolinone
MDG—methyldibromoglutaronitrile
MO—mink oil
MZ—methylisothiazolinone
PGL—propyl gallate
T—triethanolamine and derivatives that may cross-react
TG—tragacanth gum
TH—thimerosal
VE—vitamin E (tocopherol and derivatives)

*may contain [see column head]
†does contain (coal tar colors)
††formaldehyde-releasing ingredients

WATER-FREE GENERAL BODY AND FACIAL MOISTURIZERS

Product name	Form	Possible comedogenic ingredients	Possible sensitizers	Other possible sensitizers	Coal tar colors
Adrien Arpel					
Freeze-Dried Collagen Night Creme (sold with Eye Creme)	Cream	IP,PT	F,L,P	BHA	
Line Softener	Stick	IP,PT	L,PB	BHA,BHT,VE	
Body Shop					
Apricot Kernel Oil	Oil				
Body Butter Mango	Cream	PT	F,P	VE	†
Body Massage Oil	Oil			VE	
Carrot Facial Oil	Oil	OO	E,F	BHA	
Cellulite Massage Oil	Oil		E		
Cocoa Butter Suntan Lotion	Lotion	CB,S	E,P,PG	T	
Coconut Beach Oil	Oil		F		
Evening Primrose Oil	Oil				
Jojoba Oil	Oil				
Sweet Almond Oil	Oil				
Wheat Germ Oil	Oil				
Charles of the Ritz					
Revenescence Powder Glow with Encapsulated Moisturizer	Powder with oil	M	F	BO	*
Clarins					
Skin Beauty Repair Concentrate	Lotion		E,P,SA	BHT	
Clientele					
Nourishing Night Oil	Oil	OO	E,P,PG	BHA,BHT,PGL,VE	
Cosmyl					
Algae Oil Complex	Oil		P	BHA,VE	
Cuticura					
Ointment	Ointment	IM,M,PT	E		
Elizabeth Arden					
Ceramide Time Complex Capsules	Liquid		E	VE	
Orange Skin Cream	Cream	PT	F,L,P		
Special Benefit 8 Hour Cream	Cream	M,PT	F,L,P	BHA,BHT	
Erno Laszlo					
Active pHelityl Cream	Cream	IM,IP,PT	F,L	BHA,BHT	
Eutra					
Swiss Skin Creme	Cream	M,PT			

Product name	Form	Possible comedogenic ingredients	Possible sensitizers	Other possible sensitizers	Coal tar colors
Fernand Aubry					
Ligne Specifique Anti-Drying Oil	Oil	M	E	BHT	
Ligne Specifique Vitalizing Oil	Oil	M	E	BHT	
Kids William and Clarissa					
Light Oil	Oil		F,P	VE	
Lancôme					
Fluid Satine Body Silkening Dry Oil	Oil	IN	F,P,PG	BHA	
Mary Kay					
Extra Emollient Night Cream	Cream	M,PT	F,P		†
Treatment Oil	Oil		F,P,PG	BHA,VE	
Merle Norman					
Super-Lube Rich Night Time Emollient Cream	Cream	M	F		†
Nature's Family					
Vitamin E Oil	Oil			VE	
Neutrogena					
Body Oil	Oil	IM,S	F	BHT	
Body Oil (fragrance-free)	Oil	IM,S		BHT	
Orlane					
Body Slimming Sun Gel	Gel	IS,M,PT	C,F,P	VE	†
Physician's Formula					
Dry Skin Emollient Oil	Oil	LA,PT,S	F,PG	PGL	†
Emollient Oil Intensive Treatment	Oil	LA,PT,S	F,PG	PGL	†
Posner					
Coconut Moisturizing Oil	Oil	M	F,L	BHA	
Princess Marcella Borghese					
Hydro-Minerali Skin Revitalizing Extract Creme	Cream	LA,M,MM,PGS	F,L,P	BHA	†
Sally Hansen					
Rejuvia Skin Beauty Oil	Oil		E*	VE	
Sisley					
Coconut Sun Oil	Oil	IM,M	C,F	BHA,BHT,PGL	
Ultima II					
Translucent Wrinkle Cream	Cream	II,IM,M,OO,PT	F,L,P,SA	BHA	†
Vaseline					
Intensive Care Moisture Barrier Salve	Salve	M,PT	F		

109

WATER-IN-OIL GENERAL BODY AND FACIAL MOISTURIZERS

Product name	Possible comedogenic ingredients	Possible sensitizers	Other possible sensitizers	Coal tar colors
Adrien Arpel				
Bio-Cellular Night Cream	M	F,L,P,PG,PS,Q	T	
Alexandra de Markoff				
Skin Renewal Therapy				
Restorative Night Cream	II,IN	DM,P	T	†
Allercreme				
Enriched Night Cream for Dry				
Skin	M,PGS,PT	P	T	
Moisturizing Ultra Emollient				
(+ lanolin)	M,PT	L,P,Q		
Almay				
Moisture Balance Night Cream	M,OP	I,P,PG	T	†
Moisture Renew Night Cream for				
Dry Skin	M,PPG,PT	I,P,PG	T	†
Avon				
Accolade Night Treatment	IM,LA,M,MM, OP,PT	F,I,P	T	†
Moisture Touch Body				
Conditioner	II,IP,MM,OP	F,PG		†
Body Shop				
Rich Night Cream with				
Vitamin E	M,PT	BP,F,L,P	VE	†
Chanel				
Complexe Intensif Night Lift				
Cream		B,E,F,P,PG	VE,PGL	†
Charles of the Ritz				
Revenescence Moist				
Environment Night Treatment				
Cream	IM,LA,PT	F,I,L,P,PG,PS,Q		
Timeless Essence Night Recovery				
Cream	M	F,I,P	VE	
CHR				
Night Cream Concentrate	LA,M	F,I,L,P,PG	BHA	†
Christian Dior				
Hydra-Dior Creme Extra Riche				
Extra Rich Night Cream	IM	F,L,P,SA	BHT,VE	
Hydra-Dior Night Cream	IM	F,L,P	BHT,VE	
Clarins				
Gentle Night Cream	M	F,P	MCZ,MZ,VE	
Clarion				
Clarion Skin Ultra-Pure Night				
Cream	M,OS,PT	D,P	T,VE	†
Color Me Beautiful				
Night Care	DO,IP,S	E,F,I,L,P,PG,Q	T	

Product name	Possible comedogenic ingredients	Possible sensitizers	Other possible sensitizers	Coal tar colors
Coty				
Vitamin A-D Complex Cream	M	F,L,P		
Dubarry				
Moisture Petals Night Cream	M	F,I,L,P	T	
Young Promise Night Cream		F,L,P		†
Elizabeth Arden				
Micro 2000 Stressed-Skin Concentrate[1]	IM,SLS	F,P,PB,PG,Q	VE	
Millennium Night Renewal Cream	DO,IM,M	F,I,L,P,PG,Q	VE	
Nightly Recovery Cream	IP	F,L,P,PG,Q	BHA,PGL	†
Skin Basics Beauty Sleep	IM,M	F,I,L,P	BHA,BHT	
Soothing Care Overnight Soothing Cream	IM,M,PT	I,L,P,Q		
Eucerin				
Creme	M,PT		MCZ,MZ	
Moisturizing Lotion	IM,M	L,PG	BHT,MCZ,MZ	
Eutra				
Light Moisturizing Creme	M,PT	I,P		
Fashion Fair				
Dry Skin Emollient (cream)	M,PT	P,PG	BHA,PGL	†
Fragrance-Free Enriched Night Creme (with aloe vera)	IM,OP,PT	I,L,P,PG	T	†
Fernand Aubry				
Derm Aubry Equivalence Day and Night Intensive Care (cream)	IS,OP	B,C,F,P	BHA,T,VE	
Ligne Fundamentale Aubrysome Fundamental Night Cream	M	F,L,P	T,VE	
Ligne Specifique Revitalizing Night Cream	M	F,P	T,VE	
Night Cream # 2	M	E,F,L,P	BHA,T	
Germaine Monteil				
Firming Action Night Treatment	LA,M,MM,S	D,F,L,P,PG	BHA,PGL,T,VE	†
Marine Therapie Active Sea Night Cream	M,MM,PT	E		
Super Moist Night Creme	IM,LA,M,MM	D,F,L,P,PG		†
L'Oreal				
Plenitude Night Replenisher	S	F,L,P,PG,Q	BHA,BHT,MCZ, MZ,PGL,T	
Lancôme				
Noctosome Renewal Night Creme		F,I,P	MCZ,MZ,VE	
Nutrix Soothing Treatment Creme	M,PT	F,L,P		
ProgresPlus Wrinkle Creme		B,F,I,L,P,PB	MCZ,MZ,T	

[1]This product's base is cyclomethicone, making it a water-in-cyclomethicone product that also contains several oils.

Product name	Possible comedogenic ingredients	Possible sensitizers	Other possible sensitizers	Coal tar colors
La Prairie				
Cellular Wrinkle Cream	LA,M,PT	F,I,P,PG	BHT	
Mary Kay				
Extra Emollient Moisturizer	LA,S	E,F,I,P		
Max Factor				
Overnight Moisture Supplement (cream and gel layered)	IM,M,OP	I,P,PG		†
Merle Norman				
Aqualube (lotion)	M,PT	F,L,P		†
Intensive Moisturizer (cream)	DO,IP,M	F,L,P,PG	BHT	
Luxiva Night Cream with HC-12	PT	D,E,F,I,P	VE	†
Moon Drops				
Discovery Night Cream	M,MM	F,P,PG,Q		
Naomi Sims				
Revitalizing Night Cream	IM	B,I,P,PB,PG	BHA,T	
Neutrogena				
Night Cream	IS,OP,PT,S	I,P	T,VE	
Nivea				
Extra Enriched Moisturizing Lotion	M,PT	F,L	BHT,MCZ,MDG,MZ	
Moisturizing Creamy Conditioning Oil	IM,M	F,L,PG	BHT,MCZ,MZ	
Moisturizing Creme	DO,M,PT	F,L	MCZ,MZ	
Moisturizing Oil	M	F,L,PG	BHT,MCZ,MZ	
Ultra Moisturizing Creme	DO,M,PT	F,L		
Olay				
Night of Olay Night Care Cream	M	F,P		†
Orlane				
Creme à la Gelee Royale Nourishing Night Cream	M,MM,PT	F,I,L,P,PG	T,VE	
Creme Vesperale Night Cream for Sensitive Skin	IS,OP,S	E,P	T,VE	
Soothing Overnight Cream	IS,OP,S	E,I,P	BHA,T	
Physician's Formula				
Day & Night Moisture Cream for Face and Body	M,PT	I,L,P	BHA,T	†
Nourishing Night Cream	M,PT,S	L,P	BHA,BHT	
Princess Marcella Borghese				
Termi di Montecatini Dolce Notte Re-energizing Night Creme	IN,MM,PT	E,I,P	VE	
Revlon				
Maximum Moisture	IN,M,OP,OS	E,I,L,P		

Product name	Possible comedogenic ingredients	Possible sensitizers	Other possible sensitizers	Coal tar colors
Shiseido				
Facial Nourishing Cream				
Concentrate	PT	F,P	VE	
Sisley				
Arnica and Wheat Germ Night				
Cream	M,PT	F,P,PG	HS,T	
Botanical Super Night Cream	M	E,F,P,PG	T	
Tropical Resins Fluid Compound	M,O	F,P,PG,SA	MCZ,MZ	
Wood Mallow and Collagen				
Night Cream	IP,M	F,L,P,PG	MCZ,MZ,T	
Stendhal				
Maximum Moisturizing Cream	LA,M	C,F,L,P	T,VE	†
Recette Marvelleuse Revitalizing				
Night Care Cream		BP,E,F,P,PG	T	†
Recette Marvelleuse Overnight				
Firming Cream	M,PT	E,F,I,L,P	BHT,T	
Ultima II				
Advanced Formula Night Cream	M,MM	F,P,PG	BHA	
Megadose All Night Moisturizer				
(cream suspended in a gel)	IN,M	F,I,P,PG	T,VE	
Moisture Renewal Night Cream	M,MM	F,P,PG,Q		†
Vaseline				
Dermatology Formula Lotion	M,PT	DM,F,P	T	
Intensive Care Extra Strength				
Lotion	M,PT	DM,F,P	T	

OIL-IN-WATER GENERAL BODY AND FACIAL MOISTURIZING CREAMS

Product name	Possible comedogenic ingredients	Possible sensitizers	Other possible sensitizers	Coal tar colors
Adolfo				
Luxurious Body Cream	M,OP	F,L,P	T	
Adrien Arpel				
Morning After Super Moisturizer				
SPF 20	IN	B,C,D,P,PG	T,VE	
Swiss Formula #12 Day Cream	M	F,L,P,PG,PS,Q	T	
Albert Nippon				
Perfumed Body Cream	M,OP	F,L,P	T	
Alexandra de Markoff				
Skin Renewal Therapy Creme		L,P,PB,Q	T	
Allercreme				
Moisturizing Cream	M,PT	D,P		
Special Formula Lubricating				
Cream (lanolin-free/				
unscented)	M,PT,PGS	P	T	

Product name	Possible comedogenic ingredients	Possible sensitizers	Other possible sensitizers	Coal tar colors
Almay				
Anti-Irritant	PT	I,P	VE	†
Moisture Renew Cream	M	P,PG		†
Replenishing Cream	M,PO,PT	B,C,D,PB	T,VE	†
Perfect Moisture	PT	I,P	VE	
Soothing Body Cream	M,PT	D,P	T	
SPF 25 Moisture Cream for Face		B,C,I,P	VE	
Stress Cream	M,PO,PT	D,P	T,VE	†
Vitalizing Moisture Cream	M	I,P	BHA	
Avon				
Accolade Daytime Moisture Support	M,MM,PGS,PT	B,F,I,P,PB	T,VE	
Anew Facial Moisturizing Cream	IP	E,F,I,P,PG	VE	
Daily Revival:				
Continuous Nighttime Moisture Treatment		D,E,F,I,PG	T,VE	
Super Moisture Creme	OP	B,C,E,F,I,L	BHT,T,VE	†
Dramatic Firming Cream	MM	A,E,F,I,P,PG	T	
Imari Moisturizing Body Creme	MM,OP,PT	F,P	T	†
Moisture Therapy Extra Strength Creme	M,MM,PGS,PT	B,F,I,L,P	BHT,T	
Nurtura Replenishing Facial Cream	OP	B,C,F,I,L	BHT,T	†
Perfumed Body Creme (all fragrances)	M,MM,PGS,PT	F,I,P	T	†
Perfumed Skin Softener (all fragrances)	M,MM,PGS,PT	F,I,P	T	†
Pure Care Facial Creme (normal/dry)	MM,PT	B,I,P,PB	BHT,T	
Rich Moisture Face Cream	BS,S	F,L,P,PG	T	†
Vita Moist Face Cream	M,MM,PGS,PT	F,I,P,PG	T,VE	†
BalmBarr				
Hand and Body Creme (cocoa butter formula)	CB,M,PT	F,P	T	†
Biotherm				
Aqualogic Moisture Generator	OO	B,C,E,F,I,P,PG	BC,MCZ,MZ,T,VE	
Biodefense Natural All-Day Defense Treatment	MM,OO,OP	B,C,D,F,P,PS	ED,VE	
Enriched Body Treatment	M,OO	F,I,P	MCZ,MZ	
Reducteur Rides Wrinkle Smoother	OO,PT	B,C,F,I,P	MCZ,MZ,T,VE	
Soin Total Complete Daily Body Treatment	OO	D,F,P	T,VE	†
Body Shop				
Aloe Vera Moisture Cream	CB	F,P	T	
Body Butter Avocado		F,P,PS	T	†

Product name	Possible comedogenic ingredients	Possible sensitizers	Other possible sensitizers	Coal tar colors
Carrot Moisture Cream	IM	F,I,L,P	T	†
Jojoba Moisture Cream	IM	F,I,L,P	T	†
Moisture Cream with Vitamin E	IM	F,L,P	T,VE	†
Chanel				
Coco Creme Pour le Corps Perfumed Body Cream	LA,PGS	BP,F,P	T,VE	
Creme #1/Skin Recovery Cream	LA,MM,PGS	BP,F,L,P,PG	VE	
Creme Pour le Corps #5 Luxury Body Cream	M,MM	BP,F,L,P	T,VE	†
Haute Protection Naturelle Natureblock Cream SPF 15	DO	D,F,P,PG	VE	
Hydra-Systeme Maximum Moisture Cream SPF 8	LA	B,BP,C,F,P,PG	T	
Massage Raffermissant Firming Massage Cream	M,PT	E,F,I,P,PG	PGL,VE	
Charles of the Ritz				
Revenescence Cream Moisturizer	IM,M	F,L		†
Special Formula Emollient	IM,PT	L,P		†
CHR				
Creme Extraordinaire	M	F,L,P,PG	BHA	†
Moisture Creme Concentrate	IM,M	F,L,P,PG,Q		
Christian Dior				
Hydra-Dior Basic Care Cream	IM,M,ML	F,L,P,PG,Q	BHT,T,VE	
Hydra-Dior Creme Assebia Treatment	IM,M,ML	E,F,L,P,PG	BHT,T,VE	†
Hydra-Dior Creme Souveraine Firming and Moisturizing Cream	IM,M,PGS	D,F,L,P,PG	BHT,T	
Icone Secheresse Cutanee Face Cream for Dry Skin		C,F,P	VE	
Resultante Creme du Jour Pour les Rides Moisturizing Day Cream for Wrinkles	LA,M,ML,PPG,S	F,L,P,PB,PG,SA	BHT,T	†
Resultante Creme Resultante Pour les Rides Firming Wrinkle Cream	IM,LA,M,ML	F,L,P,PG	BHT,T,VE	
Resultante Creme Revitalisante Pour les Rides Revitalizing Wrinkling Cream	M,OS,PGS	F,L,P,PG	BHA,T	
Clarins				
Contouring Body Creme	M	E,F,P,PG,SA		
Gentle Day Creme	M	F,P	MCZ,MZ	
Multi-Active Day Creme		F,P	MCZ,MZ,T,VE	
Revitalizing Moisture Base with Cell Extracts	M,PT	C,E,F,P	T	

Product name	Possible comedogenic ingredients	Possible sensitizers	Other possible sensitizers	Coal tar colors
Revitalizing Tinted Moisturizer	M,MM	F,P,PG	MCZ,MZ	
Special Treatment Creme	M	E,F,L,P	MCZ,MZ	
Treatment Creme	M	F,P,PG,SA		
Clarion				
Daily Hydrating Cream	M,OS,PT	D,P	T	†
Clientele				
Preventive Age Treatment	M,OO	D,L,P		
Wrinkle Cream	M,OO,SLS	D,L,P	VE	
Clinique				
Advanced Cream Self-Repair System	M,ML	A,E,I,P	BHT,T,VE	†
Aloe Balm		C,E,I,P,PG		†
Sub-Skin Cream	OP	E,P,PG	VE	
Color Me Beautiful				
Rich Moisturizer	DO,IM,S	F,I,L,P,PG,Q	BHA,T	
Skin Care Extra Protective Hydrating Complex		B,C,E,I,P,Q	T	
Skin Care Intensive Night Care	IP	A,E,I,P,PG	T	
Skin Care Regulating Night Therapy	IP	E,I,P,PG	T	
Complex 15				
Phospholipid Moisturizing Face Cream	MM	D,PG	BHT	
Cosmyl				
Active Performance Hydrating Cream	M,MM	I,P,PG,SA	MO,T,VE	
Hydra-Cell Vital Moisture Cream	M,MM	I,L,P,PG,SA	T,VE	
Cover Girl				
Protective Skin Nourishing Creme SPF 15	M	C,I,P	T	
Curel				
Moisturizing Cream	IP,PT	F,P		
Dermablend				
Maximum Moisturizer SPF 15 (PABA-free)	DO,MM,PT	B,C,DM,L,P	MCZ,MZ,T,VE	
Dubarry				
Liquid Treasure Moisture Balm		D,F,L,P,PG		†
Paradox Creme	DO,IS,M,PT	F,L,P	BHA,BHT	
Elancyl				
Active Toning Cream with Ivy Extract	PT	E,F,P,SA	T	
Beauty Massage Cream with Extract of Ivy	PT	E,F,P,SA	T	

Product name	Possible comedogenic ingredients	Possible sensitizers	Other possible sensitizers	Coal tar colors
Elizabeth Arden				
Body Very Intensive Firming Moisturizer	PT	E,I,P	T	†
Millenium Extra Rich Renewal Creme	M,ML	F,I,L,P,Q	T	†
Millenium Hydrating Body Creme	LA,M,PT	F,I,P		
Perfection Cream for Normal to Dry Skin	PT	F,L,P	BHA,BHT	
Red Door Perfumed Body Cream	M,PT	F,I,P,PG		†
Special Benefit Active Day Protecting Moisture-Cream (untinted)	OA	D,F,PB,PG,PS,Q		†
Visible Difference Refining Moisture Cream Complex	IM,OO	F,I,P		
EPI				
Epi Lotion Hydrating Cream	M,SLS	E,I,P	T	
Erno Laszlo				
Hydra pHel Complex	M,S	D,F,P	BHA,MO,PGL,VE	
pHelityl Cream	M,PT	F,I,P		
Estee Lauder				
Advanced Night Repair		C,E,P	BHT,T,VE	†
Age Controlling Creme	M,OS,PT	I,L,P	VE	†
Gentle Action Skin Polisher	M	F,I,L,P	VE	
Re-Nutriv Creme	BS,M,OS	A,F,L,P,PG	VE	†
Re-Nutriv Firming Plus for Face and Throat	PGS	A,B,C,E,I,P	BHT,T	
Re-Nutriv Lightweight Creme	BS,M,OS,OP	A,F,L,P,PG	VE	†
Skin Defender		C,I,P	BHT,MCZ,MZ	†
Skin Perfecting Creme	IS,M,MM	A,BP,E,F,P	T,VE	
Time Zone Moisture Recharging Complex	OP,OS	B,F,I,L,P,PG	BHT,T,VE	†
Fashion Fair				
Fragrance-Free Moisturizing Creme (with aloe vera)	LA,M,OP,S	I,L,P,PG	BHA,T	
Special Beauty Creme with Collagen	M	I,L,P	T,VE	
Fernand Aubry				
Day Cream for Dry and Delicate Skins	IM,OO	F,L,P	VE	
Day Cream for Sensitive and Mixed Skins	M	F,L,P	T	
Derm Aubry Cream	IM	F,L,P	MO,T,VE	
Derm Aubry Day Cream Moisturizer	M	E,F,L,P	T,VE	

Product name	Possible comedogenic ingredients	Possible sensitizers	Other possible sensitizers	Coal tar colors
Ligne Fondamentale:				
Aubry Base Under Make-Up Moisturizer	IM,M	F,P	T	†
Hydrating Day Cream for Dry Skin	M	E,F,L,P	T	
Protective Cream for Oily Skin	IM,M	E,F,I,P,PG	T	
Soothing Day Cream for Sensitive Skin	M	C,E,F,L,P	T	
Ligne Specifique:				
Moisturizing Day Cream	M	C,E,F,L,P	T	
Slimming Cream	M	E,F,L,P	T	
Flori Roberts				
Gold/Hydrophylic Moisture Complex	DO,M	F,I,P	T	
Melanin Moisturizer	MM,PT	F,P	T	†
Formula 405				
Enriched Cream	IP,LA,M,PT	F,I,L,P	BHA,T,VE	†
Enriched Face Cream	IP,LA,M,PT	F,I,P	BHA,T,VE	†
Hand and Body Cream	IP,M	F,L,P,PG	T	
Frances Denney				
Expression Line Cream	M,PT,S	I,L,P,PG	T,VE	
FD-29 Moisture Cream Formula	PT	A,D,E,P,PG	T	†
Honey Butter Hand and Body Care	M,PT	F,L,P,PG		†
Hope Fragranced Body Cream	M,OP	F,L,P,PG	T	†
Multi-Layer Moisturizer	M	C,F,L,P,PG		
Sensitive Steady Protector	PGS	C,E,I,P,PG	T,VE	
Sensitive Time Preserver	PGS	E,I,P,PG	T,VE	
Sensitive Urgent Nourisher	PGS	C,E,I,P,PG	T,VE	
Source of Beauty Cream	M,PT	F,L,P,PG	T,VE	†
Germaine Monteil				
Acti-Vita Moisture Creme	IM,M	F,I,L,P,PG	T,VE	†
Acti-Vita Multi-Vitamin Creme	IM,M,MM,PT	D,F,L,P,PG	BHA,PGL,VE	†
Creme Satine Royal Secret Satin Body Creme	M,MM	D,F,P,PG	VE	†
Firming Action Moisture Creme	IM,M,MM	D,F,L,P,PG,SA	T,VE	†
Galore Velvet Body Creme	M,MM	D,F,I,P,PG	VE	
Line-Stop Creme Concentrate	M,PT	F,I,P,PG,SA	BHA,PGL,VE	†
Marine Therapie Active Sea Day Creme	IP,PT	E,L	VE	
Super Moist Creme Moisturizer with Line-Stop	IM,LA,M	C,D,F,L,P,PG	T,VE	†
Super Moist Creme Moisturizer with Sunscreen	IM,LA,M	C,D,F,L,P,PG	T,VE	†
Super Sensitive Moisture Creme	M,MM,SLS	E,I,P,PB,PG	T	

Product name	Possible comedogenic ingredients	Possible sensitizers	Other possible sensitizers	Coal tar colors
Supplegen All Day Moisture Creme	IM,M,MM	D,F,P,PG	T	†
Tinted Moisturizer	IM,LA,M	C,D,F,I,L,P	T,VE	
Johnson & Johnson				
Baby Cream	M	F,L,P		
L'Oreal				
Plenitude Action Liposomes	LO	A,B,BP,C,E,F,P,PG	BHA,BHT,PGL,VE	
Plenitude Wrinkle Defense Cream	PT	F,I,P	BHA,BHT,MCZ,MZ	
Lancôme				
Bienfait Multiprotective Day Creme		B,F,P,PB,PG,Q	BHT,T	
Bienfait Multiprotective Day Creme (untinted)	M	B,F,P,PB,PG,Q	T	
Creme Mousse Hydratante Continuous Hydrating Body Treatment	PT	E,I,P	T	
Forte-Vital Tissue Firming Creme	MM	A,E,F,P,Q	BHA,BHT,MCZ,MZ,T	
Hydracreme Hydrating Moisture Creme	IN,M	F,I,P	T	
Hydrix Hydrating Creme	IP,M,PT	BP,F,I,L,P		
Imanance Environmental Protection Tinted Creme SPF 8		B,C,D,E,F,P	MCZ,MZ,T,VE	
Niosome Daytime Skin Treatment		B,F,I,PB,PG	T,PGL	
Nutrix Skin Balancing Creme	M,PT	F,L,P	HS	
Renergie Double Performance Treatment for Face and Throat	MM,PT	B,BP,C,E,F,P,SA	VE	†
Trans Hydrix Multi-Action Hydrating Creme	M	A,B,BP,F,L,P,PB,PG	BHT,T	
Tresor Creme Precieuse Pour le Corps Perfumed Body Creme	PT	B,F,I,P,PG	BHA,BHT,T	†
La Prairie				
Cellular Day Cream	LA,M,PT	F,I,P,PG	T	
Sun Basics After Sun Lotion	M	F,L,P,PG	T	
Mahogany Image				
Rose Velvet Moisturizer	IM,M	F,I,L,P,PG	BHA,T	†
Mary Kay				
Moisture Renewal Treatment Cream	M,PT	F,I,L,P	T,VE	
Max Factor				
Moisture Rich Cream Moisturizer	IP,M,MM	I,P	BHA	
Ultra Rich Moisture Cream	M	P,PG		

Product name	Possible comedogenic ingredients	Possible sensitizers	Other possible sensitizers	Coal tar colors
Merle Norman				
Luxiva Day Creme with HC-12		B,C,E,F,I,P	BHA,T	
Luxiva Protein Creme	PT	DM,F,I,L,P,PG		
Luxiva Protein Body Toner	DO,PT	F,I,L,P	BHA,T	†
Moon Drops				
Enriched Moisture Balm	M,SLS	D,L,P,PG	BHA	†
Enriched Moisture Cream	IP,M	F,P,Q	BHA	†
Nature's Family				
Vitamin E Creme	M	B,D,F,L,P,PG	T,VE	
Naturessence				
Aloe Vera and Paba All Day Moisturizer	M,OP	D,F,L,P,PB,PG	T	†
Anti-UV Aging Defense Cream	M,OP	D,F,L,P,PB,PG	T	†
Collagen and Elastin Age Controlling Cream	M,MM	DM,F,F,P,PG	BHA,T	†
Neutrogena				
Norwegian Formula Emulsion	PT	F,I,P	BHA,BHT,T	
Norwegian Formula Emulsion (fragrance-free)	PT	I,P	BHA,BHT,T	
New Essentials				
Daily Hydrating Cream	M,PT	B,C,D,P	T,VE	
Daily Purifying Cream	M,PT	I,P		
Normaderm				
Cream	IP,M	F,L,P,PG	T	
Noxell				
Noxzema Skin Cream	LO	E,F,PG	T	
Olay				
Oil of Olay:				
Beauty Cream	M,MM	F,I,P,PB	BHA	†
Moisture Replenishing Cream	M,MM	F,I,P,PB	BHA	†
Sensitive Skin Moisture Replenishing Cream	M	I,P		
Water Rinsable Cold Cream	M	F	MCZ,MZ,T	
Orlane				
Anaganese Total Time-Fighting Care (+ SPF)	IS,OP	B,C,F,P	BHA,T,VE	
B-21 Points Vulnerable Creme		C,F,I,P	T	
B-21 Ultra-Light Creme for the Day	IS,OP	B,C,F,P	BHA,T,VE	
Body Slimming Creme	IP,M	F,I,L,P,PG		
Creme Integrale de Jour Protective Day Cream	M,PT	F,I,P,PB		
Day Cream	M,PT	F,I,P,PB		

Product name	Possible comedogenic ingredients	Possible sensitizers	Other possible sensitizers	Coal tar colors
Day Cream for All Skins	M,PT	F,I,P,PG	T	
Gentle Exfoliating Creme	IS,OP,S	F,P	BHA,T	
Hydro Climat Sunscreen and Skin				
Protectant Moisture Shell		B,C,F,P	BHA	
Moisturizing Day Cream	M,PT	F,I,P,PG	T	
Vital Biological Creme	IS,OP,S	F,I,P	BHA,T	
Pacquin				
Dry Skin Cream	ML	F,L,P		
Medicated Hand and Body				
Cream		F,P		
Physician's Formula				
Collagen Cream Concentrate		I,P,Q	BHA,BHT,T	
Deep Moisture Cream	M,PT	I,L,P	BHA,T	†
Enriched Dry Skin Concentrate	IS,LA	F,P,Q	BHA,BHT,T,VE	†
Ponds				
Extra-Rich Moisturizer Dry Skin				
Cream	IP,M,PT	F,I,P	T	
Prescriptives				
Extra Rich Skin Renewer Cream	IP,M,MM	E,I,L,P,PG	VE	†
Flight Cream	LA,M,ML,MM	E,I,P,PG	VE	†
Princess Marcella Borghese				
Termi de Montecatini:				
Cura di Vita per il Corpo				
Restorative Body Treatment	M,PT	E,P,PG	BHA	†
Spa Energia Daily Skin Energy				
Source	MM,PT	E,I,P,PG	VE	
Tono/Body Control Creme				
with Cura Forte Moisturizer				
Intensifier	OP	E,I,P		
Purpose				
Dry Skin Cream	M,PT	F,PG,SA		
Rachel Perry				
Bee Pollen-Jojoba Maximum				
Moisture Cream	OS	F,P,PB,Q		
Ginseng and Collagen Wrinkle				
Treatment		P,PG,Q	T,VE	
Hi Potency "E" Cellular				
Treatment	S	F,P,PG,Q	T,VE	
Lecithin-Aloe Moisture Retention				
Cream	OS	D,E,F,PB	T	
Revlon				
Charlie Moisturizing Body Cream	IM,M,OP	F,I,P,PG	T	
Eterna '27' All Day Moisture				
Cream	M,OP,OS	F,I,L,P		

Product name	Possible comedogenic ingredients	Possible sensitizers	Other possible sensitizers	Coal tar colors
Eterna '27' Cream	IM,M,PT,S	F,L,P,PG	BHA,BHT,VE	†
European Collagen Complex Cream	IM,M,OO	B,F,I,L,P,PG	BHA	†
Xi'a Xi'ang Tea Silk Body Cream	IM,M,OP	E,F,I,P,PG		†
St. Ives				
Collagen-Elastin Essential Moisturizer	M	D,E,F,P,PG	T	†
Vitamin E Enriched Facial Creme	M	E,F,P,PB,Q	T,VE	†
Sally Hansen				
Rejuvia Vitamin E Skin Beauty Cream	S	F,P,PG,Q	T,VE	†
Simplicite				
Pure 24 Hour Protection Creme	IM,M	F,I,P	VE	†
Vitalogics	IM,IP,M,PGS	D,E,P,PG	BHA,T	†
Sisley				
Special Day Cream for Dry Skin	IP,M	E,F,L,P	BHT,MCZ,MZ,T	
Super Day Cream for Mature Skin	M	C,E,P,PG,SA	MCZ,MZ,T	
Smooth Touch				
Deep Moisturizing Cream	CB,PT	F,I,L,P	T	
Stendhal				
Intense Moisture Complex Cream	IP,M	C,F,L,P	BHT,T	
Intense Nutritive Complex Cream	M	C,F,L,P	BHT,T	
Les Bio Program Creme Bio-Confort	M,PT	F,I,L,P	VE	
Pre Tan Exfoliating Creme	OP,PT	F,P	T,VE	†
Recette Marvelleuse:				
Creme Base Anti-Wrinkle Protection	M,PT	C,F,I,L,P,PG	BHT	†
Creme Anti-Rides		BP,E,F,P,PG		†
Satin Body Moisture Treatment Cream	IP,M	F,L,P	BHT,T	
Soin Bio-Reconfort Comfort Cream	M,PT	E,F,I,L,P	BHT,T,VE	
Triple Protection Tinted Cream	PGS	B,C,F,I,L,P,PG	MCZ,MZ,VE	
Sundown				
After Sun Facial Moisturizer	IP,M	F,P,PG	BHT,MCZ,MZ	
Sween				
Cream	SLS	F,L,PG,Q	BHT	
Ultima II				
The Moisturizer for Dry Skin	IN,PT	B,C,E,I,P,PG	VE	†
Under Makeup Nutrient Cream	IM,M	F,L,P,PG,Q	BHA	

Product name	Possible comedogenic ingredients	Possible sensitizers	Other possible sensitizers	Coal tar colors
Yves Saint Laurent				
Enriched Moisturizing Creme	II,IM	F,P,PB,PG,PS	T	
Intensive Skin Supplement				
Creme (with capsules)		DM,E,F,I,P,PG,Q	BHA,PGL,T,VE	

OIL-IN-WATER GENERAL BODY AND FACIAL MOISTURIZING LOTIONS

Adrien Arpel				
Bio Cellular Anti-Sebum Collagen				
Serum	IP,M	F,L,P,PG,PS,Q	T	†
Bio Cellular Hydro-Cellular				
Collagen Serum	M	F,L,P,PG,PS,Q	T	
Moisturizing Blotting Lotion	IP,M	L,P,PG,PS	T	
Swiss Formula #12 Hand &				
Body Lotion	IP,M	F,I,L,P,PG	T	†
Vital Velvet Moisturizer	M	F,L,P,PG,PS	T	
Alexandra de Markoff				
Daytime Moisture	IM	B,F,P,PG		†
Skin Renewal Therapy Lotion	II	I,L,P,PB,Q	T	†
Allercreme				
Dry Skin Lotion	M,PT	L,P	T	
Enriched Petal Lotion				
Moisturizer (normal/dry)	LA,SLS	F,I,L,P	T	†
Moisturizer for Normal/				
Combination Skin	M,PT	D,P		
Moisturizer with Collagen for				
Dry Skin SPF 8	IS,M,PT	D,E,P,PB	BHA,BHT	
Petal Lotion Moisturizer				
(unscented)	IM,M	L,P	T	
Skin Lotion	M,PT	L,P	T	
Special Formula Dry Skin Lotion				
(lanolin-free)	IP,M	P	T	†
Special Formula Skin Lotion				
(lanolin-free)	IP,M	P	T	
Almay				
All Over Body Lotion with Aloe	M,PT	I,P		†
Anti-Wrinkle Daily Moisture				
Lotion	M	C,I,P		
Moisture Balance Moisture				
Lotion (for normal skin)	M,OP,PT	P,PG	T	
Moisture Renew Moisture Lotion	M,PT	I,P,PG	T	†
Moisture Tint Sports Formula	M	C,I,P		
SPF 6 Moisturizing Lotion		B,C,I,P	VE	
Soothing Hand and Body Lotion	M,PT	I,P		†
Tinted Moisturizer	M	I,P	VE	

Product name	Possible comedogenic ingredients	Possible sensitizers	Other possible sensitizers	Coal tar colors
Alo Sun				
After Tan Moisturizing Lotion	M	F,L,P,PG	T,VE	†
Aveeno				
Moisturizing Lotion	IP,PT			
Avon				
Active Fitness System	IN,MM	F,I,P,PB,PG	T	
Bio Advance Lotion	OP,PT	I,L,P	BHT,T	
Body Beauty Silkening Body Lotion	IP,MM,S	F,I,P	BHT,T	†
Fantastique Fragranced Body Veil	IP,MM,S	F,I,P	BHT,T	†
Vivage Fragranced Body Veil	IP,MM,S	F,I,P	BHT,T	†
Care Deeply Body Lotion with Aloe	IM,S	F,I,P	T	
Care Deeply with Cocoa Butter	CB,IM	F,I,L,P	T	†
Country Classics Honey & Almond	M,MM	F,I,P,PG	T	†
Daily Revival Active Moisture Lotion	IP,M,PT	B,C,E,F,I,P	T,VE	†
Daily Revival Sensitive Skin Moisture Lotion	IP,M,PT	B,C,E,I,P	T,VE	
Dew Kiss Daytime Moisturizing Facial Lotion	S	F,L,P,PG	T	†
Dew Kiss Undermakeup	S	F,L,P,PG	T	†
Essentials Milky Balanced Moisturizer		E,F,I,P,PG	VE	
Moisture Shield SPF 15 (tinted/untinted)	M,PT	B,C,E,I,PG,PS	T,VE	
Moisture Therapy Body Lotion	M	F,I,L,P,PG	BHT,T	
Nurtura Light Replenishing Facial Moisturizer	IM	B,C,F,I,P		†
Pure Care Golden Facial Moisturizer	IP,M,PT	B,C,I,P	T	†
Rich Moisture	M,PGS	A,F,L,P,PG	T	†
Rich Moisture Light Facial Moisturizer	IP,MM	F,I,P,PG	T	†
Textone Facial Moisturizing Lotion	MM	F,I,P	T	
Visible Improvement Target Beauty Treatment	M	B,D,E,F,I,P,PG,PS	T,VE	†
Vita Moist Body Lotion	S	F,P	T	†
Vita Moist Body Mousse	M	F,I,L,P,PG	BHT,T	†
Bain de Soleil				
Tan Nourishing Facial Moisturizer	M,OP	DM,F,L,P,PG,Q		

Product name	Possible comedogenic ingredients	Possible sensitizers	Other possible sensitizers	Coal tar colors
Banana Boat				
70% Aloe Vera Skin Care Lotion	M	F,I,P,PG	T,VE	†
After-Sun Lotion	CB,M	F,I,P	T,VE	†
Ben Richert				
Benandre Moisturizing Body Lotion	LA,M	F,P,PG	T	†
Biotherm				
Lait Corporel Antidessechant Anti-Drying Body Milk	M,IP,OO	F,P,PG	BHT,T	
Skin Responsive Hydrating Lotion	M,OO	B,C,F,L,P,PG	T,VE	
Body Magic				
Baby Lotion	M	F,L,P	BC	†
Baby Lotion with Aloe	M	F,L,P	BC	
Body Shop				
Aloe Lotion	IM	F,I,P	T,VE	
Cocoa Butter Hand & Body Lotion	CB	E,P	T	†
Dewberry 5 Oils Lotion		E,F,P	VE	
Glycerin & Rosewater Lotion with Vitamin E	IM,M	E,F,I,P	T,VE	†
Unfragranced Lotion	IP	E,P,PS	T,VE	
White Musk Lotion	CB	F,I,P	T	
Bonne Bell				
Moisture Light Lotion SPF 4	M	C,F,I,L,P,PG,Q	T,VE	
Moisture Lotion	M	D,F,L,P,PG	T	
Skin Musk Body Moisturizer	M	F,I,L,P,Q	T	
10-0-6 Gentle Daily Moisturizer SPF 6 (sensitive skin)	DO,M	C,D,P	T	
Carrington				
Forever Krystle Luxurious Body Lotion	CB,M	DM,F,P,PG	BHA,T	†
Chanel				
Base Purite Total Protection Matte Lotion SPF 15		B,C,F,P,PG	PGL	
Coco Emulsion Pour le Corps Perfume Body Lotion	LA,PGS	BP,F,P	T,VE	†
Emulsion #1/Skin Recovery Emulsion SPF 8	LA	B,BP,C,F,L,P	VE	
Emulsion Hydratante Active Body Moisturizer		E,F,I,P,PG	VE	
Hydrafilm Protective Moisturizer	IM,LA	B,BP,F,I,P,PB	T,VE	
Prevention Serum/Daily Protective Complex SPF 15	LA,OS	BP,F,P,PB,PG	BHA,PGL	

Product name	Possible comedogenic ingredients	Possible sensitizers	Other possible sensitizers	Coal tar colors
Charles of the Ritz				
Measured Moisture-0 Oil-Free Lotion	IN	B,E,F,I,P,PB	VE	†
Measured Moisture-2 Emollient-Rich	IN,M	B,E,F,I,L,P,PB	VE	†
Measured Moisture-3 Emollient-Intensive	M,PGS,PT	B,D,E,F,L,P,PB	VE	†
CHR				
Pro Collagen Anti-Aging Complex for Face and Throat	M	C,E,I,P,PG	T	†
Skin Structure Lotion	DO,LA,M	B,F,P,PG		†
Christian Dior				
Hydra-Dior Base Matte (moisturizer/makeup base)	M,S	F,L,P,PB,PG	BHT,T	
Hydra-Dior Liquid Moisture Base	IM,M	C,F,L,P,PG	BHT,PGL,T,VE	
Hydra-Dior Moisture Base	IM,M	C,F,L,P,PG,Q	BHT,T,VE	
Icone Peaux Reactives		BP,C,F,P	VE	
Resultante Fluide Pour le Corps Firming Body Lotion	IM,M	D,F,L,P,PG	BHT,T	
Clarins				
Revitalizing After Sun Moisturizer	M,OS	E,F,P	BHT,MCZ,MZ,T	
Revitalizing Body Lotion with Cell Extracts	IM,M,OS	F,P,PG	MCZ,MZ,T	†
Clarion				
Nourishing Moisturizer	M,PT	D,P	VE	
Ultra Pure Moisturizer (for the face)	M	DM,P		
Clientele				
Age Defense Hand and Body Lotion	IM	D,E,P,PG	BHA,BHT,PGL,T,VE	
Anti-Aging Activator	S	B,C,PG	VE	
Aqua Protector	M,SLS	D,L,P,PG	BHA,BHT,PGL,T,VE	
Clinique				
Dramatically Different Moisturizing Lotion	M,PT,S	L,P,PG		†
Skin Texture Lotion	MM	E,I,P,PG	T,VE	
Special Hand and Body Lotion	MM	E,I,P,PG	T	†
Color Me Beautiful				
Light Moisturizer	IM,MM	F,I,L,P	T,VE	
Skin Care Lightweight Moisture Lotion	IP,MM,OP,PGS	C,E,I,P	T,VE	
Cosmyl				
Gentle Hydrating Lotion	M	C,F,I,P	T,VE	

Product name	Possible comedogenic ingredients	Possible sensitizers	Other possible sensitizers	Coal tar colors
Hydra-Cell Day Lotion		L,P,PG	BHA,BHT,T	
Moisturizing Skin Balancer	M	I,L,P,PG	T	
Silk Skin Body Lotion	M,PT	F,I,P,PG	T	
Coty				
Jovan Musk for Women: Hand & Body Moisturizing Lotion	M,PT	D,F,P,PG	BHT,T	†
Sand & Sable: Sable Body Lotion	M,PT	F,I,L,P	T	
Vitamin A-D Soft 'N' Rich Body Lotion	M,OS	DM,F,P,PG	T	†
Vitamin Moisture Balancer Emollient Daytime Lotion	M	DM,F,L,P	T,VE	†
Cover Girl				
Protective Skin Nourishing Moisturizer SPF 15		C,I,P	T	
Curel				
Moisturizing Lotion	IP,PT	F,P		
Moisturizing Lotion (fragrance-free)	IP,PT	P		
Diane Von Furstenberg				
Tatiana Moisturizing Body Lotion	IP,M,S	BP,D,F,L,P,PG	BHT,T	
Dubarry				
Moisture Petals Liquid Moisturizer	LA,SLS	F,I,L,P	T	
Paradox Moisturizing Lotion	DO,M,O,PT	F,L,P	BHA,BHT,T	
Elizabeth Arden				
Beautiful Perfumed Body Lotion	IP,PGS	F,P	T,VE	†
Daily Defense Moisture Lotion	LA,M	F,P,PG,Q	BHA,PGL	†
Extra Control Texturizing Conditioner	IM,M	P,Q		†
Immunage UV Defense Lotion for Hands and Body	OS	B,C,F,P,PG	T,VE	
Millennium Day Renewal Emulsion	IM,PGS	F,I,L,P,PG		
Moisture Rich Skin Wash		F,I,P,PG,Q		†
Red Door Perfumed Body Lotion	M,OP,OS,S	F,L,P,PB	BHA,BHT,T	†
Skin Basics Velva Moisture Film	IM,SLS	F,L,P,Q	BHA,BHT,T	
Soothing Care All Day Shielding Moisturizer SPF 4	M,OP,OS	E,I,P,PB,Q	T	
Spa for the Body: Euphorics Organic Body Moisture	OS	B,E,F,P,PG	T	†
Exhilarators Herbal Body Moisture	OS	B,E,F,P,PG	T	†

Product name	Possible comedogenic ingredients	Possible sensitizers	Other possible sensitizers	Coal tar colors
Sensual Botanical Body Moisture	OS	B,E,F,P,PG	T	†
Tranquilities Sea Body Moisture	OS	B,E,F,P,PG	T	†
Special Benefit Bye-Lines Under Makeup Lotion		F	BHA,BHT	
Visible Difference Refining Moisture Lotion SPF 4	M	F,L,P,PB	BHA,BHT,T	
EPI				
Epissentia Protective Light Moisturizer		C,D,E,P,PG	T,VE	
Erno Laszlo				
Hydra pHel Emulsion	LA,M	C,D,F,L,P	BHA,MO,PGL,T,VE	
Hydra-Therapy Hand and Body Emulsion	MM	B,C,D,F,P,PG	VE	†
pHelityl Lotion	M	F,I,P	T	
Skin Conditioner	CB,M,MM,PPG	F,I,L,P,PG		†
Total Skin Revitalizer Lotion		D,F,P,PG	BHT,VE	†
Estee Lauder				
Apres-Tan Maintainer for the Body		F,I,P		†
Maximum Care Body Lotion	II,MM	F,I,P,SA	MCZ,MZ,VE	
Night Repair Skin Recovery Complex		E,I,P,PG		†
Non-Oily Skin Supplement	ML,MM	E,F,I,P	T,VE	
Re-Nutriv Liquid	BS,M,O,PGS,S	A,F,L,P,PG	CX	†
Re-Nutriv Extra-Rich Liquid	IP,M,MM	F,I,L,P,PG	VE	†
Skin Defender Environmental Protector Lotion		C,I,P	BHT,MCZ,MZ	†
Swiss Performing Extract	M	B,E,F,L,P,PG	VE	
Tan Extender	ML	F,I,P,PG	VE	†
Fashion Fair				
Fragrance-Free Moisturzing Lotion	PT	I,L,P,PG	T	
Hand and Body Lotion	M	F,L,P,PG,Q	T	*
Moisture Lotion	M	F,I,L,P,PG	T	†
Special Formula Lotion for Extra-Dry Hands and Body	M	F,I,P,PG	T	*
Fernand Aubry				
Aubry Base Plus Under Makeup Moisturizer	IM,M	I,L,P	T	†
Ligne Specifique Body Moisturizing Milk	IM,M	F,L	T	
Toning Lotion for Dry and Delicate Skin		E,F,P	T	

Product name	Possible comedogenic ingredients	Possible sensitizers	Other possible sensitizers	Coal tar colors
Flori Roberts				
Blue Indigo Moisturizer	IP,MM,PT	F,P	T	†
Formula 405				
Body Smoothing Lotion	IP,M	F,I,L,P	T	
Light Textured Moisturizer	IM	F,I,P	BHA,VE	
Moisturizing Lotion	IP,M	F,I,L,P	T	†
Frances Denny				
Adolfo Luxurious Body Lotion	IM,M,SLS	F,I,P,PB,PG		†
Hope Body Lotion	M	F,I,L,P	T	
Interlude Body Lotion	M	F,L,P	T	
Moisture Care Lotion	IM,OO,OP,SLS	I,P,PB,PG	T	
Sensitive Body Sleek	PGS	E,I,P	T	
Sensitive Oil Balancer	PGS	C,E,I,P,PG	T	
Source of Beauty Lotion	IP,M,SLS	F,I,L,P,PG	T,VE	†
Germaine Monteil				
Acti-Vita Moisture Lotion	IM,M	F,I,L,P,PG	T,VE	†
All Weather Body Lotion	M	B,E,I,P,PB	BHA,PGL,T,VE	
Bio Miracle Lotion	M	F,I,P,PG	T	†
Body Emulsion	IM,M	F,I,P,PG,PS	T	†
Firming Action Moisture Lotion	M,OS	D,F,L,P,PG	BHA,PGL,T,VE	†
Moisture Build Triple Action Emulsion	IN,PT	B,C,E,I,P,PG	VE	
Super Moist Beauty Emulsion with Line-Stop	IM,LA,M	C,D,F,L,P,PG	T,VE	†
Super Moist Beauty Emulsion with Sunscreen	IM,LA,M	C,D,F,L,P,PG	T,VE	†
Super Sensitive Moisture Lotion	IM,M	E,I,P,PG,PS	T	
Gloria Vanderbilt				
Vanderbilt Body Lotion	IP,M	B,F,I,L,P,PG	T	†
Hawaiian Tropic				
Forever Tan Aloe After-Sun Moisturizer	CB,M	F,P,PG	MO,T,VE	†
Jergens				
Aloe and Lanolin Skin Conditioning Lotion	M	F,L,P,Q		
Eversoft Lotion	IP,M,PT	F,P,PG,Q		
Eversoft Lotion (unscented)	IP,M,PT	P,PG,Q		
Jergens Dry Skin Lotion	OS	F,L,P,Q		
Jergens Extra Dry Skin Lotion	IP,M,PT	F,P,Q		†
Vitamin E and Lanolin Skin Conditioning Lotion	M	D,F,L,P	VE	
Jheri Redding				
Caribbean Gold Suntan Extender	CB,M,MM,PT	D,F,L,P,PG,SA	T,VE	

Product name	Possible comedogenic ingredients	Possible sensitizers	Other possible sensitizers	Coal tar colors
Johnson & Johnson				
Baby Oil Pure & Gentle Body Moisturizing Mousse	M	F	MCZ,MZ	
L'Oreal				
Plenitude Active Daily Moisture Lotion		B,BP,F,P,PB		
Plenitude Active Daily Moisturizer	M,S	B,C,D,F,L,P,PG,Q	BHA,BHT,T	
Lancôme				
Clarifiance Oil-Free Hydrating Fluide		B,BP,F,P,PB	T	
Conquête du Soleil:				
Soin Apres Soleil After Sun Body Care		B,BP,C,F,I,P	BHA,BHT,MCZ,MZ	
Soin Extreme Apres Soleil Avec Systeme Niosome Suncare with Natural Botanical Extracts		E,F,I,P	BHA,BHT,MCZ,MZ,T	
Creme-Mousse Hydratante Continuous Hydrating Body Treatment	PT	E,I,P	T	
Hydrative Continuous Hydrating Resource	M	B,C,D,F,L,P,PG,PS	MCZ,MZ,T,VE	†
Niosome Daytime Age Treatment		B,F,I,P,PB,PG	PGL,T	
Nutribel Nourishing Hydrating Emulsion	M	A,F,L,P,PG	BHA,BHT,T	
Progres Texturizing Moisture Lotion for the Body	IP,M,OS	F,L,P,PG	T	
Soin Apres Soleil After Sun Body Care	PGS	B,BP,C,F,I,P	BHT,MCZ,MZ	
Soin Extreme Intensive After Sun Lotion		F,I,P	BHA,BHT,MCZ,MZ,T	
Tresor Lait Precieux Pour le Corps Perfumed Body Lotion	LO	B,E,F,I,P	T	†
La Prairie				
Cellular Body Lotion	LA,M	E,F,I,L,P	T	
Cellular Skin Conditioner	LA,M	F,I,P	T	
Suisse Sensitivity Lotion with Cellular Extracts	M	F,I,P,PG	T	
Mary Kay				
Balancing Moisturizer	M,OS	I,P,PG	T	
Enriched Moisturizer	M	I,P	T	
Exquisite Body Lotion	M	F,L,P,PG,Q	T	†
Moisturizing Lotion (body care)	IN,M	F,P,Q	T	
Nighttime Recovery System		DM,E,P,PG	T	
Skin Balancing Moisturizer	M,OS	I,P,PG	T	

Product name	Possible comedogenic ingredients	Possible sensitizers	Other possible sensitizers	Coal tar colors
Max Factor				
Moisture Equalizing Moisture Lotion	M	I,L,P	BHA	†
Moisture Rich Fluid Moisturizer (fragrance-free)	IS,M	B,P	BHA	†
Merle Norman				
Makeup Texturizer		F,P	BHA,BHT	
Moisturizer Emulsion	LA,M,ML	F,I,L,P,PG		
Moisture Lotion	M	I,P,PG	T	
Moon Drops				
Moisture Burst SPF 8	IN,PT	B,C,E,I,P,PG	VE	
Moisture Film	M,PGS,PT	F,L,P,PG,Q		
Revitalizing Moisturizer	DO,IM,SLS	F,L,P,PG,Q	T	†
Naomi Sims				
Body Conditioner	M,PT	F,L,Q	T	†
Elastin Moisturizer	M,PT	I,L,P,PB	T	†
Nature's Family				
Aloe Vera Lotion	M	B,D,F,P,PG	T,VE	
Vitamin A Lotion	M	B,F,I,P,PG	T,VE	
Vitamin E Lotion	M	B,D,F,P,PG	T,VE	
Naturessence				
NaPCA and PABA Daytime Facial Moisturizer	O,OP	F,I,P,PB		
Neutrogena				
Neutrogena Moisture Facial Moisturizer SPF 5	II,OP,PT	I,P	VE	
New Essentials				
Daily Hydrating Lotion	PT	I,P	VE	
Daily Purifying Lotion	M	I,P		
Nivea				
Original European Formula Moisturizing Lotion	IM,IP,M	F,L	MCZ,MZ	
Visage Facial Nourishing Lotion	IM,IP,M	B,C,F,L,P,PG	T,VE	
Normaderm				
Normaderm Lotion	IP,M	F,I,L,P	T	
Noxzema				
Complexion Lotion		E,F,P,PG		
Liquid Cream	LO	E,F,PG	T	
Nu Skin				
Body Smoother	S	C,D,F,P,PG	T,VE	
Olay				
Oil of Olay: Beauty Fluid	M	F,I,P		†

Product name	Possible comedogenic ingredients	Possible sensitizers	Other possible sensitizers	Coal tar colors
Intensive Moisture Complex	M	DM,F,I,P		†
Sensitive Skin Beauty Fluid	M	I,P	T,VE	
Sensitive Skin Beauty Fluid New Formula	M,PT	DM		
Orlane				
Daytime Moisturizer	MM,OP,S	E,I,P	T	
Oil-Controlling Day Creme	ML,MM	F,I,P		
Vital Biological Emulsion	M	B,E,F,I,L,P	T	
Physician's Formula				
Elastin/Collagen Moisture Lotion	IN,M,ML,SLS	D,P	BHA,BHT	†
Extra Rich Rehydrating Moisturizer	IS,LA,M,OS	D,P	BHT	†
Gentle Moisture Lotion	M,PT	I,L,P		†
Vital Defense Moisture Concentrate (PABA-free/SPF 15)	PGS	B,C,D,P	BHA,BHT,MO	
Ponds				
Cream and Cocoa Butter Lotion	CB,M	F,P,PG	T	†
Prescriptives				
Extra Firm Skin Care Concentrate		E,I	MCZ,MZ,VE	†
Multi-Moisture	MM	B,C,E,I,P,PG	BHT,VE	
Oil-Free Skin Renewer Lotion		E,I,P	T	
Simply Moisture	LA,M,MM	A,C,E,I,L,P,PG	T,VE	
Skin Refiner	LA,M	E,I,P	VE	
Skin Renewer Lotion	LA,M,MM,PGS	E,I,L,P,PG	VE	†
24 Hour Body Moisturizer	LA,M,ML,MM	E,P	VE	
Prince Matchabelli				
Aviance Night Musk Very Silky Body Lotion	LA,M	F,P,PG	T	†
Cachet Very Silky Body Lotion	LA,M	F,P	T	
Princess Marcella Borghese				
Beauty Treatment Moisturizer	IM	F,L,P,PG	BHA,VE	†
Lumina Daytime Moisturizer	IP,M,PT	F,L,P,PG		†
Termi di Montecatini:				
Concentrato de Vita "Living Water" Serum	IM,M	B,E,P,PG		†
Cura di Vita Delicata Restorative Daily Fluid with Sunscreen	PT	B,C,E,I,L,P	VE	†
Cura Forte Moisturizer Intensifier	M,OO	E,I,P,PG		
Restorative Fluid for Face	IP,M	E,P,PG,Q		†
Tono/Body Control Lotion with Cura Forte Moisturizer Intensifier	IP,M,PT	E,I,P	VE	

Product name	Possible comedogenic ingredients	Possible sensitizers	Other possible sensitizers	Coal tar colors
Pupa				
Tenderglow	IM,M,PT	F,I,L,P,PG	T,VE	
Purpose				
Dual Treatment Moisturizer SPF 12	M,OS	B,C,P,Q	BHT	
Revlon				
Anti-Aging Daily Sunscreen Moisturizer:				
For Normal Skin SPF 8	IN,IS	B,C,E,I,P,PG	VE	
For Oily Skin SPF 8	IS,PGS	B,C,E,I,P,PG	VE	
Anti-Aging Sunscreen Skin Humidifier Moisturizer SPF 6	IM,IN,LA,M	B,E,I,L,P,PB,PG	BHA,VE	
Charlie Enriched Body Silk	IP,M,PT	B,E,F,P,PG	BHA	†
Dry Skin Relief Moisture Lotion	IP,M	E,F,P,PG,Q		
Enjoli 8 Hour Hand and Body Lotion	M,PT	DM,F,L,P,PG	T	†
Enjoli Hand and Body Lotion	M,PT	DM,F,L,P,PG		†
Eterna '27' All Day Moisture Lotion	IP,LA,OO,OP,OS,SLS	F,I,P,PG	BHA	
Eterna '27' Hydracolor Tinted Moisturizer with Sunscreen	IN,OS,PGS,PT	B,C,I,P	PGL,T	
European Collagen Complex Lotion	M,PGS,PT	F,L,P,PG,Q		
Jontue Enriched Body Silk with Botanical Extracts	IP,M,PT	B,E,F,P,PG	BHA	†
Pure Skin Care Precise Moisture	IN,OP	E,I,P		
Pure Skin Care Sheer Moisture	M	E,I,P,PG		
Xi'a Xi'ang Body Silk with Peony Extract	IM,OP	F,P,PG		†
Xi'a Xi'ang Tea Silk Body Lotion	IM,L4	D,E,F,P	VE	†
Rose Milk				
Skin Care Lotion	M	D,F,P		†
St. Ives				
Aloe Vera Moisturizing Hand and Body Lotion	M	DM,E,F,P,PB,PG,Q	T	†
Collagen-Elastin Dry Skin Lotion	M	D,E,F,P,PG	MO,T,VE	†
Vitamin E Nutrient-Rich Hand and Body Lotion	M,SLS	D,E,F,P,PB,PG	VE	†
Sally Hansen				
Rejuvia Vitamin E Penetrating Moisture Formula SPF 2	M	F,I,L,P,PB,Q	VE	†
Rejuvia Vitamin E Hand and Body Lotion (with Collagen)	IP,M	F,I,P,PB,PG	T,VE	
Shiseido				
Concentrate Facial Moisturizing Lotion	PT	F,P	VE	

Product name	Possible comedogenic ingredients	Possible sensitizers	Other possible sensitizers	Coal tar colors
Simplicité				
Body Lustre Mist du Lait		DM,P	VE	
Sisley				
Cucumber Fluid Moisturizer	IM,M,O	F,P,PG,SA	HS,MCZ,MZ	
Ecological Compound for the Face	M	E,F,P,PG,SA	MCZ,MZ,T	
Soft Sense				
Aloe Formula Skin Lotion	IP,PT	F,P	VE	†
Extra Moisturizing Dry Skin Lotion	IP,PT	F,P	VE	
Stagelight				
Cucumber Moisturizer	M,S	L,P	T,TG	†
Sparkling Body Lotion	M,PT	P	T	
Stendhal				
After-Sun Face Revitalizer	IP,S	F,P	T,VE	
After-Sun Soothing Body Lotion	IP,M,S	F,P	T,VE	
Base Extreme Anti-Brilliance Anti-Shine Moisturizing Base SPF 4	IP,M	C,F,L,P,PS	BHT,MCZ,MZ,T	
Intense Moisture Concentrate SPF 4	IP,M	C,F,L,P	BHT,T	
Intensive Vitality Complex SPF 4	M	C,F,L	T	
Moisturizing Body Emulsion SPF 6 Extra Protection	IP,S	B,C,F,L	MCZ,MZ,T,VE	
Prevenance au CPF Daily Anti-Time Formula	M	B,C,F,L,P	CH,T,VE	
Recette Marvelleuse Body Emulsion Revitalizing Treatment		F,I,P,PG		†
Satin Body Moisture Treatment Lotion	IP,M	F,L,P	BHT,MCZ,MZ,T	
Suave				
Aloe Vera Skin Lotion	CB,IP,M	A,DM,F,P	T	†
Cocoa Butter Skin Lotion	CB,IP,M	A,DM,F,P	T	
Extra Relief Skin Lotion	CB,IP,M	A,DM,F,P	T	
Ultima II				
Fresh Daily Moisture	PGS,S	F,L,P,PG,Q		
Photo Aging Shield	IS,PGS	B,C,F,P,PG,Q	VE	†
ProCollagen Face and Throat Lotion with Sunscreen	M	C,E,I,P,PG	T	†
Translucent Wrinkle Lotion	IP,M	B,F,P,PG		†
Under Makeup Moisture Lotion	DO,IM,M	F,L,P,PG	BHA,T	
Vaseline Intensive Care				
Aloe and Lanolin Lotion	M	DM,F,L,P	T	†
Lotion	M	F,P,PG	T	†

Product name	Possible comedogenic ingredients	Possible sensitizers	Other possible sensitizers	Coal tar colors
Lotion for Sensitive Skin	M,PT	DM,F,P	T	
Lotion for Sensitive Skin with Vitamin E	M,PT	DM,F,P	T,VE	
Wondra				
Lotion (unscented)[2]	IP,PT	I,L,P		
Lotion for Normal to Dry Skin	IP,PT	F,I,P	T	
Yves Saint Laurent				
Intensive Serum		F,P,PG	T	

OIL-IN-WATER GENERAL BODY AND FACIAL MOISTURIZING GELS AND MOUSSES

Product name	Possible comedogenic ingredients	Possible sensitizers	Other possible sensitizers	Coal tar colors
Almay				
Stress Body Moisturizer	M,S	B,I,P		†
Avon				
Rich Moisture Facial Moisturizing Mousse	M	F,I,L,P,PG	T	
Milopa				
After-Sun Gel	M	F,I		

OIL-FREE GENERAL BODY AND FACIAL MOISTURIZERS CONTAINING EMOLLIENT ESTERS

Product name	Form	Possible comedogenic ingredients	Possible sensitizers	Other possible sensitizers	Coal tar colors
Alexandra de Markoff					
Moisture Balance Lotion	Lotion	DO,LA	F,I,P,PG	T	†
Almay					
SPF 15 Moisturizing Lotion	Lotion		B,C,I,P	T,VE	
Avon					
Adapt Facial Moisturizer	Lotion		F,P,PB,PG,SA	BHT,T	
Body Silks (all fragrances)	Lotion	OP	F,I,P	T	
Clearskin 2 Oil-Free Moisture Supplement Facial Lotion	Lotion		B,F,P,PB,PG		
Daily Revival Facial Lotion Oil Free SPF 6	Lotion	OP	B,C,D,F,I,P	T,VE	†
Fragranced Body Lotion (all fragrances)	Lotion	OP	F,I,P	T	
Momentum Facial Moisturizer	Lotion	OP	B,C,F,I,P	BHT,T,VE	†
Night Support Facial Moisturizer[3]	Lotion		F,I,P,Q	T,VE	†
Pure Care Facial Moisturizer (oily skin)	Lotion	OP	B,C,I,P	T	
Soft Musk	Mousse	IM	F,PG	BHT	

[2]This product contains a "masking fragrance."
[3]This product contains trace amounts of oil.

Product name	Form	Possible comedogenic ingredients	Possible sensitizers	Other possible sensitizers	Coal tar colors
Bonne Bell					
10-0-6 Oil-Free Moisturizer SPF 6	Lotion	DO	C,D,P	T	
Chanel					
Lift Serum Corrective Complex	Lotion	DO,OS	BP,E,F,P,PG		†
Lotion #1/Oil-Free Skin Recovery Lotion SPF 8	Lotion	MM,PGS	B,BP,C,E,F,P		†
Charles of the Ritz					
Perfumed Body Lotion	Lotion	OP	F,P		†
CHR					
Moisture Lotion Concentrate	Lotion	DO,LA	B,F,P,PG		†
Christian Dior					
Dioressence Creme Soyeuse Pour le Corps Perfumed Silk Body Cream	Cream	IM,ML	F,P,PG	T	
Miss Dior Creme Soyeuse Pour le Corps Perfumed Silk Body Cream	Cream	IM,ML	F,P,PG	T	
Clarins					
Doux Gommage Pour Lisant Visage Gentle Exfoliating Refiner	Lotion	IS	E,F,P	VE	
Clarion					
Double Defense Moisturizer	Lotion	OS	B,C,D,E,P	VE	†
Oil-Free Moisturizer	Lotion		D,P	VE	
Protective Moisturizer with SPF 6	Lotion	OS	D,P	VE	
Clientele					
Moisture Concentrate	Lotion	IP	I,P		
Oil-Free Daytime Moisture Concentrate	Lotion	IP	I,P		
Oil-Free Moisture Concentrate	Lotion	IP	I,P,PB		
Clinique					
Advanced Care Moisture Lock Body Formula	Cream	ML,MM	E,I,P,PG	BHT,T	†
Color Me Beautiful					
Skin Care Oil-Free Regulating Fluid	Lotion	MM	C,E,I,P,PG	T	
Coty					
Overnight Success: Active Strength Cream for Dry Skin	Cream	IP	F,P		

Product name	Form	Possible comedogenic ingredients	Possible sensitizers	Other possible sensitizers	Coal tar colors
Active Strength Lotion for Dry Skin	Lotion	IP	F,P		
Effective Body Lotion	Lotion	IP	F,P		
Instant Face Smoother	Lotion	LA,MM	D,F,P		
Cover Girl					
Oil-Free Pure Performing Creme	Cream	IP	DM		
Oil-Free Pure Performing Moisturizer	Lotion		DM		
Dubarry					
Hand Silk Hand and Body Cream	Cream		F,P		
Oil-Free Moisturizer	Lotion		F,I,P,PG		
Elancyl					
Hydra-2 Moisture Treatment for the Body	Lotion		F,I,P	MCZ,MZ,VE	
Elizabeth Arden					
Eau Fraiche Body Moisturizer	Lotion	LA	F,P,PG,Q		†
Estee Lauder					
Apres-Sun Cool Spray	Spray		F,I		
Re-Nutriv Firming Body Lotion	Lotion	OS	E,F,P	T,VE	†
Skin Perfecting Lotion	Lotion	MM,OS	C,E,I,P,PG	BHT,T,VE	
Fashion Fair					
Fragrance-Free Oil-Free Moisturizer	Lotion	IM,IP,PGS	D,E,P,PB,PG	T,VE	
Fernand Aubry					
Derm Aubry Cellular Renewal Complex	Lotion		F,I	MCZ,MZ	†
Flori Roberts					
Gold/Oil-Free Moisturizer	Lotion	IP,PGS	E,P,PB,PG	T,VE	
Frances Denney					
FD-29 Anti-Aging pHormula	Cream	PT	A,D,E,P,PB,PGT		
FD-29 Moisturizing pHormula	Lotion	PT	A,D,E,P,PB,PGT		
Sensitive Clean Sweep	Cream		E,I,P	T,VE	†
Sensitive Moisture Reservoir	Lotion		E,I,P	T,VE	†
Germaine Monteil					
Lift Extreme	Lotion		D,E,F,P		†
Moisture Build Triple Action Emulsion	Lotion		B,C,E,I,P	VE	
Oil-Free Moisture	Lotion	OP	F,I,L,P,PG		
Skin-Stress Relief Dual Phase Balancing System	Cream		I,P,PG	VE	

Product name	Form	Possible comedogenic ingredients	Possible sensitizers	Other possible sensitizers	Coal tar colors
Gloria Vanderbilt					
Glorious Perfumed Body Lotion	Lotion	IP	F,I,P,PG	BHA,T,VE	
Johnson & Johnson					
Baby Lotion	Lotion	IP,MM	F,P,PG	BHT	†
Kids William and Clarissa					
Lotion	Lotion	IM	D,E,F,I,P,PG	T,VE	
Lancôme					
Oglio-Major Activating Serum	Lotion		F,I,PG	MCZ,MZ,T	
Mary Kay					
Angelfire Perfumed Body Lotion	Lotion		F,P,Q	BHA,ED	†
Avenir Perfumed Body Lotion	Lotion		F,P,Q	ED	†
Genji Perfumed Body Lotion	Lotion		F,P,Q		†
Intrigue Perfumed Body Lotion	Lotion		F,P,Q		†
Oil Control Lotion	Lotion		DM,P	T	
Premonition Perfumed Body Lotion	Lotion		F,P,Q	BHA,ED	†
Max Factor					
Le Jardin Caressing Body Lotion	Lotion	OP	F,I,P		†
Merle Norman					
Protective Veil	Lotion	IP,O,PGS	DM,F,P,PG		
Sheer Tint Tinted Moisturizing Cream	Cream	ML,OP,OS	DM,P,PB,PG		
Neutrogena					
Body Lotion	Lotion	IM,SLS	F,I,P	T	
Body Lotion (fragrance-free)	Lotion	IM,SLS	I,P	T	
Neutrogena Moisture SPF 15 Formula Facial Moisturizer (tinted/untinted)	Lotion		B,C,I,P	T	
New Essentials					
Moisture Maximizer	Cream		B,I,P		
Nivea					
Visage Facial Nourishing Cream	Cream	IM,IP	B,C,F,I,L,P,PG	BHT,VE	
Nu Skin					
NaPCA Moisturizer	Lotion		C,D,F,P,PG	T,VE	
Rejuvenating Cream	Cream	OP,OS	C,D,F,P,PG	VE	

Product name	Form	Possible comedogenic ingredients	Possible sensitizers	Other possible sensitizers	Coal tar colors
Olay					
Oil of Olay:					
Daily UV Protectant 100% Color- and Fragrance-Free Beauty Fluid SPF 15[4]	Lotion		C,I,P	T	
Daily UV Protectant Beauty Fluid SPF 15[5]	Lotion		C,F,I,P	T	
Daily UV Protectant Moisture Replenishing Cream SPF 15[6]	Cream		C,F,I,P	T	
Fragrance-Free Daily UV Protectant Beauty Fluid SPF 15 Original Formula[7]	Lotion		C,I,P	T	
Oil-Free Replenishing Cream	Cream	IP	DM,F		
Oil-Free Beauty Fluid New Formula	Lotion		DM,F		
Night of Olay Night Care Cream New Formula	Cream	IP	DM,F		†
Pacquin					
Medicated Hand and Body Cream	Cream		F,P		
Physician's Formula					
Oil-Control Oil-Free Moisturizer	Lotion	IS	B,P,Q		†
Vital Defense Oil-Free Moisturizer (SPF 15/PABA-free)	Lotion	IS	B,C,P,Q		
Prescriptives					
Blemish Control (2.5% benzoyl peroxide)	Gel		E,P,PG		
Princess Marcella Borghese					
Hydro-Minerali Skin Revitalizing Extract	Lotion	IM,IS	F,I,P,PG		†
Termi di Montecatini:					
Cura di Vita Delicata Restorative Creme for Face with Sunscreen	Cream	IN	B,C,E,I,P	VE	†
Equilibrio Equalizing Spa Restorative	Lotion	IN	C,E,I,P	VE	†
Revlon					
Aquamarine Extra Moisturizing Body Lotion	Lotion	IP	F,P,PG	VE	†
Aquamarine Skin Conditioning Body Lotion	Lotion	IP	F,P,PG		†

[4]This product contains trace amounts of oil.
[5]This product contains trace amounts of oil.
[6]This product contains trace amounts of oil.
[7]This product contains trace amounts of oil.

Product name	Form	Possible comedogenic ingredients	Possible sensitizers	Other possible sensitizers	Coal tar colors
Aquamarine Soothing All-Over Body Lotion	Lotion	IP	F,P,PG		
Clean & Clear Oil-Free Facial Moisture Lotion	Lotion	IN	E,I,P,PG		†
Trouble Sensuous Body Lotion	Lotion	IM	F,P,PG		†
Sea Breeze Moisture Lotion	Lotion	PPG	DM,F,I,P	MCZ,MZ,T	
Sisley Botanical Night Complex for Mature Skin	Lotion		E,P	MCZ,MZ	
Sundown After Sun Body Moisturizer	Cream	IP,MM	F,P,PG	BHT	
Tritle's Hand and Body Lotion	Lotion	IM,IP,IS	F,I,P	T	†
Tropical Blend Tanning Accelerator	Lotion	MM,SLS,	F,I,P,PG	VE	†
Yves Saint Laurent Balancing Fluid	Lotion		F,P,PB,PG,PS		

STRICTLY OIL-FREE GENERAL BODY AND FACIAL MOISTURIZERS

Product name	Form	Possible comedogenic ingredients	Possible sensitizers	Other possible sensitizers	Coal tar colors
Adrien Arpel Clear Line Fill	Lotion		P,PG		
Allercreme Oil-Free Moisturizer	Lotion	SLS	P,PG		
Almay After Sun Soother	Lotion		I,P	VE	†
Moisture Multiplier	Cream		B,I,P		†
Oil-Control Lotion for Oily Skin	Lotion		P		
Replenishing Lotion	Lotion		B,C,I,P	VE	
Stress Moisture Supplement	Lotion		B,I,P	VE	†
Stress Tonic	Spray		I,P		
Avanza Naturessence European Elastin Firming Facial	Gel		D,F,P,PG	T	†
Avon Daily Revival Oil-Free Moisture Protector	Lotion		B,E,F	T,VE	†
Maximum Moisture Super Hydrating Complex[8]	Gel		B,E,I,P,Q	T,VE	†
Smooth Finish Facial Moisturizer	Lotion		E,P,PG		†
Time Control Facial Moisturizer	Lotion		P,PG		†

Product name	Form	Possible comedogenic ingredients	Possible sensitizers	Other possible sensitizers	Coal tar colors
Banana Boat					
Pure Collagen Gel	Gel		F,I,P,PG	T	†
Biotherm					
Symbiose Naturel Daily Care for Natural Aging	Lotion		D,F,P,PG	T	
Charles of the Ritz					
Revenescence Liquid	Lotion	SLS	F,P		
Christian Dior					
Capture Complex Liposomes	Lotion		F,P,PG	T	†
Clientele					
Ion Protector[9]	Gel		D,P,PG	BHA,BHT, PGL,VE	
Clinique					
Moisture Surge	Gel		B,E,I	MCZ,MZ,VE	†
Collastin					
Oil-Free Moisturizer for the Face	Lotion		SA		
Color Me Beautiful					
Skin Care Multi-Action Revitalizing Concentrate	Cream		C,D,E,P,PG,Q		
Cosmyl					
Vital Synergy Skin Repair Complex	Cream		C,E,P,PG	T,VE	†
Cover Girl					
Advanced Clean Moisturizing Hydrogel	Gel		DM,PG		
Estee Lauder					
Equalizer Oil-Free Hydrogel	Gel		I,PG	T	†
Fashion Fair					
Fragrance-Free All Purpose Protein Creme	Cream		I,P,PG	T	*
Fernand Aubry					
Ligne Fondamentale:					
Lotion for Dry Skin	Lotion		E,F,P,PG	T	
Lotion for Sensitive Skin	Lotion		E,F,P,PG	T	†
Ligne Specifique ISD 26					
Night Gel	Gel		E,F,P,PG	T	
Frances Denney					
FD-29 Activating pHormula	Lotion	O	D,P,PG	VE	†
Sensitive Nourishing Lotion	Lotion		E,I,P	T,VE	†
Sensitive Protecting Lotion	Lotion		E,I,P	T,VE	†
Ultimate Repair	Lotion		I,P,PG	T	†

[9]This product contains trace amounts of oil.

Product name	Form	Possible comedogenic ingredients	Possible sensitizers	Other possible sensitizers	Coal tar colors
La Prairie					
Cellular Cycle Ampules for the Body:					
Lyophilized Substance (and)	Lotion		P		
Solvent (used together)	Lotion		E,F,P,PG		†
Mary Kay					
Anti-Aging Complex	Lotion		C,DM,P,PG	T	†
Daily Defense Complex SPF 4	Lotion		DM,P,PG	T,	†
Max Factor					
Pure SPF Daily Face Protector	Lotion		C,D,P,PG	T	†
Merle Norman					
Luxiva Collagen Support	Lotion		F,I,P,PG	T	
Luxiva Energizing Concentrate	Lotion		F,I,P,PG	T	
Luxiva Moisture Mask	Cream		F,I,P,PG	TG	†
New Essentials					
Revitalizing Night Serum	Lotion		B,I,P		
Nu Skin					
Celltrex	Lotion	O	D,P,PG	VE	
NaPCA Moisture Mist	Lotion		C,D,PG		
Sunright Accel	Lotion		D,P	T,VE	
Orlane					
Extrait Vital Eye Contour	Lotion		P,PG	BHT	
Pure and Soothing Lotion	Lotion		I,P		
Princess Marcella Borghese					
Termi di Montecatini la Dolce Cura Anti-Stress Restorative Facial Creme	Cream		E,I,P,PG	BHA,T	†
Pupa					
Glitter	Lotion		F,I,P,PG	T	
Rachel Perry					
Elastin-Collagen Firming Treatment	Cream		E,F,I,P	T	
Revlon					
Anti-Aging Sunscreen Firmagel Moisturizer SPF 6[10]	Gel		E,I,P,PG	T,VE	†
Clean & Clear Moisture Firm Facial Treatment	Lotion		E,I,P,PG		
Simplicité					
Moisturin Rx	Lotion		I,P,PG		
Stagelight					
Body Jewels	Gel		F,P,PG	T	

[10]This product contains trace amounts of oil.

Product name	Form	Possible comedogenic ingredients	Possible sensitizers	Other possible sensitizers	Coal tar colors
Stendhal					
Recette Marvelleuse Anti-Wrinkle Program	Cream		E,P	HS,T	†
Self Firming Plan for the Skin	Cream		F,P,PG	MCZ,MZ,VE	†
Ultima II					
Fresh Blotting Lotion with Moisturizers	Lotion		DM,F,P,PG		

OIL-IN-WATER MOISTURIZERS CONTAINING LARGE AMOUNTS OF HUMECTANTS

Product name	Form	Possible comedogenic ingredients	Possible sensitizers	Other possible sensitizers	Coal tar colors
Aqua Care					
Cream (with 10% Urea)	Cream	M,PT	F,L		
Lotion (with 10% Urea)	Lotion	M,PT,SLS	P		
Betamide					
Lotion	Lotion	M	F		
Carmol					
10 Lotion (10% Urea)	Lotion	IP	PG		
20 Cream (20% Urea)	Cream	IM,IP	F,PG		
Epilyt					
Epilyt Lotion	Lotion	O	PG	BHT	
Gormel					
Creme (20% Urea)	Cream	M,O,SLS	P,PG	T	
Lac-Hydrin					
V-Lotion	Lotion	PT	D	MCZ,MZ	
12% Lotion[11]	Lotion	L4,M	F,P,PG,Q		
Lacticare					
Lacticare Lotion	Lotion	IP,M,ML	DM,F		
Nutraplus					
10% Urea Cream	Cream	M,ML,OP	P,PG		
10% Urea Lotion	Lotion	IP,PT	P		

SILICONE-TYPE MOISTURIZERS

Product name	Form	Possible comedogenic ingredients	Possible sensitizers	Other possible sensitizers	Coal tar colors
Estee Lauder					
Future Perfect Micro-Targeted Skin Gel	Gel		E,I,PG	MCZ,MZ,VE	†

WATER-FREE EYE AREA MOISTURIZERS

Product name	Form	Possible comedogenic ingredients	Possible sensitizers	Other possible sensitizers	Coal tar colors
Adrien Arpel					
Bio Cellular Night Eye Gelee	Cream	M,PT	C,P	VE	
Freeze-Dried Collagen Protein Eye Creme (sold with Night Creme)	Cream	IM,PT	L,P	BHA	
Almay					
Moisture Renew Eye Cream	Cream	M,PT	I,P		

[11] This product is available by doctor's prescription only.

Product name	Form	Possible comedogenic ingredients	Possible sensitizers	Other possible sensitizers	Coal tar colors
Christian Dior Hydra-Dior Gentle Eye Care Cream	Cream	IM,PT	F,L,P	BHA,BHT,PGL	
Color Me Beautiful Skin Care Fortifying Eye Cream	Cream	IP	E,I,P,PG	T	
Dermablend Wrinkle-Fix Line Smoother for Lips and Eyes	Stick	M	B,C,L,P	VE	
Elizabeth Arden Ceramide Eye Time Complex Capsules	Oil	OO	E	VE	
Kelemata Anti-Wrinkle Stick for the Eyes	Stick	IM,M,PT	B	BHT	
Nu-Skin Intensive Eye Complex	Cream	O,OP,OS	D,P	VE	
Princess Marcella Borghese Lineless for Eyes	Cream	M	E,P	BHA	
Ultima II Translucent Wrinkle Cream for the Eyes	Cream	IM,M,OP,PT	P	BHA	

OIL-BASED EYE AREA MOISTURIZERS

Almay Moisture Balance Eye Cream	Cream	IM,M,PT	I,L,P,PG	BHA,PGL	
Elizabeth Arden Special Eye Beauty Cream	Cream	CB,M,PT	F,P		
Visible Difference Eye Care Concentrate	Lotion	M,OP,OS	P,PG	BC,CH	
Fashion Fair Fragrance-Free Eye Creme	Cream	M,OP,S	D,P	BHA,T,VE	

WATER-BASED EYE AREA MOISTURIZERS

Adrien Arpel Swiss Formula #12 Day Eye Creme	Cream	M,PT,S	D,L,P,PG	BHA,T	
Alexandra de Markoff Skin Renewal Therapy Restorative Eye Creme	Cream		PG		
Allercreme Eye Cream	Cream	M,PT	D,P		
Special Help Eye Cream (+ collagen)	Cream	IS,M,PT	D,P		

Product name	Form	Possible comedogenic ingredients	Possible sensitizers	Other possible sensitizers	Coal tar colors
Almay					
Eye Protector	Cream	M,PT	I,P		
P.M. Intensive Eye Treatment	Cream	OS,PT	I,P	VE	
Avanza					
Naturessence Anti-Wrinkle Eye and Throat Cream	Cream		D,E,P	T,VE	
Avon					
Daily Revival Eye Lift Creme SPF 6	Cream	M,MM	C,E,I,P	T,VE	
Nurtura Replenishing Eye Cream	Cream	M,MM	B,C,I,P	T	
Biotherm					
Bioregard Natural Tri-Active Eye Care	Lotion	M,OO	E,I,P,PG,SA	T	
Firming Eye Cream	Cream		C,D,F,I,L,P	T,MCZ,MZ,VE	
Reducteur Rides Eyes Active Eye Smoother	Cream	MM,OO,PT	B,C,F,I,P,SA	MCZ,MZ,T,VE	
Body Shop					
Under Eye Cream	Cream	CB	P	T	
Chanel					
Creme No.1 Pour les Yeux Skin Recovery Eye Cream	Cream	BS,DO,O,M	BP,L,P,PG		
Firming Eye Cream	Cream	LA	E,I,P,PG	BHA,PGL,T	
Charles of the Ritz					
Revenescence Moist Environment Eye Cream	Cream	IM,M	I,L,P,PG	T	
CHR					
Eye Creme Concentrate	Cream	M,MM	DM,P,PG		
Christian Dior					
Resultante Creme Contour des Yeux Eye Care Cream	Cream	IM,LA	C,F,P,PG,Q	BHT,T,VE	
Clarins					
Baume "Special" Contour des Yeux Eye Contour Balm with Plant Extracts	Cream		E,P	MCZ,MZ,VE	
Clarion					
Revitalizing Eye Cream	Cream	IS,M,OS,PT	D,P	T,VE	
Clinique					
Daily Eye Benefits	Cream	MM,PT	E,I,P		
Color Me Beautiful					
Eye Care Cream	Cream	DO,IP,S	I,L,P,PG,Q	BHA,T	
Cosmyl					
Hydra-Cell Eye Creme	Cream	OP,S	D,E,P	T,VE	

Product name	Form	Possible comedogenic ingredients	Possible sensitizers	Other possible sensitizers	Coal tar colors
Cover Girl					
Invisible Lines Eye Cream	Cream	IP,M,PGS	E,P,PG	T,VE	
Dubarry					
Eye Cream	Cream		L,P		
Elizabeth Arden					
Millennium Eye Renewal Creme	Cream	M	L,P	BC,CH,BHA,BHT	
Estee Lauder					
Re-Nutriv Firming Eye Creme	Cream	BS,IM,M,O, OS,PGS	E,I,P	VE	
Fernand Aubry					
Derm Aubry Special Eye Cream	Cream	IM	F,L,P	T	
Ligne Specifique Eye Contour Gel	Gel		E,F,PG	MZ,T	
Frances Denney					
Eye Cream Concentrate	Cream	M	I,P,PG	BO,VE	
Sensitive Tender Eyes	Lotion		E,I,P	T	
Germaine Monteil					
Acti-Vita Eye Creme	Cream	IM,M	F,I,L,P,PG	BHA,PGL,T,VE	
Firming Action Eye Creme	Cream	IM,M,MM	D,F,L,P,PG	BHA,PGL,T	
Super Sensitive Moisture Eye Creme	Cream	IM,M,MM	E,I,L,P,PG	T	
L'Oreal					
Eye Defense	Cream		I,P	T	
Plenitude Eye Contour Cream	Cream		F,L,P,PG	BHA,BHT,T	
Lancôme					
Forte-Vital Firming Eye Creme	Cream	M	A,F,P		
Progres Eye Cream	Cream	PT	F	TH	
La Prairie					
Cellular Eye Contour Cream	Cream	LA,M,PT	F,I,P,PG	T	
Essence of Skin Caviar Cellular Eye Complex	Gel		B,DM,I,P,PG	T,VE	
Mary Kay					
Eye Cream Concentrate	Cream	M,PT	E,I,P,PG	BHA,T,VE	
Merle Norman					
Eye Creme Complex	Cream	LA,M,OP,OS	I,P		
Luxiva Eye Creme	Cream	MM,PT	F,I,L,P,SA	BHA,T	
Naomi Sims					
Collagen Eye Cream	Cream		D,P,PG	T	
Neutrogena					
Eye Cream	Cream	DO,M,PT	I,P	T	

Product name	Form	Possible comedogenic ingredients	Possible sensitizers	Other possible sensitizers	Coal tar colors
New Essentials					
Hydrating Eye Cream	Cream	OS,PT	I,P	VE	
Orlane					
Anaganese Eye Contour Creme	Cream	IS,OP,S	B,BP,C,E,F,P	BHA,VE	
Eye Contour Creme	Cream	IS,OP,S	B,C,F,P,PG	BHA,T,VE	
Eye Cream	Cream	IM,M	F,I,P,PG		
Physician's Formula					
Luxury Eye Cream	Cream	M,PT,S	L,P,PG	BHA,BHT,PGL	
Prescriptives					
Line Smoother (for eye area/ lips/neck)	Cream	IS,LA,ML,PT	E,P	VE	
Princess Marcella Borghese					
Termi di Montecatini:					
Hydro-Minerali Revitalizing Eye Creme	Cream	IP,M	B,P,PG,Q		
Contro Tempo Antidote for Eyes (+ SPF)	Cream	IN,M	C,E,I,P,PG	T,VE	
Restorative Eye Creme	Cream	M,PGS	E,P,PG,Q		
Simplicité					
Hydro-1 Eyecreme (sold with Gel)	Cream	IM,IP	P,PG	T	
Sisley					
Botanical Eye and Lip Contour Complex	Lotion		E,P	MCZ,MZ	
Stendhal					
Bio Contour Lift Eye Contour Creme	Cream	M	F,I,L,P	MCZ,MZ,T,VE	
RM 2 Contour Des Yeux Eye Contour Gel	Gel		F,P	CH,T,VE	

OIL-FREE EYE AREA MOISTURIZERS CONTAINING EMOLLIENT ESTERS

Product name	Form	Possible comedogenic ingredients	Possible sensitizers	Other possible sensitizers	Coal tar colors
Chanel					
Eye Lift Corrective Eye Complex	Cream	DO	D,E,P,PG	T,VE	
Estee Lauder					
Time Zone Eyes	Cream		I,P	T,VE	
Frances Denney					
FD-29 Eye Gel pHormula	Gel	O	D,P,PG	VE	†
Germaine Monteil					
Eye Rescue Gel	Gel		D,E,P,PG,SA		†
Light Years Eye Area Formula	Gel		C,I,P,PG		

Product name	Form	Possible comedogenic ingredients	Possible sensitizers	Other possible sensitizers	Coal tar colors
Kelemata					
Anti-Wrinkle Balm for the Eye	Balm		F,I	BHT,MCZ,MZ	
Merle Norman					
Eye Texturizer	Cream	MM	F,P	BHA,T	
Simplicité					
Hydro-1 Gel (sold with Eyecreme)	Gel		D,E,P,PG	T,VE	†

STRICTLY OIL-FREE EYE AREA MOISTURIZERS

Product name	Form	Possible comedogenic ingredients	Possible sensitizers	Other possible sensitizers	Coal tar colors
Almay					
Stress Eye Gel	Gel		B,D,P,PG		
CHR					
Anti-Aging Complex Especially for Eyes			C,E,I,P,PG		
Color Me Beautiful					
Skin Primers Eye Care Gel	Gel		E,I,P,PG,Q	T	
Elizabeth Arden					
Special Benefit Puffiness Calming Eye Gel	Gel		E,P,PG	T	
Estee Lauder					
Eyezone Repair Gel	Gel		I,PG	MCZ,MZ	
Kelemata					
Herb Eye Gelee for the Eye Area	Gelee		E,I,P,PG		
Herb Eye Mask	Cream		E,I,P,PG		
Max Factor					
Puffy Eye Minimizer	Gel		D,P,PG	T	
Merle Norman					
Luxiva Triple Action Eye Gel[12]	Gel		D,E,F,P	BO,T	
Princess Marcella Borghese					
Termi di Montecatini Restorative Eye Balm	Gel		C,E,P,PG,Q		
Revlon					
Anti-Aging Firming Eye Gel	Gel		C,I,P,PG		
Sisley					
Botanical Eye and Lip Balm	Gel		P,PG	MCZ,MZ,T	†
Ultima II					
Megadose for Eyes	Gel		I,P,PG		

[12]This product contains trace amounts of oil.

Product name	Form	Possible comedogenic ingredients	Possible sensitizers	Other possible sensitizers	Coal tar colors
Yves Saint Laurent					
Instant Smoothing Eye Contour Gel	Gel	P,PG			

FOOT MOISTURIZERS[13]

Product name	Form	Possible comedogenic ingredients	Possible sensitizers	Other possible sensitizers	Coal tar colors
Avon					
Essentials Peppermint Foot Lotion	Lotion	IM,S	B,E,F,I,P	T	†
Fancy Feet Deep Moisture Cream	Cream	M,SLS	F,I,P		
Fancy Feet Double Action Cream	Cream		F,I,P	T	
Barielle					
Total Foot Care Cream	Cream	M,PT,S,SLS	F,I,L,P	VE	†
Body Shop					
Peppermint Foot Lotion	Lotion	CB	E,L,P	T	†
EPI					
EPI Ped Revitalizing Moisture Gel for Feet	Gel	M	D,F,P	T	
Mary Kay					
Energizing Foot and Leg Treatment	Lotion	M	I,P,PG,Q	T	†
Pretty Feet & Hands					
Pretty Feet & Hands	Lotion		F,P		
Smooth Touch					
Smooth Touch Foot and Leg Lotion	Lotion	CB,M	F,I,P,PG	T	†

WATER-BASED HAND MOISTURIZERS

Product name	Form	Possible comedogenic ingredients	Possible sensitizers	Other possible sensitizers	Coal tar colors
Adrien Arpel					
Swiss Formula #12 Hand & Body Lotion	Lotion	IP,M	F,I,L,P,PG	T	†
Almay					
Intensive Moisture Mask for Hands	Cream	PT	I,P	VE	†
Intensive Therapy for Hands	Cream	M,OS,PT	I,P	VE	†
Moisture Repair for Hands, Nails and Cuticles	Cream	M,OS,PT	I,P	VE	
Soothing Hand and Body Lotion	Lotion	M,PT	I,P		†
Avon					
Care Deeply: With Aloe	Cream	IM,M,MM,S	F,L,P,PG	T	

[13]Products in this chart are water-based unless otherwise noted.

Product name	Form	Possible comedogenic ingredients	Possible sensitizers	Other possible sensitizers	Coal tar colors
Cocoa Butter	Cream	CB,IM,M, MM,S	F,L,P,PG	T	
for Pump Decanters	Lotion	IM,S	F,I,L,P	T	
Hand and Body with Aloe	Lotion	IM,S	F,I,P	T	
Hand and Body with Cocoa Butter	Lotion	CB,IM	F,I,L,P	T	†
Essentials Hand and Body Lotion	Lotion	IP,PT	B,E,F,I,P	T,VE	†
Fragranced Hand Cream	Cream	IP	F,P,PG	BHT,T	
Moisture Therapy SPF 8	Cream		B,C,F,I,L	BHT	
Rich Moisture Hand Cream	Cream	M,S	F,I,L	BHA	†
Silicone Glove Silicone Hand Cream	Cream	M,SLS	F,I,P		
Skin-So-Soft Hand and Body Cream	Cream	IP	F,P,PG	BHT,T	
Vita Moist Hand Cream	Cream	IP,M,MM	F,I,P	T	†
BalmBarr					
Hand and Body Creme (cocoa butter formula)	Cream	CB,M,PT	F,P	T	†
Barielle					
Professional Protective Hand Cream	Cream	IP,M	F,I,L,P,PB,PG	VE	†
Biotherm					
Bio Main Protective Hand Treatment	Cream	M,OO	F,L,P	BHT,T	
CHR					
Hand Creme Concentrate	Cream	IM,IS,M	F,P,PG		†
Christian Dior					
Resultante Creme Soin des Mains Treatment for Hands	Cream	M,ML,PPG	F,P,PB,PG,SA	BHT,T,VE	
Clarins					
Creme Jeunesse des Mains Hand and Nail Treatment Cream	Cream	IM	E,F,PG	MCZ,MZ,T	
Clinique					
Special Hand and Body Lotion	Lotion	MM	E,I,P,PG	T	†
Complex 15					
Phospholipid Hand and Body Cream	Cream	M,MM	D	BHT	
Phospholipid Hand and Body Lotion	Lotion	MM	D	BHT	
Cosmyl					
Silk Skin Hand Creme	Cream	M,OP	F,I,L,P	T	
Silk Skin Hand Lotion	Lotion	M,OP	F,I,L,P	T	

Product name	Form	Possible comedogenic ingredients	Possible sensitizers	Other possible sensitizers	Coal tar colors
Cutex					
Complete Care for Nails and Hands	Lotion	CB,MM,PPG, PT	DM,F,P,PG	VE	
Delore					
Hand Saver Moisturizing Creme	Cream	IP,M,PT	D,F,P		†
Elizabeth Arden					
Immunage UV Defense Lotion for Hands and Body	Lotion	OS	B,C,F,P,PG	T,VE	
Estee Lauder					
Maximum Care Hand Cream	Cream	IP,OP,OS	F,I,P,PG	MCZ,MZ,VE	†
Re-Nutriv Extra-Rich Lotion for Hands and Arms	Lotion	M,MM	B,F,L,P,PB		†
Fashion Fair					
Hand and Body Lotion	Lotion	M	F,L,P,PG,Q	T	*
Special Formula Lotion for Extra-Dry Hands and Body	Lotion	M	F,I,P,PG	T	*
Formula 405					
Hand and Body Cream	Cream	IP,M	F,L,P,PG	T	
Frances Denney					
Honey Butter Hand and Body Care	Cream	M,PT	F,L,P,PG		†
Sensitive Hand Rescue	Cream	PGS	B,E,I,P,PG	T,VE	†
Germaine Monteil					
Protective Hand Treatment	Lotion	IM,M,MM,OP	F,I,L,P,PS	BHA,PGL	†
Lancôme					
Nutrix Hand Treatment Cream	Cream	IP,M,OS	BP,F,I,L,P,PB		
La Prairie					
Cellular Hand Cream	Cream	M	E,F,I,P,PG	T	
Mary Kay					
Hand Cream	Cream	LA,S	C,F,I,P,Q	VE	†
Mavala					
Hand Cream	Cream	IM	A,F,P	T	
Max Factor					
Age Shield Moisture Treatment for Hands SPF 4	Lotion	M,OP	C,I,P		
Merle Norman					
Extra Rich Hand Creme	Cream	M	F,P,PG	T	
Nu Skin					
Hand Lotion	Lotion	S	C,D,F,P	VE	
Pretty Feet & Hands					
Pretty Feet & Hands	Lotion		F,P		

Product name	Form	Possible comedogenic ingredients	Possible sensitizers	Other possible sensitizers	Coal tar colors
Princess Marcella Borghese					
Termi di Montecatini Splendide Mani Smoothing Hand Cream with Sunscreen	Lotion		C,E,I,P	VE	
St. Ives					
Aloe Vera Moisturizing Hand and Body Lotion	Lotion	M	DM,E,F,P, PG,Q	T	†
Vitamin E Nutrient-Rich Hand and Body Lotion	Lotion	M,SLS	D,E,F,P,PB, PG	VE	†
Sally Hansen					
Rejuvia Hand & Nail Therapy Moisturizing Lotion	Lotion	M	B,DM,F,I,P, PG	VE	*
Rejuvia Vitamin E Hand and Body Lotion	Lotion	IP,M	F,I,P,PB,PG	T,VE	
Rejuvia Vitamin E Hand Cream	Cream	IP	F,I,P,PB	T,VE	
Stendhal					
Satin Soft Hand Cream SPF 3	Cream	IP,MM,OP	C,I,F,P,PG	VE	
Suave					
Hand & Nail Lotion	Lotion	CB,IP,M	A,DM,F,P	T,VE	†
Vaseline Intensive Care					
Hand & Nail Formula Lotion	Lotion	M	DM,F,P,PG	T,VE	†
Hand & Nail Formula Lotion (fragrance-free)	Lotion	M	DM,E,P,PG	T,VE	†

OIL-FREE HAND MOISTURIZERS CONTAINING EMOLLIENT ESTERS

Product name	Form	Possible comedogenic ingredients	Possible sensitizers	Other possible sensitizers	Coal tar colors
Blistex					
Tritle's Hand and Body Lotion	Lotion	IM,IP,IS	F,I,P	T	†
Body Shop					
Hawthorne Hand Cream	Cream	IM	E,F,P		†
Clinique					
Advanced Care Hand Repair SPF 6	Lotion		I,P,PG	BHT,T,VE	†
Estee Lauder					
Hand Perfecting Treatment	Cream		A,B,C,F,I,P	BHT,VE	†
Neutrogena					
Norwegian Formula Hand Cream	Cream		F,P		
Norwegian Formula Hand Cream (fragrance-free)	Cream		F,P		

STRICTLY OIL-FREE HAND MOISTURIZERS

Product name	Form	Possible comedogenic ingredients	Possible sensitizers	Other possible sensitizers	Coal tar colors
Avon					
Moisture Therapy Hand Cream	Cream		F,I,P		
Mavala					
Eau Active Hand Lotion	Lotion		F,I,P	MCZ,T	†

WATER-FREE LIP MOISTURIZERS

Product name	Form	Possible comedogenic ingredients	Possible sensitizers	Other possible sensitizers	Coal tar colors
Adrien Arpel					
Lip Problem Repair	Stick		B,C,L,P	BHA,VE	
Almay					
Lip Concentrate	Stick	PT	B,C,I,P	T,VE	†
Moisturizing Lip Protector	Ointment	M,PT	B,C,P	BHA,VE	
Avon					
Care Deeply with Aloe/ Sunscreen	Ointment	M,PT	C,F	BHT	
Citrus Tinglers Flavor Savers	Stick	I,P	C,F,L	BHT	†
Lip Dew	Stick	I,P	F,L	BHT	†
Moisture Therapy	Ointment	PT	B,C,L	BHT	†
Sunseekers Protective Lip Balm SPF 15	Stick	CB,M,PT	B,C	BHT,VE	
Body Shop					
Honey Stick	Stick		B,C,E,L,P,SA		
Lip Balm	Ointment	PT	E,F,P		*
Dermablend					
Wrinkle-Fix Line Smoother for Lips and Eyes	Stick	M	B,C,L,P	VE	
Elizabeth Arden					
Special Benefit 8 Hour Cream Lip Protectant Stick SPF 15	Stick	PT	F,L,P,PB	BHT,R,VE	
Fashion Fair					
Perfect Primer Lip Moisturizer	Stick	OP	F,PG	BHA,PGL	*
Germaine Monteil					
Traitement Continuelle Lip Conditioner with Sunscreen SPF 6	Compact	OP,OS	B,C,E,P	BHA,VE	†
Lancôme					
Nutrix Lip Balm	Ointment	LA,PT,S	B,C,F,L	BHA,BHT	*
Max Factor					
Pure Magic Restorative Lip Care	Stick	OA,OP	C,F,P	BHA,BO,VE	†

Product name	Form	Possible comedogenic ingredients	Possible sensitizers	Other possible sensitizers	Coal tar colors
Merle Norman					
Lip Moisture	Compact		F,L	BHA,BHT	†
Moon Drops					
All Weather Lip Moisturizer	Stick	LA,M,OA	F,L,P,PB	BHA	*
Neutrogena					
Lip Moisturizer SPF 15	Stick	M,OP,PT	B,C,L		
Pfeiffer					
Petroleum Jelly Lip Treatment	Ointment	PT			

WATER-BASED LIP MOISTURIZERS

Product name	Form	Possible comedogenic ingredients	Possible sensitizers	Other possible sensitizers	Coal tar colors
Adrien Arpel					
Bio Cellular Lip Line Cream Line Softener	Cream	M,PT,S	F,I,L,P,PG	T	
Almay					
Stress Lip Treatment	Cream		B,C,I,P	T,VE	
Avon					
Advanced Foundation Lip Conditioner	Cream	M,MM	C,I,P		
Care Deeply Medicated Lip Relief	Cream	M,MM,PGS, PT	B,P,PB		
Elizabeth Arden					
Visible Difference Lip-Fix Creme	Cream	IM,M	A,I,P,Q		
Fernand Aubry					
Derm Aubry Special Lip Cream	Cream	M	F,L,P	T	
New Essentials					
Soothing Lip Treatment	Cream	PT	B,C,I,P	VE	
Prescriptives					
Line Smoother (for eye area/ lips/neck)	Cream	IS,LA,ML,PT	E,P	VE	
Simplicité					
Lip Comfort Treatment	Stick	IM,M	P	BHA,VE	
Sisley					
Botanical Eye and Lip Contour Complex	Lotion		E,P	MCZ,MZ	
Stendhal					
Recette Marvelleuse Smoothing Lip Care	Cream	M,PT,S	F,I,L,P,PG	BHT,T	
RM 2 Tour des Levres Lip Contour Creme	Cream	IP,S	F,P	CH	†

Product name	Form	Possible comedogenic ingredients	Possible sensitizers	Other possible sensitizers	Coal tar colors
STRICTLY OIL-FREE LIP MOISTURIZERS					
Sisley					
Botanical Eye and Lip Balm	Gel		P,PG	MCZ,MZ,T	†
WATER-FREE NAIL MOISTURIZERS					
Almay					
Hot Oil Therapy for Nails and Cuticles	Oil	M,O	P	BHA,VE	
Barielle					
Intensive Nighttime Nail Renewal	Cream	M,O,S	F,P	VE	
Chanel					
Huile Fortifiante Pour les Ongles Strengthening Nail Oil	Oil		E	BHT,VE	
Cutex					
Medicated Cuticle Rescue	Cream	IM,M,OA,OS	E,P	VE	
Le Ponte					
Precious Organic Nail Treatment	Cream	O		VE	
Sally Hansen					
Apricot Extract Cuticle Cream Groomer	Cream	OP	F,P,PG	BHA,PGL	
Vitamin E Moisturizing Nail and Cuticle Oil	Oil		P	VE	
OIL-BASED NAIL MOISTURIZERS					
Chanel					
Creme Fortifiante de L'Ongle Nail Repair Creme	Cream	DO	E,F,P,PG	VE	
Christian Dior					
Creme Abricot Pour les Ongles Apricot Nail Cream	Cream	M	BP,F,L,P	BHT	†
Mavala					
Cuticle Cream	Cream	M,PT	BP,F,L,P,PG		
WATER-BASED NAIL MOISTURIZERS					
Almay					
Daily Cuticle Therapy	Cream	M,O	I,P	VE	
Moisture Repair for Hands, Nails and Cuticles	Cream	M,OS,PT	I,P	VE	
Nail Refinishing Buffing Cream	Cream	M	I,P	VE	†

Product name	Form	Possible comedogenic ingredients	Possible sensitizers	Other possible sensitizers	Coal tar colors
Barielle					
Nail Strengthener Cream	Cream	M,PT,SLS	F,I,L,P	VE	
Clarins					
Creme Jeunesse des Mains Hand and Nail Treatment Cream	Cream	IM	E,F,PG	MCZ,MZ,T	
Clarion					
Nail Resiliance Cream	Cream	M,OP,PT	D,P		
Clinique					
Nail Treatment Cream	Cream	OP,OS	A,E,I,P	BHT	
Cosmyl					
Cuticare Cuticle Cream	Cream	IM	I,P,PB,PG	VE	*
Cutex					
Complete Care for Nails and Hands	Lotion	CB,MM,PPG, PT	DM,F,P,PG	VE	
Time Drops Nail Renewal Complex	Lotion	S	B,I,P,PG	BHA,T,VE	†
Mavala					
Nailactan Nutritive Nail Cream	Cream	IM,OA	F,I,P	MCZ,MZ,VE	
Merle Norman					
Nail Treatment Creme	Cream	M	F,I,L,P,PG	T	†
Pro-Cute					
Cream	Cream		F	T	
Lotion	Lotion		F,SA	T	
Revlon					
Cuticle Massage Night Cream	Cream		E,F,I,L,P,PG		†
Sally Hansen					
Apricot Extract Cuticle Massage Cream	Cream	IP,M	F,I,L,P,PG,SA		†
Nail Therapy	Gel	IP,MM	F,I,PG	MZ,MCZ,T,VE	†
No More Dry Cuticles	Lotion	M	D,F,P,PG	T,VE	*
Rejuvia Hand & Nail Therapy Moisturizing Lotion	Lotion	M	B,DM,F,I,P, PG	VE	
Renew-A-Nail Night Time Nail Therapy	Lotion	S	B,E,F,I,P,PG	BHA,T,VE	*
Suave					
Hand & Nail Lotion	Lotion	CB,IP,M	A,DM,F,P	T,VE	†
Vaseline Intensive Care					
Hand & Nail Formula Lotion	Lotion	M	DM,F,P,PG	T,VE	†
Hand & Nail Formula Lotion (fragrance-free)	Lotion	M	DM,E,P,PG	T,VE	†

Product name	Form	Possible comedogenic ingredients	Possible sensitizers	Other possible sensitizers	Coal tar colors
OIL-FREE NAIL MOISTURIZERS CONTAINING EMOLLIENT ESTERS					
Clarion					
Conditioning Strengthening Gel	Gel		DM	T	†
Estee Lauder					
Nail Perfecting Treatment	Cream	SLS	B,C,F,I,P,SA	T,VE	
Revlon					
Daily Diet Nail Grow Cream	Cream	IP,MM,O	E,F,I,P,PG	VE	†
STRICTLY OIL-FREE NAIL MOISTURIZERS					
Almay					
Conditioning Nail Concentrate	Liquid	O	B,I,P	VE	†
NECK AND THROAT MOISTURIZERS[14]					
Alexandra de Markoff					
Throat Creme	Cream	IM,M	F,I,L,P,PG		†
Avon					
Anew Perfecting Complex for Chest and Neck (oil-free)	Lotion		E,I,P,PG		
Body Shop					
Neck Gel	Gel	CB	E,F,P	T	
CHR					
Pro Collagen Anti-Aging Complex for Face and Throat	Lotion	M	C,E,I,P,PG	T	†
Christian Dior					
Resultante Creme Pour le Cou Throat Cream	Cream	IM,OA	C,F,L,P,PG, SA	BHT,CH	
Elizabeth Arden					
Ceramide Time Complex Capsules (water-free)	Liquid		E	VE	
Millennium Throat Renewal Creme	Cream	PT	F,P		
Fernand Aubry					
Derm Aubry Beauty Gel for the Neck	Gel		E,F,P,PG	T	†
Frances Denney					
Neck & Throat Care Cream	Cream	IP,M	F,I,L,P,PG		

[14]All products in this chart are water-based preparations unless otherwise noted.

Product name	Form	Possible comedogenic ingredients	Possible sensitizers	Other possible sensitizers	Coal tar colors
Germaine Monteil					
Contour Throat Creme	Cream	M,ML	B,C,D,F,I,P,PG	T,VE	†
Lancôme					
Progres Throat Creme	Cream	IM,PO	F,P,PB,PG,Q	BHA,BHT	
Renergie Double Performance Treatment for Face and Throat	Cream	MM,PT	B,BP,C,E,F,P,SA	VE	†
La Prairie					
Cellular Neck Cream	Cream	LA,M,PT	F,I,P,PG	T	
Merle Norman					
Luxiva Neck Creme	Cream	IP	E,F,I,P,PG,SA	BHA,VE	
Naturessence					
Anti-Wrinkle Eye and Throat Cream	Cream		D,E,P	T,VE	
Prescriptives					
Line Smoother (for eye area/ lips/neck)	Cream	IS,LA,ML,PT	E,P	VE	
Stendhal					
Recette Marvelleuse Neck and Decolette Treatment	Cream	IM,M	C,F,P		†
Ultima II					
ProCollagen Face and Throat Lotion with Sunscreen	Lotion	M	C,E,I,P,PG	T	†

Soaps and Cleansers, Abrasive Scrubs, and Masks

HOW CLEANSERS WORK

Cleansers are products that remove excess sebum (skin oils), dirt, and other undesirable substances from the skin. They may be applied with the fingers, a wash cloth, or a puff with equal results.

Some data show that soaps may remove oil from the skin better than detergents. Otherwise, there is no convincing data showing one type of cleanser to be superior to another. Cleansing ability is usually not a major factor in choosing a skin cleanser.

Cleansers range from very moisturizing to very drying. It is important to know your skin type in order to choose the best type of skin cleanser for your skin (see Chapter 5). Use the following chart to find out which cleansers are best suited to your skin type.

Soaps and Cleansers	Moisturization	Skin Type
lipid cleansers or cleansing creams	very moisturizing	dry, dry/sensitive
lipid-free	mildly moisturizing	sensitive; any skin type
surfactant with oil	probably mildly moisturizing	moderately dry
surfactant with oil-free moisturizing ingredients	probably neutral	normal
surfactant, plain	drying	oily
deodorant soaps or acne cleansers	drying	oily

Abrasive Scrubs	Moisturization	Skin Type
plain	drying	oily
with oil-free moisturizing ingredients	neutral, reduces oil	any skin type
oil-containing	moisturizing	dry

Masks	Moisturization	Skin Type
powder	drying	oily
vinyl, plain	mildly drying	normal to oily
vinyl with humectants	neutral, reduces oil	any skin type
gel type	mildly moisturizing	any skin type
lipid type	moisturizing	dry

LIPID CLEANSERS AND CLEANSING CREAMS

The simplest cleansers are oils and water. Sebum and other oily materials will dissolve in oil and dirt can be removed by water. Since the combination of rinsing with water and using an oil is an effective way to clean the skin, a number of cosmetics companies market lipid cleansers. These products are very effective at removing oily cosmetics. Moreover, they leave an oily residue and are excellent for dry skin. They are also very gentle and effective for dry to normal sensitive skin. Some of these products may be water-free oils; others are oil-based or water-based creams or lotions. Water-free products are the most moisturizing and water-based products are the least moisturizing. The oiliness of any of these products is enough to aggravate pimples; they should be avoided by people with oily or acne-prone skin.

Cleansing creams are traditionally lipid cleansers with sodium borate added. Sodium borate is no longer believed to have strong antiseptic and cleansing effects, and is used today primarily as a buffering ingredient (i.e., an ingredient used to control the pH of a product). Lipid cleansers, cleansing creams, lipid makeup removers, and oily moisturizers are virtually identical types of products.

LIPID-FREE CLEANSERS

Lipid-free cleansers contain water and mild solvents such as glycerin and propylene glycol and no oils, soaps, or detergents. They are minimally irritating products and are probably the best cleansers to use for sensitive skin that is normal to oily. The solvents used are also humectants that act as mild moisturizing agents. These products are designed for sensitive skin and can be used by all skin types.

SURFACTANTS, SOAPS, DETERGENTS, AND SOAP-FREE CLEANSERS

Many cleansers use surfactants to clean the skin. Surfactants are complex substances that are able to dissolve both oil- and water-soluble substances.

Soaps are surfactants that are salts derived from plant and animal oils or fats. The two most common soaps used in cosmetic products are sodium cocoate and sodium tallowate.

Synthetic detergents are surfactants, but are not derived from plant or animal oils or fats. Soap-free cleansers are detergent cleansers with no soap. Some products contain both detergent and soap.

Surfactant cleansers (soaps, soap-free cleansers, and soap/detergent combinations) can be made with added oil to produce a mildly moisturizing product for slightly dry skin. Alternatively, they can be made with added oil-free moisturizing ingredients such as humectants, emollient esters, or fatty acids (soaps containing the latter are called superfatted soaps). These oil-free products are probably relatively neutral products (or slightly drying) most suitable for normal skin. Some superfatted soaps claim to be for dry skin; however, lipid cleansers are certainly more effective for moisturizing very dry skin. Surfactant cleansers without added moisturizing ingredients are somewhat drying because they remove oil from the skin without replacing it and are therefore best for oilier skin.

Soaps and Skin Irritation
The irritancy of soaps has been a rather controversial subject. The pH of the skin reflects whether the skin is acidic or basic. A pH of 7.0 is neutral, values above 7.0 are basic, and values below 7.0 are acidic. The normal skin pH is around 5 to 6, which is slightly acidic. The least irritating cleansers will have a pH that is close to the normal skin pH. Plain soaps have a higher (basic) pH and will be irritating if left on the skin for extended periods of time. In contrast, most soap-free cleansers and soap/detergent combinations have been modified chemically to have a lower pH so that they will be less intrinsically irritating.

The Finn chamber test is the standard laboratory test done to measure the irritancy of cleansers. Unfortunately, this test leaves cleansers on the skin for lengths of time far exceeding normal washing and therefore soaps appear extremely irritating. If rinsed thoroughly from the skin after use, most soaps will not irritate normal skin. When using any cleanser, it is important to rinse off as much residue as possible. Some cleansers rinse off more easily than others. If hard water is used for bathing, soap residue will be more difficult to rinse off thoroughly and irritation is more likely to occur. In these cases, a soap-free cleanser may be less irritating.

Skin Cleansers for Sensitive Skin
Soap-free cleansers or soap-detergent combinations are modified so that the pH is closer to normal skin pH and may be sufficiently mild to use on sensitive skin. Lipid-free cleansers or lipid cleansers are usually even less prone to causing irritation.

Cleansers for Acne
Acne cleansers may be soaps and/or detergents with the addition of therapeutic agents used in acne medications (benzoyl peroxide, sulfur). Alternatively, they may be alcohol or witch hazel solutions that are essentially astringents or skin toners (see Chapter 13) but are marketed to be used as cleansers. Also, some exfoliants are marketed as acne cleansers to help unplug skin pores. Any of these products are certainly helpful for acne; however, the less expensive deodorant soaps probably work just as well.

Abrasive scrubs marketed for acne can actually aggravate acne by irritating skin follicles if used too aggressively. In addition, not all abrasive scrubs are appropriate for use with acne.

Deodorant Soaps
Deodorant soaps are usually plain soaps with added antibacterial agents, such as triclocarban or triclosan, to kill the bacteria responsible for body odors. Deodorant soaps are also very effective cleansers for acne because they are also active against bacteria that play a role in acne.

ABRASIVE SCRUBS

Abrasive scrubs contain particulate matter that abrades the skin. They have been marketed as mechanical exfoliating products that peel off dead skin or for use by people with acne to unplug the skin pores. Plain abrasive scrubs are probably able to remove some skin oils, are mildly drying, and are therefore best for oily skin. They will remove dead surface skin cells but are usually not too successful at unplugging skin pores. They can irritate follicles and aggravate acne further. Since they are only mildly drying, they can probably be used without problem except on very dry skin.

Some abrasive scrubs have added humectants, emollient esters, or oils. Products with added oil-free moisturizing ingredients such as humectants or emollient esters are probably neither drying nor moisturizing and can be used on any skin type. Oil-containing products are probably moisturizing and are best for dry skin; they should not be used by people with oily skin or acne.

Some abrasive scrubs also contain surfactants (soaps and/or detergents) for extra cleansing. Some products contain chemical exfoliants, such as salicylic acid, that provide an additional peeling effect.

Many abrasive scrubs extol the benefits of removing dead surface skin cells; however, it is debatable whether these benefits are significant or whether the appearance of the skin is improved. The danger of these products is that abrasive scrubbing may actually do more harm than good by creating inflammation.

Abrasive ingredients commonly used in abrasive cleansers include aluminum oxide and ground fruit pits or nut shells, which are purportedly more abrasive than polyethylene beads, which are in turn more abrasive than sodium tetraborate decahydrate granules.

Chart 12-1
SOAPS, CLEANSERS, AND ABRASIVE SCRUBS

The charts are designed to help you minimize adverse reactions and choose products with the proper oil content for your skin type. If you have cosmetics-related acne, you should also choose products with the least amounts of potentially comedogenic ingredients.

Although most cosmetics contain potentially sensitizing ingredients, there is no reason to avoid any ingredient unless you are experiencing adverse reactions to cosmetic products. If you know you are allergic to certain ingredients, the charts will show you which products to avoid. If you are experiencing reactions to a certain cosmetic product, the charts can help you select alternative products that do not contain the same potentially sensitizing ingredients. To choose new products that are least likely to cause allergic reactions, keep in mind that fragrance is by far the most frequent cause of allergic reactions to cosmetics, followed by ingredients listed as "possible sensitizers." The ingredients listed as "other possible sensitizers" cause allergic reactions less frequently. Using these charts should help solve many cosmetics-related skin problems; however, if a problem persists, consult a dermatologist for advice and possible patch testing.

The products listed in these charts include many

of the nationally advertised and distributed brands that have the largest market share of cosmetics sales; an extensive sampling of other brands available in the Chicago area is also included.

After locating several suitable products, use the pricing information on pages 18–19 for comparison shopping.

> Names of products and product lines, and ingredients, are continually changing. Read the labels carefully before purchasing any beauty or skin-care product.

KEY

Possible Comedogenic Ingredients

BS—butyl stearate
CB—cocoa butter
DO—decyl oleate and derivatives
II—isopropyl isostearate
IM—isopropyl myristate
IN—isostearyl neopentanoate
IP—isopropyl palmitate
IS—isocetyl stearate and derivatives
LA—lanolin, acetylated
L4—laureth-4
M—mineral oil
ML—myristyl lactate
MM—myristyl myristate
O—oleic acid
OA—oleyl alcohol
OO—olive oil
OP—octyl palmitate
OS—octyl stearate and derivatives
PO—peanut oil
PGS—propylene glycol stearate
PT—petrolatum
S—sesame oil/extract
SLS—sodium lauryl sulfate

Possible Sensitizers

A—and other ingredients
B—benzophenones
BP—bronopol (2-bromo-2-nitropropane-1,3-diol)‡
C—cinnamates

D—diazolidinyl urea‡
DM—DMDM hydantoin‡
E—essential oils and biological additives
F—fragrances
I—imidazolidinyl urea‡
L—lanolin and derivatives that may cross-react with lanolin
P—parabens
PG—propylene glycol
PS—potassium sorbate
Q—quaternium-15‡
SA—sorbic acid
THN—tris (hydroxymethyl) nitromethane‡

Other Possible Sensitizers

BC—benzalkonium chloride
BHA—butylated hydroxyanisole
BHT—butylated hydroxytoluene
CH—chlorhexidine and derivatives
CX—chloroxylenol
HQ—hydroquinone and derivatives
MCZ—methylchloroisothiazolinone
MO—mink oil
MZ—methylisothiazolinone
PGL—propyl gallate
T—triethanolamine and derivatives that may cross-react
TH—thimerosol
VE—vitamin E (tocopherol and derivatives)
Z—zinc pyrithione

* may contain [see column head]
† does contain (coal tar colors)
‡ formaldehyde-releasing ingredients

WATER-FREE LIPID CLEANSERS AND CLEANSING CREAMS

Product name	Possible comedogenic ingredients	Possible sensitizers	Other possible sensitizers	Coal tar colors
Body Shop				
Honeyed Beeswax, Almond & Jojoba Oil Cleanser		E,P		
Clinique				
Crystal Clear Cleansing Oil	M		VE	
Elizabeth Arden				
Ardena Cleansing Cream (extra dry)	M,PT	F,L,P		
Special Benefit Cleansing Cream	M,PT	F,L,P		
Erno Laszlo				
Hydra pHel Cleansing Treatment (lotion)	M,PT	F,P	BHA,BHT,MO,PGL	
Germaine Monteil				
Marine Therapie Active Sea Cleanser	M	E		

OIL-BASED LIPID CLEANSERS AND CLEANSING CREAMS

Product name	Possible comedogenic ingredients	Possible sensitizers	Other possible sensitizers	Coal tar colors
Adrien Arpel				
Coconut Cleanser (makeup melt) (cream)	DO,IS	E,F,L,P,PG,PS	T	
Foam Cleanser	DO	E,F,P,Q		
Alexandra de Markoff				
Skin Renewal Therapy Conditioning Lotion Cleanser	M,PGS	DM,P	T	†
Allercreme				
Cleansing Cream for Dry Skin	M			
Almay				
Deep Cleansing Cold Cream	M	P		
Avon				
Cold Cream	M	F,I,P		
Rich Moisture Cold Cream	M	F,I,P		
Charles of the Ritz				
Revenescence Feather Touch Cleanser (lotion)	M,PT	F,I,L,P,PG	BHA,PGL	
CHR				
Extraordinary Creme Cleanser	M,OP	F,P,PG	BHA	†
Clinique				
Extremely Gentle Cleansing Cream	M,PT	L,P		†

Product name	Possible comedogenic ingredients	Possible sensitizers	Other possible sensitizers	Coal tar colors
Coty				
Overnight Success Refining				
Cream Cleanser	M	DM,F,P,PG	T	
Dubarry				
Cleansing Cream	CB,M,PT	F		†
Moisture Petals Whipped				
Cleansing Cream	M	F,L,P,THN		†
Paradox Creme Cleanser	M	D,F,L,P		†
Estee Lauder				
Re-Nutriv Extremely Delicate				
Skin Cleanser	M,PT	A,F,L,P		†
Fashion Fair				
Cleansing Creme Concentrate	M,PT	P		
Deep Cleansing Lotion	IP,M	F,L,P	T	
Frances Denney				
Satin Cleansing Cream	M,PT	DM,P		
Germaine Monteil				
Non-Liquefying Cleansing				
Creme	M	F,I,P		
Lancôme				
Douceur Demaquillante Nutrix				
Cleansing Emulsion	IP,M	F,P,PG	BHT,T	
Mary Kay				
Extra Emollient Cleansing				
Cream	M,PT	F,P		
Gentle Cleansing Cream	M,PT	I,P	T	
Max Factor				
Moisture Equalizing Cleansing				
Liquid	IM,M	B,I,L,P	BHA	†
Ultra Rich Cleansing Cream	M	L,P		
Merle Norman				
Cleansing Cream	CB,M	F		†
Physician's Formula				
Gentle Cleansing Cream	M,PT	I,L,P	BHA	
Ponds				
Cold Cream Deep Cleanser	M	F		
Lemon Cold Cream Deep				
Cleanser	M	F		

WATER-BASED LIPID CLEANSERS AND CLEANSING CREAMS

Product name	Possible comedogenic ingredients	Possible sensitizers	Other possible sensitizers	Coal tar colors
Adrien Arpel				
Sea Kelp Cleanser	M,PT	F,P,PS,Q	T	†

Product name	Possible comedogenic ingredients	Possible sensitizers	Other possible sensitizers	Coal tar colors
Albolene				
Liquefying Cleanser (cream)	M,PT			
Alexandra de Markoff				
Skin Renewal Therapy Conditioning Creme Cleanser	M	DM,P,PG	T	†
Almay				
Deep Cleansing Cold Cream (water-rinsable formula)	M,PT	I,P		
Moisture Balance Cleansing Lotion	M,OS,PT	I,P,PG	T	†
Avon				
Accolade Cleanser	DO,M,PT,S	F,I,P	BHT,T	
Daily Revival Gentle Cream Cleanser	M,PT	B,E,F,I,P	T	†
Nurtura Creamy Wash-Off Cleanser	PT	F,I,L,P	T	
Pure Care Cleanser (normal to dry)	DO,M,PT	I,P	T	
Rich Moisture Rinsable Cold Cream	DO,M,PT,S	F,I,P	T	
Biotherm				
Lait Purifiant Oligo-Thermal Cleansing Milk	M,OO	F,I,L,P,PG	T,VE	
Savon Creme Purifiant Oligo-Thermal Cream Wash	M,OO	F,I,P	BHA, BHT, T, VE	
Body Shop				
Cucumber Cleansing Milk	M	BP,F,L,P	T	†
Chanel				
Demaquillant Creme Gentle Cleansing Cream	M,MM	BP,F,P	VE	
Demaquillant Fluide Cleansing Milk	IM,IN,M,PGS	BP,F,P	VE	
Gentle Exfoliating Cleanser (cream)	M,MM	BP,F,P	VE	†
Charles of the Ritz				
Revenescence Moisture Cream Cleanser	M	I,P		
Christian Dior				
Hydra-Dior:				
Cleansing Emulsion (lotion)	IM,M	F,P,PG	BHA, BHT, T, VE	
Demaquillant Fluide Cleanser for Oily Skin	IM,M	F,P,PG	BHT,PGL,T,VE	
Demaquillant Cleansing Milk	IM,M	F,P,PG	T	

Product name	Possible comedogenic ingredients	Possible sensitizers	Other possible sensitizers	Coal tar colors
Clarins				
Cleansing Milk with Alpine Herbs	IM,M	E,F,L,P,PG	T,VE	†
Cleansing Milk with Gentian	IM,M	E,F,L,P	T,VE	†
Clinique				
Gentle Exfoliator Rinse-Off Formula	M	E,I,P	T,VE	
Color Me Beautiful				
Cleanser I (cream)	M	F,I,L,P	T	*
Skin Care Extra Gentle Cleansing Cream	IP,M,PT	E,I,P,PG	BHA,T	
Cosmyl				
Deep Pore Cleansing Milk		I,P	T	
Delicate Cleansing Milk	M	I,P	MO,T	
Cover Girl				
Moisture-Rich Gentle Cleansing Beauty Wash		F,I,P	T	
Dubarry				
Penetrating Cleanser (lotion)	M	F,L,P,PG,THN	T	
Elizabeth Arden				
Extra Control Oil Removing Cleanser	M	P	T,Z	†
Fluffy Cleansing Cream (normal to dry)	M,PT	F,L,P		
Skin Basics Skin Deep Milky Cleanser	M	F,P	T	
Estee Lauder				
Rich Results Hydrating Cleanser (souffle)	II,IM,IN,M	E,I,P,PG		†
Tender Creme Cleanser (lotion)	IS,M	F,I	VE	
Fashion Fair				
Fragrance-Free Cleansing Creme (with Aloe Vera)	M	I,P	T	
Fernand Aubry				
Ligne Fondamentale:				
Cleansing Milk for Dry Skin	IM,M	F,I,P,PG	T	
Cleansing Milk for Sensitive Skin	M	E,F,P	T	
Flori Roberts				
Kind-Cleans	DO,M,PT	F,L,P,Q	T	
Melanin Cleanser	M,PGS	F,I,L,P	T	†

Product name	Possible comedogenic ingredients	Possible sensitizers	Other possible sensitizers	Coal tar colors
Frances Denney				
FD-29 Cleansing pHormula (lotion)	IM,M	D,P,PG	T	
Sensitive Gentle Cream Wash		E,I,P	T	
Germaine Monteil				
Fresher Skin Scrub (lotion)	IM,M	D,E,F,I,L,P,PG	T,VE	
Rich Whipped Cleanser (cream)	M	F,I,L,P,PG	BHA,PGL,T,VE	†
Super Sensitive Cleanser	LA,M	E,I,L,P,PG	T	
L'Oreal				
Hydrating Cleansing Cream	M	D,F	BHA,BHT,T	
Plenitude Aqua Cleansing Cream	PT	BP,E,F,I,L,P	MCZ,MZ	
Lancôme				
Galatee Milky Creme Cleanser	IM,M,PGS	A,F,P,PG	BHT,T	
La Prairie				
Purifying Cream Cleanser	M,PT	F,I,P,PG	BHA,MO,T	
Mary Kay				
Creamy Cleanser	M	DM,P,PG	T	
Max Factor				
Moisture Rich Cleansing Cream	M	B,I,P		†
Merle Norman				
Cleansing Lotion	IP,M,PT	C,I,L,P	T	
Luxiva Collagen Cleanser (lotion)	LA,M,PT	F,I,L,P,PG	T	
Moon Drops				
Moisture Enriched Cream Cleanser	IM,M,MM,PT	F,P,PG,Q		†
Moisturizing Cleanser (lotion)	M,OP	F,P,PG,Q	BHA	†
Revitalizing Skin Cleanser (lotion)	M,OP	F,P,PG		†
Mustela				
Cleansing Lotion	PO	F,P		
Naturessence				
Citrus and Aloe Vera Rinse-Off Cleansing Milk	OP	F,I,P,PG		
Nu Skin				
Cleansing Lotion	S	D,F,P,PG	T	
Olay				
Oil of Olay Daily Facial Cleansing Lotion		F,I,P	T	†
Orlane				
Gentle Cleansing Milk	M,ML,OS	F,L,P,PG	T	
Wash-Off Cleansing Creme	IP,SLS	F,L,P,PG	T	

Product name	Possible comedogenic ingredients	Possible sensitizers	Other possible sensitizers	Coal tar colors
Physician's Formula				
Enriched Cleansing Concentrate	M,PT	F,I,L,P	BC,BHA,BHT	†
Gentle Cleansing Lotion	M,PT	I,L,P	BC	
Ponds				
Cold Cream Water Rinsable Cleanser	M	F,P		
Cold Cream Water Rinsable Cleanser for Sensitive Skin	M	P		
Prescriptives				
Soothing Cream Cleanser	IS,M	I,P	VE	†
Princess Marcella Borghese				
Termi di Montacatini Cleansing Creme	M	F,I,P,PG		†
Pupa				
Face and Eyes Cleansing Milk	IM,LA,M	E,F,I,P	T	†
Rachel Perry				
Citrus-Aloe Cleanser and Face Wash (cream)	DO,MM	E,P,PG		
Revlon				
Milk Plus 6 Moisturizing Cleanser	IM,M,PT,S	F,P,PG,Q	BHA	
Sea Breeze				
Whipped Facial Cleanser (cream)		DM,F,I,P	T	
Stendhal				
Bio Demaquillant Gentle Cleansing Cream	M,PT	BP,E,F,L,P,PG	T	
Ultima II				
Creamy Cleansing Concentrate (cream)	M,MM,PT	F,P,PG,Q		†
Fresh Gentle Cleanser (lotion)	M	F,P,PG,Q		
THE Cleanser for Dry Skin	IM,IP,M,PGS	B,E,I,P,PG	BHA	†
Yves Saint Laurent				
Gentle Cleanser (lotion)	II,M	F,P,PG	BHA,T	

LIPID-FREE CLEANSERS

Product name	Form	Possible comedogenic ingredients	Possible sensitizers	Other possible sensitizers	Coal tar colors
Body Shop					
Glycerin & Oatmeal Facial Lather	Lotion		F,I,P	T	

Product name	Form	Possible comedogenic ingredients	Possible sensitizers	Other possible sensitizers	Coal tar colors
Clarion					
Purifying Cleanser	Lotion	IS,OS	DM,P	T	
Estee Lauder					
Instant Action Rinse-Off Cleanser	Lotion	PGS	F,I,P	MCZ,MZ	
Flori Roberts					
Gold/Double O Soap	Bar		E	BHT	†

SURFACTANTS CONTAINING OILS: SOAPS

Product name	Form	Possible comedogenic ingredients	Possible sensitizers	Other possible sensitizers	Coal tar colors
Allercreme					
Hand Soap	Bar	PT	F	BHT	
Almay					
Anti-Bacterial Cleansing Bar	Bar				†
Cold Cream Cleansing Bar	Bar	M	P		
Moisture Balance Facial Soap	Bar	M	P	BHT	
Moisture Renew Facial Soap	Bar	M	PG	BHT	†
Alpha Keri					
Moisture-Rich Cleansing Bar	Bar	M	F,L	BHT*	*
Avon					
Aloe Vera Complexion Soap	Bar	BS,S	F,L	BHT	†
Daily Revival Oil Balancing Bar	Bar	M	E,F	BHT	†
Rich Moisture Soap	Bar	BS,S	F,L	BHT	
Clientele					
Gentle Cleansing Bar for Normal and Oily Skin	Bar	M	Q		
Cuticura					
Mildly Medicated Bar	Bar	M,PT	F		
Elancyl					
Beauty Massage Soap with Ivy Extract	Bar		E,F		
Elizabeth Arden					
One Great Soap	Bar			VE	
Spa for the Bath:					
Euphorics Soap	Bar		E,F	VE	*
Exhilarators Soap	Bar		E,F	VE	*
Sensual Soap	Bar		E,F	VE	*
Tranquilities Soap	Bar		E,F	VE	*
Erno Laszlo					
Active pHelityl Soap	Bar	IP	F		
Hydra pHel Cleansing Bar	Bar	OS	F	BHT	
Estee Lauder					
Micro-Moisture Bar Cleanser	Bar		E		†
Micro-Refining Bar Cleanser	Bar		F		†

Product name	Form	Possible comedogenic ingredients	Possible sensitizers	Other possible sensitizers	Coal tar colors
Fabergé					
Fabergé Organics Bar Soap	Bar		F	BHT	
Irish Spring					
Bar Soap (deodorant soap)	Bar		F,L	BHT	†
Jergens					
Aloe and Lanolin Skin Conditioning Bar	Bar		F,L	BHT	
Gentle Touch Bar Soap	Bar	M	F		
Lancôme					
Bienfait Savon Cleansing Bar	Bar	IM,M	F	BHT	
Mary Kay					
Premonition Perfumed Soap	Bar	M	F		†
Merle Norman					
Bath Oil Soap	Bar	IP	F,L	BHT	
Mustela					
Almond Oil Bar Soap for Babies and Children	Bar		F		
Oilatum					
Superfatted Bar Soap	Bar	OS	PG	HQ	†
Palmolive					
Gold Bar Soap (deodorant soap)	Bar	OO	F		†
Revlon					
Pure Skin Care Wash-Up	Bar	M	E,I,P		
Shepards					
Moisturizing Bar Soap for Dry Skin	Bar	M	F,L		
Stendhal					
Recette Marvelleuse Gentle Cleansing Cream	Cream	DO	F,I,L,P,PG		
Tone					
Skin Care Bar (with cocoa butter)	Bar	CB	F	BHT	†
Yardley					
Baby Bar Soap	Bar		F		
Cocoa Butter Bar Soap	Bar	CB	F	BHT	†

SURFACTANTS CONTAINING OILS: SOAP-FREE CLEANSERS

Product name	Form	Possible comedogenic ingredients	Possible sensitizers	Other possible sensitizers	Coal tar colors
Almay					
Moisture Renew Cleansing Cream for Dry Skin	Cream	M,PT	I,P,PG		†
Sensitive Cleanser	Cream	M,PT	I,P,PT		†

Product name	Form	Possible comedogenic ingredients	Possible sensitizers	Other possible sensitizers	Coal tar colors
Aveeno					
Cleansing Bar for Normal to Oily Skin	Bar	PT			
Cleansing Bar for Dry Skin	Bar		SA		
Avon					
Moisture Therapy Body Cleanser	Lotion		F,I,L,P	BHT	†
Moisture Therapy Liquid Soap	Lotion		F,L	BHT	†
Body Shop					
Pineapple Facial Wash	Lotion		E,F,P,PG	T	
Chanel					
Demaquillant Aquapurifiant Purifying Clay Cleanser	Lotion	M	BP,E,F,P,PG		
Gel Demaquillant Moussant Foaming Gel Cleanser	Lotion		D,E,F,P,PG	PGL	†
Gel Fraicheur Refreshing Body Cleanser	Lotion		D,E,F,P,PG	VE	†
Buf Puf					
Daily Cleanser (cream formula)	Cream	L4,OS	D,F,P,PG		
CHR					
Extraordinary Lotion Cleanser	Lotion	IM,LA,M,SLS	F,P,PG		†
Christian Dior					
Equite Pain Velours Gentle Cleansing Bar	Bar	SLS	E,F		
Clarins					
Gentle Foaming Cleanser	Cream	OS	F,P,SA		
Color Me Beautiful					
Skin Care Skin Conditioning Cleanser	Cream	IP,PT	E,I,P,PG	T	
Elizabeth Arden					
Millennium Hydrating Cleanser	Lotion	M	F,I,P,PG		
Soothing Care Gentle Cleansing Emulsion	Cream		I,P,PG,Q		
Eucerin					
Cleansing Bar	Bar		L		
Fernand Aubry					
Cleansing Milk (Dry/Delicate Skin)	Lotion	IM,M	F,P	T	
Cream Soap	Lotion	M	E,F,P,PG	T	
Frances Denney					
Creamy Cleansing Lotion	Lotion	IM,M	P,PG	BC	†
Source of Beauty Cleanser	Lotion	SLS	F,I,PG	MCZ,MZ,T,VE	†

Product name	Form	Possible comedogenic ingredients	Possible sensitizers	Other possible sensitizers	Coal tar colors
Germaine Monteil					
Decongestant Cleanser for Combination Dry/Oily Skin	Lotion	IM,IS,SLS	E,DM,P,PG	T,VE	†
Decongestant Cleanser for Oily Skin	Lotion	IM,IS,SLS	E,DM,P,PG	T,VE	†
Jheri Redding					
Extra Enriched Beauty Bar Soap	Bar	M,SLS	E,F,PB		†
Kids William and Clarissa					
Liquid Soap	Lotion	M	D,E,F,PG		
Lancôme					
Savon Amincissant Slimming Body Bar	Bar		E,F,PG		
Nu Skin					
Body Bar	Bar		E,P,Q	VE	
Olay					
Oil of Olay Daily Cleansing Lotion	Lotion		F,I,P	T	†
pHisoDerm					
Skin Cleanser and Conditioner:					
Oily Skin Formula	Lotion	M,OA,PT	A,I		
Regular Formula	Lotion	M,OA,PT	I,L		
Skin Cleanser for Baby	Lotion	M,OA,PT	F,I,L		
Physician's Formula					
Deep Cleanser	Lotion	SLS	D,P	BHA,BHT	†
Ponds					
Daily Cleanser Facial Cleansing Foam	Lotion	M	P		
Prescriptives					
Lotion Cleanser	Lotion	M,OS	E,I,P,PG		
Princess Marcella Borghese					
Termi di Montecatini:					
Bagno di Vita Revitalizing Body Cleanser	Lotion	OO	D,E,P,PG	T,VE	†
Esfoliante Delicato Gentle Cleanser Exfoliant	Lotion	SLS	E,I,P,PG		†
Revlon					
European Collagen Complex Moisture Nourishing Cleanser	Lotion	IM,IP,M,PGS	F,P,PG,SA	BHA	†
Simplicité					
Pure Performer Vitamin Cleanser	Lotion	M	F,I,P	VE	†
Westwood					
Lowila Cake Soap	Bar	M	F		

SURFACTANTS CONTAINING OILS: SOAP/DETERGENT COMBINATIONS

Product name	Form	Possible comedogenic ingredients	Possible sensitizers	Other possible sensitizers	Coal tar colors
Avon					
Daily Revival Mild Cleansing Bar	Bar	BS,S	E,F,L	BHT	†
Witch Hazel and Lyme Soap	Bar	BS,S	F,L	BHT	†
Caress					
Bar Soap	Bar	M	F	BHT	†
Clientele					
Gentle Cleansing Bar for					
Normal-Dry/Sensitive Skin	Bar	PO	PG,Q	HQ	†
Erno Laszlo					
Special Skin Soap	Bar	SLS	F	BHT	
Jergens					
Liquid Soap	Liquid	M	DM,F,L,P,Q		
Vitamin E and Lanolin Skin					
Conditioning Bar	Bar		F,L	BHT,VE	
Keri					
Facial Bar Soap	Bar	M,OS	F,L,P	BHT	
Lournay					
Sensitive Skin Cleansing Bar	Bar		E		
Olay					
Oil of Olay Daily Cleansing Bar	Bar	OS	F,P		†
Oil of Olay Facial Cleansing Bar	Bar	OS	F,P		†
Revlon					
Xi'a Xi'ang Tea Gel Body					
Cleanser	Gel	IS,M	B,E,F,I,P,PG		†

SURFACTANTS CONTAINING OIL-FREE MOISTURIZING INGREDIENTS: SOAPS

Product name	Form	Possible comedogenic ingredients	Possible sensitizers	Other possible sensitizers	Coal tar colors
Allercreme					
Glycerin Cleansing Bar	Bar		F	BHT	†
Hand and Body Soap	Bar		F	BHT	
Almay					
Clean-Up Cleansing Bar					
(deodorant soap)	Bar				†
Artra					
Medicated Complexion Soap					
(deodorant soap)	Bar		F	BHT,VE	
Body Shop					
Aloe Soap	Bar		E		
Wheatgerm Oil Soap with					
Vitamin E	Bar		E	VE	
Camay					
Bar Soap	Bar		F		†

Product name	Form	Possible comedogenic ingredients	Possible sensitizers	Other possible sensitizers	Coal tar colors
Chattem Ultra Swim Bar Soap	Bar	OS	F		
Coast Deodorant Soap	Bar		F	BHT	
Dial Deodorant Bar Soap	Bar		F	BHT	
Dickinson's Pure & Mild Transparent Cleansing Bar with Aloe	Bar	OS	F		†
Erno Laszlo Sea Mud Soap	Bar		F	BHT	
L'Oreal Deep Cleansing Bar	Bar		F	BHT	†
Lifebuoy Antibacterial Soap (deodorant soap)	Bar		F	BHT	
Olay Oil of Olay Facial Cleansing Bar	Bar	OS	F,P		†
Purpose Gentle Cleansing Bar Soap	Bar		F	BHT	†
Princess Marcella Borghese Termi di Montecatini Crema Saponetta Clarifying Cleansing Creme	Cream		E,P		†
Revlon Clean and Clear Complexion Bar	Bar		F	BHT	†
Safeguard Safeguard Deodorant Soap	Bar		F	BHT	†
Sardo Dry Skin Care Bar Soap	Bar		F	BHT	†
Shield Bar Soap	Bar		F	BHT	†
Spirit Deodorant Soap	Bar		F	BHT	
Zest Deodorant Soap	Bar		F		

SURFACTANTS CONTAINING OIL-FREE MOISTURIZING INGREDIENTS: SOAP-FREE CLEANSERS

Product name	Form	Possible comedogenic ingredients	Possible sensitizers	Other possible sensitizers	Coal tar colors
Adrien Arpel Freeze-Dried Collagen Protein Cleanser	Lotion	IP,MM,SLS	F,P	MCZ,MZ	†

Product name	Form	Possible comedogenic ingredients	Possible sensitizers	Other possible sensitizers	Coal tar colors
Allercreme					
Cleansing Lotion	Lotion	SLS	P,PG		
Combination Skin Cleanser		SLS	F,P,PG		
Petal Lotion Skin Cleanser	Lotion	SLS	F,P,PG		†
Almay					
Anti-Bacterial Foaming Cleanser (deodorant cleanser)	Lotion		I,P		†
Foaming cleanser	Gel		B,I,P		†
Oil Control Cleansing Sponges	Lotion		I,P,PG		
Sensitive Skin Foaming Cleanser	Lotion		I,P		†
Totally Clean Face Cleanser	Lotion		I,P		†
Wake-Up Cleansing Gel	Gel		B,I,P		†
Aquanil					
Lotion	Lotion	SLS			
Avon					
Essentials Cleansing Lotion	Lotion		B,D,E,F,I	T	†
Fancy Feet Double Action Foot Soak	Lotion	MM	A,F	BHT	†
Gentle Everyday Face Wash	Lotion		F		†
Pure Care Oil-Clearing Cleanser	Lotion		I,P,PG	T	
Biotherm					
Foaming Cleansing Gel	Gel		B,F,I,P		
Body Shop					
Passion Fruit Cleansing Gel	Gel		E,F,P	T	†
Strawberry Body Shampoo	Lotion	SLS	BP,E,P		†
Tea Rose Shower Gel	Lotion		E,P		†
Tropics Shower Gel	Lotion		E,P		
White Musk Shower & Bath Gel	Lotion		E,F,P		
Bonne Bell					
10-0-6 Soap-Free Cleansing Gel	Gel	SLS	D,P		
Shower 2000 Liquid Body Cleanser	Lotion		F,I,P,PG	VE	†
Skin Musk Bath and Shower Gelee	Gelee		F,I,P,PG	VE	†
Buf Puf					
Buf Puf Daily Cleanser (gel formula)	Gel	OS	D,F,P,PG		†
Cetaphil					
Gentle Skin Cleanser	Lotion	SLS	P,PG		
Chanel					
Demaquillant Vivifiant Refreshing Cleansing Bar	Bar		E,F,P,PG		
Charles of the Ritz					
Deep Cleansing Complex	Lotion		DM,I,P		

Product name	Form	Possible comedogenic ingredients	Possible sensitizers	Other possible sensitizers	Coal tar colors
Clarion					
Gentle Action Cleanser	Lotion	OP	DM,P	T	
Color Me Beautiful					
Cleanser II	Gel	SLS	F,I,P,PG,Q		†
Skin Care Very Effective					
Cleansing Gel	Gel	SLS	E,I,P,PG,Q		
Cover Girl					
Clearly Different Deep Cleansing					
Face Wash (deodorant					
cleanser)	Lotion		F		
Dial					
Liquid Dial Antibacterial Soap					
(deodorant cleanser)	Lotion		DM,F		†
Elizabeth Arden					
Visible Difference Deep					
Cleansing Lotion	Lotion	IM	F,P,PG		
EPI					
EPIssentia Purifying Gel Cleanser	Gel	SLS	E,P		
EPIssentia Gentle Cleansing Gel	Gel		E,P,PG	VE	
Estee Lauder					
Facewash Self-Foaming System	Gel	SLS	E,I,P,PG		†
Eucerin					
Cleansing Lotion	Lotion	SLS	I,L		
Fashion Fair					
Facial Shampoo (regular					
formula)	Lotion	SLS	F,P,PG,Q		†
Gentle Facial Shampoo	Lotion		F,I,P,PG	BHA,PGL	*
Fernand Aubry					
Ligne Specifique Satin Body					
Exfoliant	Gel	SLS	F,PG		
Flori Roberts					
Gold/Optima Gel Cleanser	Gel		P	T	
Optima Gel Cleanser (oil-free)	Gel		P	T	
Formula 405					
Soapless Cleansing Lotion	Lotion		F,P,PG		†
Frances Denney					
Sensitive Body Smoother	Cream		E,I,P		
Germaine Monteil					
Cleanser Actif (oil-control)	Lotion		D,F,I,P		†
L'Oreal					
Deep Cleansing Gel with					
Lipoprotein	Lotion		B,F,I,P	T	†
Plenitude Active Cleansing Gel	Gel		B,F,I,P	T	†

Product name	Form	Possible comedogenic ingredients	Possible sensitizers	Other possible sensitizers	Coal tar colors
Lancôme					
Ablutia Foaming Gel Cleanser	Gel		B,F,I,P	T	
Ablutia Foaming Oil Cleanser	Lotion		B,D,F,P,PG		†
Clarifiance Oil-Free Gel Cleanser	Gel		B,F,I,P	T	†
Savon Fraichelle Daily Cleansing Gel	Gel		B,E,F,P,PG,Q		†
La Prairie					
Essential Purifying Gel	Gel		D,DM,E,F,P,PG	T	
Mahogany Image					
Fluid Float	Lotion	SLS	F,P,PG		
Foam Wash	Lotion	SLS	F,P		†
Mary Kay					
Cleansing Gel (body care)	Gel		F,PG,Q		
Deep Cleanser	Lotion		DM,E,P,PG		
Purifying Bar	Bar		E		
Max Factor					
Cleanse-A-Gel Cleanser and Toner	Lotion		B,E,F,I,P		†
Le Jardin Caressing Shower/Bath Gelee	Gelee		B,F,P		†
Merle Norman					
Gel Cleanser	Gel	L4	B,F,I,P	T	†
Naturessence					
Elastin and NaPCA Creamy Facial Wash	Lotion		F,I,P		
New Essentials					
Extra Gentle Purifying Gel	Lotion		I,P		
Nu Skin					
Body Cleansing Gel	Gelee	SLS	D,E,PG		
Olay					
Oil of Olay:					
Foaming Face Wash	Lotion	SLS	DM,F		
Foaming Face Wash New Advanced Formula	Lotion	SLS	DM,F		
Sensitive Skin Foaming Face Wash	Lotion	SLS	DM		
Sensitive Skin Foaming Face Wash New Formula	Lotion	SLS	DM		
Pears					
Facial Cleansing Liquid	Lotion		D,F	VE	†
pHresh					
pHresh 3.5 Finnish Cleansing Formula	Lotion		F,P		

Product name	Form	Possible comedogenic ingredients	Possible sensitizers	Other possible sensitizers	Coal tar colors
Prescriptives					
Essential Cleansing Bar	Bar				†
Essential Cleansing Gel	Gel		E,I,P,PG		†
Rachel Perry					
Aloe Vera All-Over Body Washes	Lotion	SLS	F,I,P		
Spearmint Leaf Revitalizing Body Wash	Lotion		E,P,PG,Q		
Revlon					
Clean and Clear Facial Cleansing Liquid	Lotion		F,I,P		
Sea Breeze					
Facial Cleansing Gel	Gel		D,F,P		†
Soft Soap					
Soft Soap Antibacterial Moisturizing Soap	Lotion		DM,F	CX	†
Soft Soap Liquid Soap	Lotion	SLS	DM,F		†
Soft Soap Original Formula	Lotion	SLS	DM,F		
Stendhal					
Active Cleansing Mousse	Mousse	SLS	F,P	BHT,T	
Ultima II					
Fresh Liquid Facial Soap	Lotion	SLS	DM,F,P		
Yardley					
Liquid Aloe Vera Soap	Lotion		A,F,P		†
Liquid English Lavender Soap	Lotion		A,F,P		
Yves St. Laurent					
Foaming Cleanser	Lotion	OS	F,I,P,Q		

SURFACTANTS CONTAINING OIL-FREE MOISTURIZING INGREDIENTS: SOAP/DETERGENT COMBINATIONS

Product name	Form	Possible comedogenic ingredients	Possible sensitizers	Other possible sensitizers	Coal tar colors
Almay					
Oil Control Facial Soap	Bar		PG	BHT	†
Sensitive Skin Cleansing Bar	Bar				†
Clarion					
Gentle Action Facial Bar	Bar				
Purifying Facial Bar	Bar	LA			
Clearasil					
Antibacterial Bar (deodorant soap)	Bar		F		
Dove					
Bar Soap (white)	Bar		F	BHT	
Bar Soap (white/unscented)[1]	Bar			BHT	

[1]This product contains a "masking" fragrance.

Product name	Form	Possible comedogenic ingredients	Possible sensitizers	Other possible sensitizers	Coal tar colors
Lubriderm					
Body Bar (unscented)	Bar		F		
Neutrogena					
Baby Cleansing Bar	Bar		F	T,VE	
Cleansing Bar for Acne Prone Skin	Bar		F	T,VE	
Cleansing Wash	Lotion			BHA, BHT, T	
Dry Skin Cleansing Bar	Bar		F	T,VE	
Dry Skin Cleansing Bar (fragrance-free)	Bar			T,VE	
Liquid Neutrogena Facial Cleansing Formula	Lotion		P	BHA,BHT,T	†
Liquid Neutrogena Facial Cleansing Formula (fragrance-free)	Lotion		P	BHA,BHT,T	†
Oily Skin Cleansing Bar	Bar		F	T,VE	
Original Formula Cleansing Bar	Bar		F	T,VE	
Original Formula Cleansing Bar (fragrance-free)	Bar			T,VE	
Revlon					
Clean and Clear Acne Cleansing Bar	Bar	SLS	E		†
Shiseido					
Facial Cleansing Foam	Foam		F,PG		

PLAIN SURFACTANTS: SOAPS

Product name	Form	Possible comedogenic ingredients	Possible sensitizers	Other possible sensitizers	Coal tar colors
Acne Aid					
Cleaning Bar	Bar				
Body Shop					
Coconut Milk Soap	Bar				
Estee Lauder					
Basic Cleansing Bar	Bar		F		†
Yardley					
Aloe Vera Soap	Bar		B,F	BHT	†
English Lavender Fragranced Soap	Bar		F	BHT	
Oatmeal Soap	Bar		F	BHT	

PLAIN SURFACTANTS: SOAP-FREE CLEANSERS

Product name	Form	Possible comedogenic ingredients	Possible sensitizers	Other possible sensitizers	Coal tar colors
Almay					
Oil-Control Cleansing Lotion	Lotion		I,P		†
Amino Pon					
Conditioning Beauty Bar	Bar		F		†

Product name	Form	Possible comedogenic ingredients	Possible sensitizers	Other possible sensitizers	Coal tar colors
Avon					
Clearskin Foaming Cleanser	Lotion		F,I,P		
Body Shop					
Dewberry Body Shampoo	Lotion		E,F,P		
Herb Body Shampoo	Lotion		E,F,P		†
Buf Puf					
Singles	Pads				†
Dermablend					
Corrective Cosmetics Cleanser	Lotion		D,P,PG		
Estee Lauder					
Solid Milk Cleansing Grains	Powder	SLS	A,F,P,SA		
Frances Denney					
Quick Foam Cleanser	Lotion		PG,Q		†
Germaine Monteil					
Cleanser Actif	Lotion		A,B,D,F,I,P	T	†
Johnson & Johnson					
Baby Bar Soap	Bar		F		
Lancôme					
Effacil Cleansing Lotion for the Eyes	Lotion		F	TH	
Moisturel					
Sensitive Skin Cleanser	Lotion		DM	MCZ,MZ	
Naomi Sims					
Chamomile Cream Soap for Normal/Oily Skin	Cream		E,F	MCZ,MZ	
Chamomile Cream Soap for Dry/Sensitive Skin	Cream		E,F	MCZ,MZ	
Physician's Formula					
Oil-Control Deep Pore Cleansing Gel	Gel		P,Q	BHA	
Princess Marcella Borghese					
Hydro Minerali Revitalizing Cleansing Treamtent	Lotion	SLS	F,P,SA		†
Sisley					
Lotion Opaline Special Cleanser for Eyes and Lips	Lotion		E,P	MCZ,MZ	

PLAIN SURFACTANTS: SOAP/DETERGENT COMBINATIONS

Product name	Form	Possible comedogenic ingredients	Possible sensitizers	Other possible sensitizers	Coal tar colors
Lancôme					
Tresor Savon Parfume Pour le Corps Perfumed Bath Soap	Bar		F	BHT	†

ACNE AND ANTISEPTIC SOAPS AND CLEANSERS

Product name	Form	Possible comedogenic ingredients	Possible sensitizers	Other possible sensitizers	Coal tar colors
Almay					
Clear-Out Cleansing Pads	Pads		B		
Extra Clear Skin Astringent	Lotion		B		†
Aveeno					
Cleansing Bar for Acne	Bar	IM	F,P,PG		
Avon					
Clearskin Wipes	Pads		F	VE	
Bonne Bell					
10-0-6 Antiseptic Deep Cleansing					
Skin Lotion	Lotion		F		†
Buf Puf					
Antiseptic Cleanser	Lotion		E,F	BC,VE	†
Acne Cleansing Bar	Bar			T,VE	
Clairol					
Sea Breeze Antiseptic Cleanser	Lotion		E		†
Clear by Design					
Medicated Cleansing Pads	Pads		F		
Clearasil					
Double Clear Dual Textured					
Pads:					
Maximum Strength	Pads		F		
Regular Strength	Pads		F		
Cover Girl					
Clear Skin Clarifying Pads	Pads		E,F		
Dickinson's					
Witch Hazel Astringent Cleanser:					
Lotion	Lotion				
Pads	Pads				
Towelettes	Towelettes				
Estee Lauder					
Trouble-Shooter Anti-Blemish					
Solution	Lotion		A,E,I,P	T	
Fostex					
Super Strength 10% BPO					
Cleansing Bar	Bar				
Medicated Cleansing Bar	Bar		F		
10% BPO Wash (super strength)	Lotion				
Naturessence					
Antiseptic Clarifying Deep					
Cleansing Lotion	Lotion		C,F	T	†

Product name	Form	Possible comedogenic ingredients	Possible sensitizers	Other possible sensitizers	Coal tar colors
Neutrogena					
Antiseptic Cleanser for Acne Prone Skin	Lotion		E,P		
Noxzema					
Antiseptic Skin Cleanser (extra strength formula)	Lotion		E,F		†
Antiseptic Skin Cleanser (regular formula)	Lotion		E,F		†
Antiseptic Skin Cleanser (sensitive skin formula)	Lotion		DM,E,F	BC	†
Clear-Ups Medicated Pads (maximum strength)	Pads		E,F		
Clear-Ups Medicated Pads (regular strength)	Pads		E,F		
Oxy Clean					
Medicated Cleanser	Lotion	SLS	PG		
Oxy 10					
Daily Face Wash	Lotion		D,P		
Medicated Bar Soap	Bar		F	T	†
PanOxyl					
BPO 5% Acne Wash Bar	Bar	BS,M,SLS			
BPO 10% Acne Wash Bar	Bar	BS,M,SLS			
Pernox					
Abraidant Scrub Cleanser	Lotion		F		
Propa pH					
Medicated Cleansing Pads	Pads		B,F,PG		
Perfectly Clear Skin Cleanser for Normal/Combination Skin	Lotion		B,F		
Perfectly Clear Skin Cleanser for Sensitive Skin	Lotion		B,F		
Rachel Perry					
Herbal Antiseptic Skin Cleanser	Lotion		E,F		
Revlon					
Clean & Clear Antiseptic Skin Cleansing Lotion	Lotion		E,F		†
Sal Ac					
Cleanser	Lotion				
Seba Nil					
Skin Cleanser	Lotion		F		

Product name	Added ingredients	Possible comedogenic ingredients	Possible sensitizers	Other possible sensitizers	Coal tar colors
PLAIN ABRASIVE SCRUBS					
Body Shop Pumice Foot Scrub Seaweed and Loofah Soap (bar) Japanese Washing Grains	Surfactant		E,P		
Erno Laszlo Sea Mud Body Skin Polisher	Surfactant		D,F,P,PG	T	
Lancôme Exfoliant Doux Gentle Body Skin Polisher	Surfactant		F,P,Q		†
Mary Kay Buffing Cream (body care)	Surfactant		F,P,Q		
Pernox Abraidant Scrub Cleanser	Exfoliant		F		
Princess Marcella Borghese Termi di Montecatini Massagio per il Corpo Stimulating Body Refiner	Surfactant		E,P,PG		†
ABRASIVE SCRUBS WITH OIL-FREE MOISTURIZING INGREDIENTS					
Almay Oil Control Complexion Scrub Skin Smoothing Scrub	Surfactant Surfactant		I,P I,P		†
Biotherm Gel Exfoliant Smoothing Body Scrub Gel Nettoyant Profond Gentle Facial Scrub			B,F,I,P B,F,I,P		† †
Brasivol Facial Cleanser and Conditioner: Fine Rough	Surfactant Surfactant	SLS SLS	F,Q F,Q	BHT BHT	† †
Chanel Gommage Corporel Active Body Polisher	Surfactant	SLS	E,F,P,PG	VE	†
Color Me Beautiful Scrub Skin Care Exfoliating Scrub Skin Care Gentle Sloughing Cream	Surfactant	OP	E,F,I,P,PG E,I,P,PG,Q E,I,P,PG	T	†

Product name	Added ingredients	Possible comedogenic ingredients	Possible sensitizers	Other possible sensitizers	Coal tar colors
Coty					
Emergency Facial Energizing Scrub	Exfoliant		D,E,F,P		†
Elizabeth Arden					
Visible Difference Gentle Scrub Cream for the Body	Surfactant	SLS	F,P,PG	BC,CH	†
EPI					
EPI Ped Exfoliating Massage Cream for Feet		M	DM,F,P,SA	T,VE	
EPIssentia Refining Scrub Mask	Surfactant	O	B,D,DM,E,P,SA	VE	
Fashion Fair					
Deep Pore Cleansing Mask	Surfactant		I,P,PG		†
Fragrance-Free Gentle Facial Polisher	Surfactant		E,I,P		
Listerex					
Scrub Herbal Medicated Lotion	Exfoliant		F,P	T	†
Mahogany Image					
Facial Scrub			F,P,PG		
Merle Norman					
Luxiva Skin Refining Cleanser (cream)			I,P		
Naomi Sims					
Honey and Almond Facial Scrub			E,F,P,PG	MCZ,MZ	†
Naturessence					
Non-Chemical Skin Peel (gel)	Surfactant	SLS	DM,P	T	†
New Essentials					
Exfoliating Facial Scrub	Surfactant		I,P		
Nu Skin					
Liquid Body Lufra	Surfactant		D,E,P,PG	T	
Princess Marcella Borghese					
Hydro-Minerali Revitalizing Cleansing Scrub	Surfactant		F,PG	BHT	
Rachel Perry					
Sea Kelp Herbal Facial Scrub			D,E,F,P		
Simplicité					
Scrub 'Spirit' Brilliant			F,P,PG		
Smooth Touch					
Buffing Cream		IM,MM	F,I,P	BC,T	
Ultima II					
30-Second Refining Scrub Mask			E,I,P		

ABRASIVE SCRUBS CONTAINING OILS

Product name	Added ingredients	Possible comedogenic ingredients	Possible sensitizers	Other possible sensitizers	Coal tar colors
Aapri					
Aapri Apricot Facial Scrub		SLS	I,L,P	VE	
Adrien Arpel					
Honey & Almond Scrub			E,F,P,PS,Q		
Avon					
Body Beauty Cleansing Scrub		M	F,P	T	†
Clearskin 2 Cleansing Scrub	Surfactant	M	F,SA	BHA	
Essentials Gentle Skin Polisher		IM,OP,PT,S	E,F,I,P	T	
Skin Refiner Gentle Action					
Scrub		M	F,P	T	†
Body Shop					
Rice Bran Body Scrub			D,E,P,PG		
Viennese Chalk Facial Wash		DO	F,L		†
Wheat Scrub Soap			E	VE	
Christian Dior					
Exfoliating Gel			D,F,P		†
Cosmyl					
Vital Exfoliating Scrub	Surfactant	M	I,P	T	
Elizabeth Arden					
Visible Difference Gentle Scrub					
Cream for the Face	Surfactant	M,PT	F,P		
EPI					
EPIssentia Mild Exfoliating					
Cream		SLS	E,I,P,PG	BHA,BHT	
Fernand Aubry					
Derm Aubry Facial Scrub					
Cream			E,F,P,PG	T	
Frances Denney					
Gentle Cleansing Scrub		M,OA	F,I,L,P,PG	BHA,PGL,T	†
Gentle Body Exfoliator		M,OA	F,I,L,P,PG	BHA,PGL,T	†
L'Oreal					
Plenitude Gentle Exfoliating					
Cream		M	F,P		
Lancôme					
Exfoliance Delicate Facial Buff	Exfoliant	M	A,F,P		
La Prairie					
Essential Exfoliator	Surfactant	M	A,E,F,P,PG	T	†
Max Factor					
Pumice Cream			P,Q		
Naturessence					
Apricot and Kelp Facial Scrub		M	DM,F,P,PG	BHA	†

Product name	Added ingredients	Possible comedogenic ingredients	Possible sensitizers	Other possible sensitizers	Coal tar colors
Nu Skin					
Exfoliant Scrub		PGS,S	D,E,P	T,VE	
Facial Scrub		PGS,S,	D,E,P	T,VE	
Orlane					
Scrub Creme (exfoliant)		M	F,I,P,PG	T	†
Revlon					
Pure Skin Care Scrub Mask			E,I,P		
Sea Breeze					
Facial Scrub			DM,F,I,P	T	
Simplicité					
Scrub du Menthe		M	DM,E,P,PG	VE	†
St. Ives					
Apricot Scrub with Elderflower (cream)		SLS	E,F,L,P,PG,Q	T	

MASK CLEANSERS

Masks are products designed to be applied to the face, left on the skin for 20 to 30 minutes, and then washed or peeled off. Like other cosmetics, there are versions appropriate to each skin type.

Powder masks are designed to decrease facial oiliness as do astringents. These products usually contain oil-free liquids and absorbing powders that are mixed to make a paste. Most powder masks have been premixed and are sold in paste form. Powder masks are drying because of the absorbing powders and the evaporation of the water in the paste. Some powder masks also contain abrasives or chemical exfoliants; the purpose of these abrasives is the same as abrasive scrubs. Humectants are sometimes added to replenish skin moisture without replacing oil to the skin. Some powder masks contain oil and the purpose of such products is not clear.

Vinyl masks form a plastic film on the face; the film is then peeled off. These products contain alcohol, which creates a mild drying effect as it evaporates. Some also contain moisturizing humectant ingredients, such as glycerin or propylene glycol. Products containing alcohol without humectants are mildly drying and most suitable for normal to oily skin. Vinyl masks with added humectants attempt to decrease oiliness through the use of alcohol and then to replace moisture through the use of a non-oily humectant. The desired result is a reduction in skin oiliness. They can be used on all skin types.

There are also a few gel-type and lipid-type masks that are actually moisturizers designed to be worn as masks, and then washed off. Gel-type products are oil-free, humectant-rich products that are slightly moisturizing and can be used on any type of skin. Lipid products are more strongly moisturizing and best for drier skin.

Chart 12-2
MASKS

The charts are designed to help you minimize adverse reactions and choose products with the proper oil content for your skin type. If you have cosmetics-related acne, you should also choose products with the least amounts of potentially comedogenic ingredients.

Although most cosmetics contain potentially sensitizing ingredients, there is no reason to avoid any ingredient unless you are experiencing adverse reactions to cosmetic products. If you know you are allergic to certain ingredients, the charts will show you which products to avoid. If you are experiencing reactions to a certain cosmetics product, the charts can help you select alternative products that do not contain the same potentially sensitizing ingredients. To choose new products that are least likely to cause allergic reactions, keep in mind that fragrance is by far the most frequent cause of allergic reactions to cosmetics, followed by ingredients listed as "possible sensitizers." The ingredients listed as "other possible sensitizers" cause allergic reactions less frequently. Using these charts should help solve many cosmetics-related skin problems; however, if a problem persists, consult a dermatologist for advice and possible patch testing.

The products listed in these charts include many of the nationally advertised and distributed brands that have the largest market share of cosmetics sales; an extensive sampling of other brands available in the Chicago area is also included.

After locating several suitable products, use the pricing information on pages 18–19 for comparison shopping.

KEY

Possible Comedogenic Ingredients

BS—butyl stearate
II—isopropyl isostearate
IM—isopropyl myristate
IN—isostearyl neopentanoate
IP—isopropyl palmitate
LA—lanolin, acetylated
M—mineral oil
MM—myristyl myristate

O—oleic acid
OA—oleyl alcohol
OO—olive oil
OP—octyl palmitate
OS—octyl stearate and derivatives
PGS—propylene glycol stearate
PT—petrolatum
S—sesame oil/extract
SLS—sodium lauryl sulfate

Possible Sensitizers

A—and other ingredients
B—benzophenones
BP—bronopol (2-bromo-2-nitropropane-1,3-diol)‡
D—diazolidinyl urea‡
DM—DMDM hydantoin‡
E—essential oils and biological additives
F—fragrances
I—imidazolidinyl urea‡
L—lanolin and derivatives that may cross-react with lanolin
P—parabens
PB—PABA
PG—propylene glycol
PS—potassium sorbate
Q—quaternium-15‡

Other Possible Sensitizers

BHA—butylated hydroxyanisole
BHT—butylated hydroxytoluene
BO—bismuth oxychloride
CH—chlorhexidine and derivatives
MCZ—methylchloroisothiazolinone
MO—mink oil
MZ—methylisothiazolinone
PGL—propyl gallate

> Names of products and product lines, and ingredients are continually changing. Read the labels carefully before purchasing any beauty or skin-care product.

T—triethanolamine and derivatives that may cross-react

TG—tragacanth gum

VE—vitamin E (tocopherol and derivatives)

* may contain [see column head]

† does contain (coal tar colors)

‡ formaldehyde-releasing ingredients

POWDER MASKS					
Product name	Form	Possible comedogenic ingredients	Possible sensitizers	Other possible sensitizers	Coal tar colors
Adrien Arpel					
Flower Petal & Milk Protein 3 Minute Pick-Me-Up Masque	Plain		E,F,P,Q	TG	
Sea Mud Pack	Plain		F,P,PG,PS		
Allercreme					
Scrub Masque for Oily Skin	Abrasive		P		
Almay					
Moisture Balance Cleansing Mask	Abrasive		P,PG		
Oil-Control Clay Mask	Abrasive		I,P		
Avon					
Pore Reducer Facial Mask	Exfoliant		D,E,F,I,P,PG		†
Pure Care Mask (normal/dry)	Plain		I,PG		
VIP Pore Reducer	Plain		D,E,F,I,P,PG		†
Biotherm					
Deep Cleansing Mineral Masque	Plain	OO	BP,F,P,PG		
Body Shop					
Chamomile Face Mask	Plain	SLS	E,I,P,PG		†
Honey & Oatmeal Scrub Mask	Plain		F,P		†
Chanel					
Masque Lumiere Cleansing Mask	Plain		BP,F,P,PG		
Charles of the Ritz					
Special Refiner Cleansing Masque	Abrasive		P		
Chattem					
Mudd Mask	Abrasive		F,I,P		
Mudd Scrub & Mask	Abrasive		F,I,P,PG	BHA,PGL,T	
Christian Dior					
Cleansing Masque (for Oily Skin)	Plain		F,P		
Hydra-Dior Masque Adoucissant Wash Off Moisturizing Mask	Plain		BP,F,P,PG		
Clarins					
Doux Peeling Visage Gentle Facial Peeling with Plant Extracts	Plain		E,P	T	

Product name	Form	Possible comedogenic ingredients	Possible sensitizers	Other possible sensitizers	Coal tar colors
Clientele					
Facial Masque (normal-dry/ sensitive)	Plain				
Facial Masque (normal/oily)	Plain				
Color Me Beautiful					
Honey Mask	Plain	IM	E,I,P	BHA,T	†
Mud Mask	Plain		F,I,P		†
Skin Care Regulating Mask	Plain		E,I,P,PG		
Cosmyl					
Honey and Clay Purifying Mask	Plain		F,P,PG		†
Hydra-Cell Wheat Germ Mask	Plain	M,S	D,P,PG	MO,T	†
Coty					
Sweet Earth Mud Mineral China Clay Facial Mask	Plain		F,P,PG	VE	
Dead Sea					
Mud from the Dead Sea Natural Face Mask	Plain				
Elizabeth Arden					
Millennium Hydra-Exfoliating Mask	Plain		F,P,PG		
Skin Basics Velva Cream Mask	Plain		F,P		
Spa Intensives Streamliner Contouring Mud	Plain	M	E,F,L,P,PG,PS		†
Estee Lauder					
Almond Clay Pack	Abrasive		F,I,P		
Fernand Aubry					
Cleansing Mask for Oily Skin	Plain	IM,OA	F,P,PG		†
Ligne Fondamentale: Clarifying Mask for Oily Skin	Plain	IM,OA	F,P,PG		
Soothing Mask for Sensitive Skin	Plain	PT	E,P		†
Mask for Sensitive and Mixed Skins	Plain	OA,PT	F,P		
Flori Roberts					
Derma-Pure Facial	Plain		E,F,I,P,PG		*
Frances Denney					
Deep Cleansing Facial Mask	Plain		D,P,PG		
Sensitive Texture Treatment	Plain		E,I,P,PG	VE	
Germaine Monteil					
Masque Clarité	Plain		D,F,I,P,PG		†
Masque Satine	Plain		D,F,P,PG	VE	†
Lancôme					
Empriente de Beaute Deep Cleaning Clay Masque	Plain		F,P,PG		

Product name	Form	Possible comedogenic ingredients	Possible sensitizers	Other possible sensitizers	Coal tar colors
La Prairie					
Suisse Purifying Clay Masque with Cellular Extracts	Plain		E,I,P	T	
Mahogany Image					
Sea Kelp Mask	Plain	S	F,P,PG	BHA,PGL	
Mary Kay					
Revitalizing Mask	Abrasive		I,P,PG	T	
Max Factor					
The Incredible Blue Mask	Plain		P,Q	T	
Naomi Sims					
Rose Tonic Mask	Plain		E,F,P		
New Essentials					
Energizing Face Mask	Plain		P		
Nu Skin					
Clay Pack	Plain		D,P,PG	T,VE	
Face Lift/Lift Activator	Plain		P		
Glacial Marine Mud	Plain		BP,P		
Orlane					
Masque Bleu Pore Cleaning Mask	Plain		F,P,Q		†
Masque Rose Clay Mask	Plain	M,PT	F,I,L,P	MCZ,MZ,T	†
Owen					
Seba Nil Cleansing Mask	Plain		F,P		
Physician's Formula					
Deep Cleaning Clay Mask	Plain				
Princess Marcella Borghese					
Hydro Minerali 3 Minute Energy Masque	Plain		B,E,F,P,PG		†
Termi di Montecatini Fango Active Mud for Face and Body	Plain		E,P,PG	BO	
Rachel Perry					
Clay and Ginseng Texturizing Mask	Plain		D,E,F,P	VE	
St. Ives					
Firming Masque (with pure mineral clay)	Plain	SLS	E,F,P,Q		†
Simplicité					
Masque Resplendent Nutrient	Plain	S	F,P,PG	BHA,PGL	
Stendhal					
Active Clarifying Masque (gel)	Abrasive		F,P	T	†
Ultima II					
Deep Pore Scrub Mask	Abrasive		F,P,PG		
Mineral Mask Concentrate	Plain		F,P,PG		†

VINYL MASKS

Product name	Form	Possible comedogenic ingredients	Possible sensitizers	Other possible sensitizers	Coal tar colors
Avon					
Clearskin 2 Clarifying Mask	Plain		F,P		†
Peel-Off Masks (all fragrances)	Plain		B,F,P		†
Biotherm					
Aqualogic Masque Moisture Generating Mask	Humectant		F,I,P	T,VE	†
Body Shop					
Aloe Vera Peel-Off Face Mask	Plain		E,L,P,PS		†
Bonne Bell					
Orange Peel Masque	Humectant		F,P,PG	T	†
Clarion					
Clarifying Masque	Humectant		DM,P,PG		†
Coty					
Sweet Earth Peel-Away Apricot Facial Mask	Plain			BHA	
Moon Drops					
Moisturizing Honey Mask	Humectant		F,P,PG		†
Re-Texturizing Whole Egg Masque	Plain		F,I,P,Q		
Noxell					
Noxzema Clear-Ups Peel Off Mask	Plain		DM,E,F,P		†
Princess Marcella Borghese					
Hydro Minerali Revitalizing Deep Hydration Facial	Humectant	SLS	F,P,Q		
West Cabot					
Cabot's Vitamin E Peel-Off Facial Masque	Humectant		F,I,P,PG	VE	†

GEL MASKS

Product name	Possible comedogenic ingredients	Possible sensitizers	Other possible sensitizers	Coal tar colors
Avon				
Pure Care Mask (oily)		T		
Clinique				
Moisture Surge		B,E,I	MCZ,MZ,VE	†
Lancôme				
Masque #10 Hydrating Masque[1]		A,F,P	TG	†

[1]This product appears to be a gel and claims to be hydrating; however, this cannot be verified from the incomplete list of ingredients found on the package.

Product name	Possible comedogenic ingredients	Possible sensitizers	Other possible sensitizers	Coal tar colors
La Prairie				
Sun Basics After-Sun Masque		E,F,I,P,PG	T	†
Princess Marcella Borghese				
Termi di Montecatini Formula Energia Spa				
Eye Energizing Masque		E,I,P,PG	VE	
Yves Saint Laurent				
Intensive Treatment Masque (Phase 2)		E,F,P,PG		

LIPID MASKS

Product name	Possible comedogenic ingredients	Possible sensitizers	Other possible sensitizers	Coal tar colors
Adrien Arpel				
Freeze-Dried Collagen Moisture Lock				
Masque	IP	F,P	MCZ,MZ,T	†
Vegetable Peel Off		E,F,L,P		
Almay				
Moisture Renew Hydrating Mask	M	I,P		†
Avon				
Accolade Rinse-Off Mask	IM,LA,OP,PT	F,I,L,P	T	
Deep Cleansing Mud Mask	M,PT	I,P	BHT,T	†
Moisturizing Sea Mineral Mask	M,PT	I,P	BHT,T	†
Nurtura Rinse-Off Mask	IM,LA,OP,PGS,PT	F,I,L,P,PG	T	†
Refreshing Herbal Mask	M,PT	E,I,P,PG,PS	BHT,T	†
Clarins				
Masque Hydratant Revitalizing Moisture				
Mask with "Cell Extracts"	BS	E,F,P	T,VE	
Color Me Beautiful				
Skin Care Hydrating Mask	O,PT	I,P,PG,Q	T,VE	
Elizabeth Arden				
Extra Control Deep Oil Removing Masque	IM,M	E,I,L,P		†
Estee Lauder				
Re-Nutriv Firming Moisture Mask	II,IN,M	F,I,P	T	†
Rose Refining Mask	M,MM,PT	F,I,L,P		†
Triple Creme Hydrating Mask	II,IM,IN,M	F,I,P		†
Fernand Aubry				
Derm Aubry Eye Contour Masque	M		T	
Ligne Fondamentale Hydrating Mask for				
Dry Skin	M,PT	E,F,P		
Frances Denney				
Sensitive Moisture Infusion	PGS	E,I,P	T	†
Germaine Monteil				
High Fiber Facial	MM,PGS	E,I,P,PG	VE	
Lancôme				
Hydra-Bleu Cool Hydrating Masque	M	B,F,I,L,P,PB,PG	PGL,T	

Product name	Possible comedogenic ingredients	Possible sensitizers	Other possible sensitizers	Coal tar colors
La Prairie				
Cellular Masque	M	F,I,P,PG	T	
Suisse Moisture Masque with Cellular				
Extracts	M	F,I,P,PG	T	
Mary Kay				
Moisture Rich Mask	M,OS,PT,S	I,P	T,VE	†
New Essentials				
Soothing Face Mask	PT	I,P	VE	
Stendhal				
Les Bio Program Masque Bio Hydratante	PPG,PT	F,L,P,PG	MCZ,MZ,VE	
Masque Aqua Purifiant Aqua Purifying				
Mask	OP,PT	F,I,P,PG	VE	†
Recette Marvelleuse:				
Eye Area Beauty Masque	M,PT	E,F,I,L,P	BHT	
Firming Beauty Masque	PPG,PT	BP,E,F,L,P,PG	MCZ,MZ	
RM 2 Masque Contour des Yeux Eye				
Contour Mask	M,OP	F,P	CH,T,VE	
Ultima II				
5-Minute Rehydrating Moisture Mask		D,E,P		†
Yves Saint Laurent				
Intensive Treatment Masque (Phase 1)		E,F,P,PG	BHA,PGL,VE	

CHAPTER 13

Toners, Refiners, and Exfoliants

These products are probably the most carelessly named cosmetics on the market, with names that do not accurately describe their function. Some have been placed in more appropriate charts.

Toners, refiners, and exfoliants come in several forms designed for different skin types (see Chapter 5). The chart below will help you find the products that can be used with your type of skin.

TONERS, ASTRINGENTS, SKIN FRESHENERS, AND CLARIFIERS

Toners, astringents, skin fresheners, and clarifiers are all names for the same products. In their usual form, these products are useful for oily skin or for the oily T-zone with normal combination skin. Despite claims to the contrary, these products do not tighten the skin (except by drying it),

neither do they decrease oil production nor shrink oil glands. They are solutions consisting primarily of alcohol and/or witch hazel that evaporate and have a drying effect on the skin. They are used after washing oily skin. Similar products have been marketed as acne cleansers.

Toners for Normal to Dry Skin
Some manufacturers market toners specifically for normal and dry skin. Like other toners, these products are solutions of alcohol or witch hazel. Additionally they contain humectant ingredients, such as glycerin, that act as moisturizers. These products are intended to decrease oiliness through the use of a toner and then replace moisture through the use of a non-oily humectant. The desired result is a reduction in skin oiliness. They can be used by all skin types.

Type of Product	Skin Type	Effect
toner	oily	drying
toner for normal to dry skin	any skin type	reduces oil; not drying or moisturizing
refiner	any skin type	moisturizing
exfoliant	see text	removes dead skin cells
T-zone controller	normal	drying

Refiners

For lack of a better name, the term *refiner* will be used to refer to products that are water-containing solutions usually with humectants or fatty acids but without drying ingredients such as alcohol or witch hazel. These weak oil-free moisturizers can be used by all skin types but are designed for normal to dry skin. A few of these products contain very small amounts of oil; these are noted in the charts.

A few refiners are water-based solutions without any moisturizing humectants. These products are pleasant-smelling rinses but do not have any other obvious benefits. Refiners without humectants are noted in the charts.

Exfoliants

A toner or refiner is called an exfoliant when peeling agents such as salicylic acid or resorcinol are added to the product. Salicylic acid and resorcinol unplug skin pores and are definitely beneficial in treating acne when blackheads and whiteheads are present. Many of these products also extol the benefits of removing dead surface skin cells; however, it is debatable whether these additional claims are significant or whether the appearance of the skin is improved. Exfoliating ingredients have also been added to some facial masks and abrasive scrubs to try to achieve the same results.

T-zone Controllers

T-zone controllers are toners for normal combination skin that are marketed for use on the T-zone; however, they may also contain some absorbing powder. (Normal skin tends to be a little dry except on the forehead and central face—the T-zone—where it is a little oily.) T-zone controllers are listed with other toners on pages 197–203. Makeup will often work better on combination skin if the skin is made more uniform prior to makeup application. This can be accomplished by washing the face, applying a toner to the oily T-zone, and applying a moisturizer to the remainder of the face, if necessary.

Chart 13–1
TONERS, REFINERS, AND EXFOLIANTS

The charts are designed to help you minimize adverse reactions and choose products with the proper oil content for your skin type. If you have cosmetics-related acne, you should also choose products with the least amounts of potentially comedogenic ingredients.

Although most cosmetics contain potentially sensitizing ingredients, there is no reason to avoid any ingredient unless you are experiencing adverse reactions to cosmetic products. If you know you are allergic to certain ingredients, the charts will show you which products to avoid. If you are experiencing reactions to a certain cosmetics product, the charts can help you select alternative products that do not contain the same potentially sensitizing ingredients. To choose new products that are least likely to cause allergic reactions, keep in mind that fragrance is by far the most frequent cause of allergic reactions to cosmetics, followed by ingredients listed as "possible sensitizers." The ingredients listed as "other possible sensitizers" cause allergic reactions less frequently. Using these charts should help solve many cosmetics-related skin problems; however, if a problem persists, consult a dermatologist for advice and possible patch testing.

The products listed in these charts include many of the nationally advertised and distributed brands that have the largest market share of cosmetics sales; an extensive sampling of other brands available in the Chicago area is also included. After locating several suitable products, use the pricing information on pages 18–19 for comparison shopping.

> **Names of products and product lines, and ingredients, are continually changing. Read the labels carefully before purchasing any beauty or skin-care product.**

KEY

Possible Comedogenic Ingredients

IM—isopropyl myristate
IP—isopropyl palmitate
L4—laureth-4
M—mineral oil
OP—octyl palmitate
OS—octyl stearate and derivatives
SLS—sodium lauryl sulfate

Possible Sensitizers

A—and other ingredients
B—benzophenones
BP—bronopol (2-bromo-2-nitropropane-1,3-diol)††
C—cinnamates
D—diazolidinyl urea‡
DM—DMDM hydantoin‡

E—essential oils and biological additives
F—fragrances
I—imidazolidinyl urea‡
P—parabens
PB—PABA
PG—propylene glycol
PS—potassium sorbate
Q—quaternium-15‡
SA—sorbic acid

Other Possible Sensitizers

BC—benzalkonium chloride
BHT—butylated hydroxytoluene
BO—bismuth oxychloride
BZ—benzoin, gum benzoin
CH—chlorhexidine and derivatives
MCZ—methylchloroisothiazolinone
MZ—methylisothiazolinone
PGL—propyl gallate
T—triethanolamine and derivatives that may cross-react
VE—vitamin E (tocopherol and derivatives)

*may contain [see column head]
† does contain (coal tar colors)
‡ formaldehyde-releasing ingredients

TONERS

Product name	Possible comedogenic ingredients	Possible sensitizers	Other possible sensitizers	Coal tar colors
Allercreme				
Astringent for Oily Skin				†
Almay				
Oil-Control Toner				†
Body Shop				
Carrot Soothing Gel		E,I	T	†
Elderflower Water		E,F,I,P		†
Sage & Comfrey Open Pore Cream		E,F,P	T	†

Product name	Possible comedogenic ingredients	Possible sensitizers	Other possible sensitizers	Coal tar colors
Charles of the Ritz				
Activating Skin Cleanser (clarifier)		DM,P,PS		
Revenescence Softening Lotion		I		†
T-Zone Controller				
Christian Dior				
Equité Tonique Vitalite Vitalizing Toner		B,E,F,P		†
Clarins				
Gel Contour des Yeux Eye Contour Gel				
with Plant Extracts		E,P	MCZ,MZ,T	
Color Me Beautiful				
Skin Care Purifying Tonic		E,I,P,PG,Q		
Cosmyl				
Pore Minimizing Skin Refreshener		P,PG		†
Dermalab				
Skin Cleanser		F		†
Dubarry				
Special Astringent		F	BZ	†
Elancyl				
Active Toning Gel		E,F	T	
Elizabeth Arden				
Extra Control Clearing Astringent[1]		PG		†
Extra Control Oil Control Lotion				
Millennium Revitalizing Tonic		F,I,P		
Refreshing Skin Rinse		P	CH	†
Skin Basics Skin Lotion		E,F		
Visible Difference Refining Toner		F	BC,CH	†
Estee Lauder				
Counter Blemish Lotion (for acne)[2]				
Full Strength Protection Tonic		B		†
Mild Action Protection Tonic		F,I,P		†
Fashion Fair				
Deep Pore Astringent		F,PG		†
Fernand Aubry				
Camphorated Lotion				†
Ligne Fondamentale Balancing Lotion				
for Oily and Sensitive Skin				†
Flori Roberts				
Gold/Double O Complex		E		†
Oil-Free Astringent '40'		F,I,P,PG		†

[1]This product contains salicylic acid.
[2]This product contains phenylephrine, which may temporarily decrease facial redness.

Product name	Possible comedogenic ingredients	Possible sensitizers	Other possible sensitizers	Coal tar colors
Frances Denney				
Clarifying Astringent Plus		B,F,I,P		†
Germaine Monteil				
Decongestant Toner for Oily Skin		B,E,I,P		†
Toner Actif		F,I,P		†
Lancôme				
Controle Regulating Liquide			T	
Tonique Fraicheur Mild Astringent		B,E,F,P		†
Max Factor				
Moisture Equalizing Astringent			BZ	†
Merle Norman				
Miracol Booster Revitalizing Lotion				
Concentrate	P			
Oil-Control Lotion	PG		BO	
Noxell				
Noxzema Astringent		E,F		†
Princess Marcella Borghese				
Termi di Montecatini Botanico				
Restorative Eye Compresses		E,I,P,PG,Q	T	
Physician's Formula				
Invigorating Facial Masque		I	BZ	†
Oil-Control Antiseptic Skin Conditioner		B		†
Ultima II				
Fresh Purifying Toner		B,F		†

TONERS FOR NORMAL-TO-DRY SKIN AND T-ZONE CONTROLLERS

Product name	Possible comedogenic ingredients	Possible sensitizers	Other possible sensitizers	Coal tar colors
Alexandra de Markoff				
Skin Renewal Therapy Conditioning				
Toner (contains oil)		B,P	T	†
Allercreme				
Oil Regulating Lotion			T	†
Skin Freshener for Normal/				
Combination Skin		PG		†
Almay				
Clear-Off Skin Astringent				†
Moisture Balance Toner				†
Moisture Renew Toner for Dry Skin		P		†
Oil Relief Gel		B,I,P		†
Avanza				
Naturessence Water Lily Pore Lotion				
Astringent		F,I,P		

Product name	Possible comedogenic ingredients	Possible sensitizers	Other possible sensitizers	Coal tar colors
Avon				
Clearskin 2 Medicated Astringent Cleansing Lotion	IM	B,F,PG		†
Collagen Booster Line Controlling Lotion		F,PG	BHT	†
Daily Revival Pore Refiner		E,F,PG		†
Eye Perfector Soothing Eye Gel		E,I,P,PG	T	†
Fragranced Body Refreshers (all fragrances)	M	F,P,PG		†
Nurtura	IP,OP,OS	B,F		†
Pure Care Oily		PG		†
Skin Reviving Liquid		B,E,F,I,P,PG,PS	T,VE	†
Sparkling Finish		B,F		†
Visible Advantage Skin Reviving Liquid		B,E,F,I,P,PG	T,VE	*
Biotherm				
Invigorating Toner (5% alcohol)		B,F,I,PG	MCZ,MZ	†
Oil-Free Hydrating Liquide				†
Bonne Bell				
10-0-6 Light Cleanser/Toner for Dry Skin		F		†
Chanel				
Refining Toner		D,E,F,P,PG		†
Charles of the Ritz				
Revenescence Firmessence 770 Wrinkle Lotion		B,E,P		†
CHR				
Extraordinary Firming Toner		B,F,P,PG		†
Pro Collagen After-Sun Skin Repair Pack		F,I,P,PG	VE	†
Christian Dior				
Hydra-Dior All Day Refresher		E,F,P,PG		
Hydra-Dior Lotion de Fraicheur Skin Freshener		E,F,P,PG		
Hydra-Dior Lotion Purifiante Astringent for Oily Skin		E,F,P,PG		†
Hydra-Dior Lotion Stimulante Stimulating Lotion		E,F,P,PG		†
Clairol				
Sea Breeze Astringent for Sensitive Skin		E,F		†
Clarion				
Oil Zone Toner		E,P		†
Clientele				
Surface Refining Lotion-40				
Surface Refining Lotion-60				

Product name	Possible comedogenic ingredients	Possible sensitizers	Other possible sensitizers	Coal tar colors
Clinique				
Clarifying Lotion # 1 (sensitive)		P,PG		†
Clarifying Lotion # 2 (normal/oily)				†
Color Me Beautiful				
Skin Care Balancing Toner		E,I,P,PG,Q		
Skin Care Blemish Zapper		E,I,P,PG		
Tonic I		E,F,I,P,PG		
Tonic II		E,F,I,P,PG		†
Cosmyl				
Natural Rosewater Mist		E,I,P		
Cover Girl				
Extra Fresh Purifying Astringent		DM,F		
Extremely Gentle Refining Toner		F		†
Dubarry				
Moisture Petals Gel Freshener		F,PG		†
Skin Firming Lotion		F	BZ	†
Elizabeth Arden				
Spa for the Body:				
Sensual Body Splash		E,F	VE	†
Exhilarators Body Splash		E,F	VE	†
Euphorics Body Splash		E,F	VE	†
Tranquilities Body Splash		E,F	VE	†
Erno Laszlo				
Light Controlling Lotion		F		
Regular Controlling Lotion		F		
Estee Lauder				
In-Control T-Zone Solution			PGL	†
Fashion Fair				
Fragrance-Free Skin Freshener I		I,P,PG		†
Fragrance-Free Skin Freshener II (dry/ sensitive)		I,P,PG		†
Toning Lotion		F,PG		†
Flori Roberts				
Oil-Free Skin Freshener		F,I,P,PG		†
Gold/Optima Refining Lotion		F,I,P,PG,Q		†
Frances Denney				
FD-29 Priming pHormula		DM,E,I,P,PG		†
Mild Skin Lotion		B,F,I,P,PG		†
pHormula ABC		P		†
Protective Oil Control Lotion		F,I,P,PB	BO,T	
Sensitive Balancing Lotion		E,I,P		†
Sensitive Oil Terminator		C,E,I,P	T,VE	
Source of Beauty Alcohol-Free Freshener		B,I,P,PG		†

Product name	Possible comedogenic ingredients	Possible sensitizers	Other possible sensitizers	Coal tar colors
Germaine Monteil				
Decongestant Toner for Combination Skin		E,I,P		†
Freshener Actif		B,D,F,I,P,PG		†
T-Zone Oil-Control		D,PG		
Kelemata				
Wake Up Lotion for the Eye Area		I,PG	BHT,MCZ,MZ	
La Prairie				
Skin Caviar		E,P,PG	T	
Lancôme				
Clarifiance Alcohol-Free Natural Astringent		E,F,I,P	MCZ,MZ	
Mahogany Image				
Golden Honey Water		F,P,PG		†
Mary Kay				
Blemish Control Toner		E,PG		
Gentle Action Freshener		I,P,PG		†
Refining Freshener		PG		†
Max Factor				
Moisture Rich Skin Freshener		B,PG		†
Merle Norman				
Fresh 'N' Fair Skin Freshener		F,I,P,PG,SA		†
Nail Conditioner		F		
Refining Lotion		DM,E,I,P,PG		†
Moon Drops				
Moisture Enriched Skin Freshener		B,F,P		†
Moisturizing Skin Toner	IM,L4	F,P	VE	†
Revitalizing Skin Toner		F,P,PG,Q		†
Naomi Sims				
Body Polisher		F	MCZ,MZ,T	
Primrose Rinsing Lotion:				
For Dry/Sensitive Skin		E,F,I,P		†
For Normal/Combination Skin		E,F,I,P		†
For Oily Skin		E,F,I,P		†
Neutrogena				
Drying Gel		B,P,PG	T	†
New Essentials				
Clarifying Skin Tonic				
Oil Balancing Gel		B,I,P		
Refreshing Skin Tonic		I,P		
Nu Skin				
pH Balance		D,PG		

Product name	Possible comedogenic ingredients	Possible sensitizers	Other possible sensitizers	Coal tar colors
Olay				
Oil of Olay Refreshing Toner		F		†
L'Oreal				
Plenitude Hydrating Floral Toner		B,DM,E,F	MDG	†
Orlane				
Purifying Lotion for Mixed and Problem Skin		E,F,P,PG	T	
Reviving Toner		E,F,P,PG	T	†
Physician's Formula				
Pore-Refining Skin Freshener		F		†
Prescriptives				
Skin Refining Gel		I,P		†
Princess Marcella Borghese				
Termi di Montecatini Stimulating Tonic		E,P,PG		†
Pupa				
Tonic Lotion		E,F,I,PG	MCZ,MZ	†
Rachel Perry				
Lemon-Mint Astringent		E,F,P		
Violet Rose Skin Toner		E,F,P,PG		
Revlon				
Eterna '27' Gentle Toning Lotion		F,P,PG		†
Eterna '27' Intensified Skin Recharger	OS	D,F,P,PG		
Shiseido				
Facial Astringent Lotion Mild		B,F,P		†
Facial Softening Lotion		B,F,P,PG		†
Simplicité				
Texturizing Purifier pH		F		†
Stagelight				
Water Toner		F,P		†
Stendhal				
Bio-2 Beauty Energizer		F,P,PG	T	
Ultima II				
Lotion Refreshant		B,F,PG		†
THE Toner for Dry Skin		E,I,P,PG		†
THE Toner for Normal/Combination Skin		B,D,E,P,PG		†

REFINERS

Product name	Possible comedogenic ingredients	Possible sensitizers	Other possible sensitizers	Coal tar colors
Adrien Arpel				
Herbal Astringent		F,P,PG,PS	T	†
Lemon and Lime Freshener		E,F,P,PG,PS		

Product name	Possible comedogenic ingredients	Possible sensitizers	Other possible sensitizers	Coal tar colors
Alexandra de Markoff				
Skin Renewal Therapy:				
Conditioning Freshener (trace oil)		I,P,PG	T	†
Oxygenation Booster	L4	B,DM,I,P		†
Allercreme				
Alcohol-Free Moisturizing Toner		E,P		†
Avon				
Accolade		B,F,I,P		†
Daily Revival Softening Toner		B,E,F,I,P		†
Pure Care Normal/Dry[3]		B,I,P		†
Biotherm				
Invigorating Toner (alcohol-free)		B,F,I,P,PG	MCZ,MZ	†
Body Shop				
Aloe Body Spray[3]		PS		
Aloe Gel[3]		I,P,PS		
Cucumber Water		E,F,PS		
Honey Water[3]		E,F,P	BZ	
Orange Flower Water[3]		BP,E,P		†
Bonne Bell				
Good Nature Gel		F,I,P	BO,T	†
Chanel				
Lotion Douce Firming Freshener		F,P,PG	PGL	†
Charles of the Ritz				
Gentle Clarifier (100% alcohol-free)		DM,P		†
Revenescence Softening Lotion (alcohol-free)		B,DM,E,P		†
CHR				
Extraordinary Gentle Clarifier		B,F,I,P,PG		†
Christian Dior				
Equite Lotion Douceur Sans Alcool Alcohol Free Softening Lotion[3]		B,E,F,P		†
Clarins				
Toning Lotion (yellow)		E,F,P	CH,T,VE	†
Toning Lotion (green)		E,F,P	CH	†
Color Me Beautiful				
Renaissance Liquid		D,P,PG,Q		
Skin Care Hydrating Mist		E,I,P,PG,Q		
Skin Care Hydrating Tonic		E,I,P,PG		
Skin Care Refreshing Eye Treat (pads)		E,I,P,PG		
Cosmyl				
Extra Gentle Refining Toner		DM,E,I,P,PG	T	†

[3]This product contains no humectants.

Product name	Possible comedogenic ingredients	Possible sensitizers	Other possible sensitizers	Coal tar colors
Elizabeth Arden				
Soothing Care Calming Skin Refreshener		I,P	T	
EPI				
EPIssentia Moisturizing Toning Gel		D,E,P,PG	T	
Estee Lauder				
Gentle Protection Tonic (alcohol-free)[3]		D,P		†
Re-Nutriv Gentle Skin Toner		F,I	BC	†
Fernand Aubry				
Ligne Specifique ISD 26 Intensive Complex		F		
Toning Lotion (sensitive/mixed skin)		F,P,PG	T	
Germaine Monteil				
Nutri-Collagen Concentrate		D,F,P,PG		†
Super Sensitive Freshener		E,I,PG		
Kelemata				
Recovery Complex for the Eye Area		I	BHT,MCZ,MZ	†
L'Oreal				
Plenitude Floral Tonic		B,E,F,I	MCZ,MZ	†
Lancôme				
Tonique Douceur:				
Non-Alcoholic Freshener		E,F,P		†
Soothing Lotion		E,F,P		†
La Prairie				
Cellular Refining Lotion		B,E,F,P,PG,SA		†
Suisse Synergel		E,P		†
Max Factor				
Pure SPF 12 Invisible Face Protector		C,D,P	T	†
Merle Norman				
Luxiva Collagen Clarifier		DM,F,I,P,PG		†
Milky Freshener		F,I,P		
Miracol Revitalizing Cream		E,F,I,P		†
Miracol Revitalizing Lotion		E,F,I,P		†
Nu Skin				
Enhancer		C,D,E,P		
Physician's Formula				
Gentle Refreshing Toner				
Prescriptives				
Line Preventer		A,E,I,P,PG	BHT,VE	†
Skin Balancer		E,I,P,PG		
Simplicité				
Sheer Botanical Activizer		DM,E,PG	VE	†

Product name	Possible comedogenic ingredients	Possible sensitizers	Other possible sensitizers	Coal tar colors
Stendhal				
Les Bio Program:				
Bio 2 Vitality Accelerator		F,P,PG	MCZ,MZ,T	
Eau Bio Tonic		BP,F,I	MCZ,MZ	
Recette Marvelleuse:				
Alcohol-Free Vivifying Lotion		F,I		†
Alcohol-Free Revitalizing Eye Gel		F,P	T	†
Ultima II				
Gentle Skin Balancing Lotion		F,P,PG		†
Yves Saint Laurent				
Soft Tonique (lotion)		F,P,PG	T	

EXFOLIANTS

Product name	Possible comedogenic ingredients	Possible sensitizers	Other possible sensitizers	Coal tar colors
Almay				
Regulating Toner		B		†
Avon				
Blemish Solver		E,PG		
Clearskin Overnight Treatment			T	
Shine Solution			T	†
Bonne Bell				
10-0-6:				
Deep Cleansing Softening Lotion				
(normal/oily)		F		†
Deep Cleansing Softening Lotion				
(sensitive)				
Charles of the Ritz				
T-Zone Controller				
Clinique				
Body Sloughing Cream	SLS	I,P,PG		†
Clarifying Lotion # 3 (oily/very oily)		PG	BC	†
Clarifying Lotion # 4 (excessively oily)		PG	BC	†
Turnaround Cream		P	VE	
Cover Girl				
Clear Skin Clarifying Pads		E,F		
Dubarry				
Paradox Skin Freshener		F		†
Elizabeth Arden				
Special Benefit Complexion Renewal				
Lotion		E,PG		
La Prairie				
Suisse Emergency Tonic		E,PG		

Product name	Possible comedogenic ingredients	Possible sensitizers	Other possible sensitizers	Coal tar colors
Merle Norman				
Dab-O-Matic Toning Lotion		B,I,P		†
Naomi Sims				
Clearing Citrus Lotion		F		†
New Essentials				
Extra Strength Tonic				
Orlane				
Gentle Astringent	L4	B,F		†
Oxy				
Oxy Clean Medicated Pads (for sensitive skin)		F		
Oxy Clean Medicated Pads (maximum strength)	SLS	F,PG		
Oxy Clean Medicated Pads (regular strength)	SLS	F,PG		
Oxy Night Watch	SLS	P,PG		
Prescriptives				
Anti-Bac Antibacterial Lotion		B	BC	
Skin Reviver			PGL	†
Propa pH				
Extra Strength Medicated Acne Cream	IM	E	T	
Stendhal				
Lotion Purifiante Active Toning Lotion with Alcohol	L4	B,F	T	†

PART THREE

SKIN: THE BODY

CHAPTER 14

The Effects of Sunlight on the Skin

SUN EXPOSURE AND SKIN CANCER

In recent years, there has been an alarming increase in the incidence of skin cancers. Most common skin cancers are caused by the cumulative effects of the sun. As the total amount of sunlight on the skin increases over a lifetime, precancerous areas and/or basal and squamous cell skin cancers become more likely to occur. Moreover, potentially lethal but less common skin cancers called melanomas occur more frequently in individuals who have had extensive sunburn during their lifetime.

Skin Color

The darker the color of an individual's skin, the more sunlight will be tolerated in a lifetime without the appearance of sun-related skin damage and the less likely that skin cancer will develop. Thus, many women of color who have never used sunscreens will probably never have sun-related skin problems. On the other hand, light-skinned persons of Irish or other Northern European ancestry have a very low lifetime threshold of sun exposure before sun damage will occur. These people are most likely to de-velop skin cancers such as basal and squamous cell cancers with increasing cumulative sun exposure.

Increase in Skin Cancers

In the recent past, when we were less knowledgeable about the effects of the sun, sunbathing became fashionable. Since the effects of sun exposure are delayed, we are only now becoming aware of the damage that was done by this activity. Frequent sunbathing without sunscreens by persons with lighter skin color during teenage years and early adulthood has caused the skin of many adults to look prematurely wrinkled and discolored as they enter middle age. These people also tend to develop skin cancers at an earlier age than others.

In addition, there has been a population shift in our country, either part-time or full-time, to the sunbelt states where there is more exposure to the sun. This has contributed to the increase in the incidence of skin cancers in this country.

Finally, our environment has changed. The amount of airborne pollutants has increased and has reduced the ozone layer of Earth's atmosphere. At one time this protective layer filtered out most of the sun's potentially damaging radiation before it reached our skin. With the reduction of this protective layer, we have been exposed to higher levels of harmful radiation without altering our sun-loving habits. This may prove to be the most important reason for the dramatic increase in skin cancer today.

The Importance of Using
Sunscreens Regularly
The regular use of sunscreens provides a way to shield the skin from the damaging effects of the sun. Sunscreens not only prevent sunburn, but also slow down the development of skin damage associated with cumulative sun exposure, such as wrinkles and skin cancers.

CHAPTER 15

Sunscreens

A sunscreen is a product designed to filter out a portion of the damaging sunlight so that it will not reach the skin. Regular use of these products will slow down the rate of total accumulated sun exposure and delay or help prevent the appearance of sun-related wrinkles, discoloration, and skin cancers.

STRENGTH OF PROTECTION

The amount of protection from ultraviolet B in sunlight that a sunscreen will give is stated on the label in the form of a sun protection factor (SPF) number. Ultraviolet B is the part of sunlight most responsible for sunburn. The higher the number, the more sun protection given by the product. A person who is normally able to stay in the sun for only 15 minutes without developing sunburn will be able to stay in the sun for 15 times longer or 225 minutes (3 hours and 45 minutes) when wearing an SPF-15 sunscreen. With an SPF-2 sunscreen, the same person would be able to remain in the sun for only 2 times as long (30 minutes) without burning.

Sunscreens with an SPF number lower than 15 are used for mild sun protection when a person is primarily trying to get a suntan. When using these products, keep in mind that a significant amount of sunlight will reach the skin. Therefore, most dermatologists recommend using at least an SPF-15 sunscreen to obtain good protection from the sun. It is possible to get a suntan with an SPF-15 sunscreen, but it will be a slower process.

Other Factors
Altitude, too, affects the time it takes for your skin to show the sun's effects. The intensity of UV (ultraviolet) radiation at 5,000 feet, for example, is about 20 percent greater than at sea level; for every 1,000-foot increase in altitude, the intensity of ultraviolet light increases about 4 percent. And if you're skiing in the mountains, you'll also be exposed to reflected light from snow. Beachgoers are similarly vulnerable to reflected light from sand and water, which can strike the skin where the overhead sun doesn't normally shine, such as the underarms.

Ultraviolet A and Ultraviolet B Light
Sunlight contains both ultraviolet A (UVA) and ultraviolet B (UVB) light. The SPF number measures only the amount of protection from ultraviolet B light—the part of sunlight that causes the most immediate

skin damage. Some individuals have skin conditions that require ultraviolet A protection. Most sunscreens that protect from UVB also offer at least partial UVA protection.

Although several sunscreen ingredients offer some protection against part of the ultraviolet A light spectrum, this protection is usually unsatisfactory for people who are unable to tolerate ultraviolet A light. Currently, sunscreens with avobenzone (butylmethoxydibenzoylmethane) are the best at providing broad-spectrum ultraviolet A protection. People who need to avoid ultraviolet A light are advised to discuss this issue with their dermatologist.

Application of Sunscreens

Sunscreens are most effective when applied about 30 minutes before exposure to the sun, and many will specifically state this in the directions. That's because sunscreens need time to penetrate the skin. Others just instruct you to apply prior to sun exposure.

Whatever product you use, be sure to apply a medium-size palmful—about 1 ounce for an average-size person, the standard dose on which SPF Ratings are based—and spread it over every exposed part of your body. You can also estimate the dose on the basis of the bottle's total contents.

Be especially careful to reapply sunscreen if you towel down after swimming. However, reapplying sunscreen does not extend the period of protection. It just renews the protection that you already had. An SPF 8, for example, extends your time

---

> **CAUTION: POTENT FORMULAS**
> Be aware that sunscreens can stain. Many leave their mark on bathing suits and towels.

---

before sunburn by about eight times. If you turn pink in 15 minutes, the SPF protects you for 2 hours and only 2 hours, no matter how many times you apply the sunscreen.

TYPES OF SUNSCREEN PRODUCTS

Sunscreens contain many of the same ingredients and have many of the same properties found in other skin-care products. Most sunscreens contain oils, but there are also oil-free lotion and gel sunscreens available for people with oilier skin. It is important to know your skin type to choose the best sunscreen for your needs (see Chapter 5). The chart below will help you quickly locate the type of sunscreen best for your skin type.

Sunscreen Type	Skin Type
oil-containing	normal to dry
oil-free	oily

Oil-containing Sunscreens

Oil-containing sunscreens may be water-free, oil-based, or water-based products. All of these are suitable for normal to dry skin but contain oil and are not the best choice for oily skin.

Oil-free Sunscreens

There are now a number of oil-free cream, lotion, spray, and gel sunscreens on the market. These are slightly drying products and are the best choice for oily skin or acne. They can also be used on normal skin but are probably too drying for dry skin. Some of the products contain oil-like emollient esters and other products are strictly oil-free. The latter are the very best choice for people with significant acne.

Sunblock Products

The term *sunblock* is used in two ways by cosmetics companies. Some sunscreen products with a very high SPF number are called sunblocks because they prevent a high percentage of sunlight from reaching the skin. These products, however, should really be called sunscreens. The term sunblock should be reserved for products that physically block the sun because they are opaque. The more sunblock applied, the more protection received. A very thick layer will block out almost all sunlight while a standard application gives an estimated protection of approximately SPF 6.

These products are thick white creams and are less cosmetically appealing than sunscreens because they are visible on the surface of the skin. Zinc oxide paste is the best known example; however, there are many other sunblocks available. They are usually water-free but are made with enough added powder that the net product may not be very oily. Most of these products can therefore be used by all skin types.

Many of these products are made in "fun" colors and are used as beachside fashion accessories in addition to supplying sun protection.

This year, a new type of physical sunblock has been developed in which titanium dioxide particles are finely ground in order to make a product that is as cosmetically appealing as chemical sunscreens. Neutrogena has marketed one such product, which is rated SPF 17.

SKIN CANCER FOUNDATION (SCF) SEAL OF APPROVAL

While the SCF seal is a good validation of a sunscreen's quality, absence of the seal does *not* necessarily indicate an inferior product. For one thing, some products that are authorized to use the SCF seal may not have displayed it on their packaging by the time you're shopping for a sunscreen. In addition, some products simply don't go through the process of obtaining the Skin Cancer Foundation's approval. Limited tests at *Consumer Reports* show that even without the SCF seal, most sunscreens do live up to their label claims.

PROTECTING THE SKIN OF CHILDREN

Sunscreens for infants and children are usually formulated with few potentially irritating chemicals and often with a highly emollient lotion base. That also makes them attractive to adults with sensitive skin. Nevertheless, since most sunscreens advise against use on children under six months old, an infant is best protected by being kept out of direct sunlight.

It's also especially important to educate children at an early age about the benefits of sunscreens. There is a direct correlation between severe sunburns in childhood and the development of melanoma later in life.

By one estimate, regular use of an SPF-15 sunscreen between the ages of 1 and 18 will reduce the lifetime risk of nonmelanoma skin cancer by roughly four-fifths.

ALLERGIES TO SUNSCREEN

Allergic reactions to sunscreen ingredients are not uncommon. Many people develop a reaction to PABA (para-aminobenzoic acid) and its derivatives (glyceryl PABA and octyl dimethyl PABA, or Padimate O), but other sunscreen ingredients, notably benzophenones, cinnamates, and avobenzone, can also sometimes cause allergic reactions. Other sunscreen ingredients such as salicylates, menthyl anthranilate, titanium dioxide, and red petrolatum do not commonly cause allergic reactions.

Unfortunately, there are products on the market that claim to be PABA-free but contain PABA derivatives. This is somewhat misleading. In this book, products with PABA derivatives such as octyl dimethyl PABA (Padimate O) and glyceryl PABA are listed as containing PABA.

The benzophenones include oxybenzone and dioxybenzone and may cause allergic reactions more commonly than PABA. Numerous cases of allergic reactions to benzophenones have been reported by people who assumed they were allergic to PABA and switched to another PABA-free sunscreen only to discover a poor reaction to the substitute because it also contained benzophenones.

Cinnamates are occasionally photosensitizers—they can cause allergic reactions when the product is worn in the sun. Since sunscreens are only worn in the sun these reactions appear identical to those seen with PABA, PABA derivatives, and benzophenone.

Keep in mind that sunscreens also have many of the same potential sensitizers found in other cosmetics that may also cause allergic reactions. The chart shows the presence of any additional possible sensitizing ingredients in sunscreen products.

Chart 15–1
SUNSCREENS

The charts are designed to help you minimize adverse reactions and choose products with the proper oil content for your skin type. If you have cosmetics-related acne, you should also choose products with the least amounts of potentially comedogenic ingredients.

Although most cosmetics have potentially sensitizing ingredients, there is no reason to avoid any ingredient unless you are experiencing adverse reactions to cosmetic products. If you know you are allergic to certain ingredients the charts will show you which products to avoid. If you are experiencing reactions to a certain cosmetic product, the charts can help you select alternative products that do not contain the same potentially sensitizing ingredients. To choose new products that are least likely to cause allergic reactions, keep in mind that fragrance is by far the most frequent cause of allergic reactions to cosmetics, followed by ingredients listed as "possible sensitizers." The ingredients listed as "other possible sensitizers" cause allergic reactions less frequently. Using these charts should help solve many

> Names of products and product lines, and ingredients, are continually changing. Read the labels carefully before purchasing any beauty or skin-care product.

cosmetics-related skin problems; however, if a problem persists, consult a dermatologist for advice and possible patch testing.

The products listed in these charts include many of the nationally advertised and distributed brands that have the largest market share of cosmetics sales; an extensive sampling of other brands available in the Chicago area is also included. After locating several suitable products, use the pricing information on pages 18–19 for comparison shopping.

KEY

Sunscreen Ingredients Found in Sunscreen Products

B—benzophenones
BM—butylmethoxydibenzoylmethane
  (avobenzone)
C—cinnamates
ECD—2-ethylhexyl-2-cyano-3, 3-diphenyl acrylate§
MA—menthyl anthranilate
OC—octocrylene§
PB—PABA and derivatives
PS—2-phenylbenzimidazole-5-sulfonic acid
SL—salicylates
TI—titanium dioxide

Possible Comedogenic Ingredients

BS—butyl stearate
CB—cocoa butter
DO—decyl oleate and derivatives
II—isopropyl isostearate
IM—isopropyl myristate
IN—isostearyl neopentanoate
IS—isocetyl stearate and derivatives
M—mineral oil
ML—myristyl lactate
MM—myristyl myristate

OA—oleyl alcohol
OO—olive oil
OP—octyl palmitate
OS—octyl stearate and derivatives
PGS—propylene glycol stearate
PPG—myristyl ether propionate
PT—petrolatum
SLS—sodium lauryl sulfate

Possible Sensitizers

A—and other ingredients
B—benzophenones
BP—bronopol (2-bromo-2-nitropropane-1,3-diol)‡
C—cinnamates
D—diazolidinyl urea‡
DM—DMDM hydantoin‡
E—essential oils and biological additives
F—fragrances
I—imidazolidinyl urea‡
L—lanolin and derivatives that may cross-react with
  lanolin
P—parabens
PB—PABA
PG—propylene glycol
PS—potassium sorbate
Q—quaternium-15‡
SA—sorbic acid

Other Possible Sensitizers

BC—benzalkonium chloride
BHA—butylated hydroxyanisole
BHT—butylated hydroxytoluene
ED—ethylenediamines
MCZ—methylchloroisothiazolinone
MO—mink oil
MZ—methylisothiazolinone
PGL—propyl gallate
R—rosin (colophony) and derivatives‡
T—triethanolamine and derivatives that may cross-
  react
VE—vitamin E (tocopherol and derivatives)

* may contain [see column head]
† does contain (coal tar colors)
§ These ingredients are the same.
‡ formaldehyde-releasing ingredients

OIL-CONTAINING SUNSCREENS

Product name	SPF	Form	Active sunscreen ingredients	Possible comedogenic ingredients	Possible sensitizers	Other possible sensitizers	Coal tar colors
Avon							
Sunseekers Dark Tanning Gelee	4	Cream	PB	CB,IM,M,PT	E,F,P,PB	VE	†
Sunseekers Sun Block Stick	15	Stick	B,PB	CB,M	B,F,L,PB	BHA,VE	
Sunseekers Sunblocking Lotion	23	Lotion	B,C,PB	CB	B,C,F,I,PB	BHT,VE	†
Tanning Lotion	4	Lotion	B,PB	CB	B,F,P,PB		
Tanning Lotion	8	Lotion	B,PB	CB	B,F,I,P,PB		
Tanning Lotion	15	Lotion	B,PB	CB	B,F,I,P,PB		
Bain de Soleil							
Body Silkening Golden Tanning Spray Oil	4	Spray	C,PB	IM,M	C,F,P,PB		†
Body Silkening Stick	25	Stick	B,C,PB	PT	B,C,F,P,PB	VE	†
Classique Suntan Gelee Orange	4	Cream	C,PB	IM,M,PT	C,F,P,PB		†
Classique Suntan Gelee Orange	4	Stick	C,PB	IM,M,PT	C,F,P,PB		
Classique Suntan Gelee Orange	10	Cream	C,PB,SL	IM,M,PT	BP,C,F,P,PB		
Banana Boat							
Dark Tanning Lotion	6	Lotion	PB	CB,M	F,I,P,PB,Q	MO,T,VE	
Dark Tanning Oil with Sunscreen	2	Oil	PB	CB,M	F,L,PB		
Lotion	15	Lotion	B,C,PB	CB,M	B,C,F,P,PB,Q	MO,T,VE	
Lotion	34	Lotion	B,PB,SL,TI	CB,M	B,I,P,PB,Q	MO,T,VE	
Supreme Tanning Blend Oil	2	Oil	PB	CB,M	E,F,L,PB	MO	
Biotherm							
Stick Solaire Tri-Protection Sun Stick	15	Stick	B,C	CB,M,OA,OO	B,C,F,L	BHA,BHT,VE	
Body Shop							
Carrot Sun Milk	12	Lotion	B,PB		B,E,I,P,PB	T	†
Carrot Sun Oil	6	Oil	B,PB	CB,M	B,E,PB	VE	†
Bullfrog							
Body Gel	9	Cream	B,C		B,C,F	VE	
Body Gel	18	Cream	B,C,OC		B,C,F	VE	
Gel Concentrate	18	Cream	B,C,OC		B,C,F	VE	
Gel Concentrate	36	Cream	B,C,OC		B,C,F	VE	
Chanel							
Protection Intense Spot Protector	30	Stick	B,C,PB,SL	IS,M	B,BP,C E,P,PB,PG	PGL,VE	
Clarins							
Moisturizing Sun Care Milk	8	Lotion	B,C,PS	M	B,C,E,F	MCZ,MZ,T	
Moisturizing Sun Care Oil	4	Oil		M	F,E,P	BHT	†

Product	SPF	Form					+
Coppertone							
All Day Protection Lotion	30+	Lotion	B,C,PB,SL	CB	B,C,F,I,P,PB	T,VE	
Broad Spectrum Lotion	25	Lotion	B,C,PB	IM	B,C,D,F,P,PB	T,VE	
Lite Tanning Oil	2	Oil	SL	CB,M	F,L,PG	BHA,PGL	+
Lotion with Vitamin E and Aloe	8	Lotion	B,PB	CB,IM	B,F,L,P,PB	T,VE	
Moisturizing Suntan Lotion	4	Lotion	B,PB	CB,IM	B,F,L,P,PB	T,VE	
Moisturizing Suntan Oil	2	Oil	B,SL	CB,M,OO	B,F,L	BHA,PGL,VE	+
Sun Sense Towelettes	15	Towels	B,C,SL		B,C,I,P	T,VE	
Suntan Oil	2	Oil	SL	CB,M	F,L	BHA,PGL,VE	+
Ultra Protection Lotion	15	Lotion	B,PB	IM,CB	B,F,I,L,P,PB	T,VE	
Eclipse							
Original Eclipse Lotion	10	Lotion	B,PB,SL	M	B,F,PB		
Total Eclipse Lotion	15	Lotion	B,PB,SL	M	B,I,F,PB		
Total Eclipse Lotion	25	Lotion	B,C,SL,TI	M	A,B,C,D,P	T	
Elizabeth Arden							
Immunage UV Defense Cream	15	Cream	B,PB	M	B,DM,F,L,P,PB	BHA,BHT,T,VE	
Immunage UV Defense Lotion	15	Lotion	B,C	M	B,C,F,I,L,P,PB	T,VE	
Spa for the Sun Sheltering Sun Block (waterproof)	35	Cream	B,PB	IM,M	B,F,P,PB		
SunScience:							
Gentle Tanning Cream	6	Cream	B,PB	IM,M	B,F,L,P,PB,Q	BHA,BHT,T	
Spot-Protection Sunblock	15	Stick	B,PB	ML,PT	B,F,L,P,PB	BHA,BHT,R	
Superblock Cream	34	Cream	B,PB	IM,M	B,F,I,P,PB	BC,BHT	
Superblock Cream	35	Cream	B,PB	BS,IM,M	B,F,I,P,PB	BC,BHT	
Waterproof	35	Lotion	B,PB	IM,M	B,F,P,PB	BC,BHT	
Erno Laszlo							
Sensitive Area Protector	18	Powder	B,C	IS,M	B,C,D,P,PG	BHA,VE	
Sun Control Mist	10	Lotion	B,C,SL		B,C,E,F	VE	
Sun Shield Emulsion	18	Lotion	BC		B,C,DM,E,F,P	T,VE	
Estee Lauder							
Gentle Tanning Creme	8	Cream	B,C	IM,M	B,C,F,I,P	BHT,T,VE	+
Golden Bronzing Oil	3	Oil	B,C	IM	B,C,F,P	VE	+
Oil-Free Tanning Formula (has oil)	6	Cream	B,C	IM	A,B,C,F,I,P	BHT,VE	
Perfect Climate Sportwear Tint	12	Cream	C	MM	A,C,F,I,P	BHT,T,VE	
Sun-Out for Sensitive Skin	30+	Cream	B,C,PB,SL		A,B,C,E,I,P,PB	BHT,MCZ,MZ,VE	
Super Sunblock	20	Cream	B,C,SL	IM	A,B,C,F,I,P	BHT,MCZ,MZ	
Tinted Sunscreen	8	Cream	B,C	M	B,C,F,I,P,PG	VE	
Waterworld Sunscreen	15	Cream	B,C,SL	IM,PGS	A,B,C,F,I,P	BHT	+
Eutra							
Block Sunblock	18	Oint.	B,C	M,PT	B,C		
Block Sunblock and Moisturizer	32	Cream	B,C,SL	M,PT	B,C,I,P		
Swiss Sun Creme	8	Cream	C,PB	M,PT	C,PB		

Product name	SPF	Form	Active sunscreen ingredients	Possible comedogenic ingredients	Possible sensitizers	Other possible sensitizers	Coal tar colors
Frances Denney							
Sun Care Sun Block	15	Lotion	B,PB,SL	M	B,F,I,PB		
Sun Care Suntan Lotion	10	Lotion	PB	PT	F,PB		
Sun Care Suntan Oil Spray	4	Spray	C	CB,IN,IS	C,P,PG		
Jheri Redding							
Caribbean Gold Suntan Intensifier	4	Lotion	B,C	CB	B,C,D,F,P,SA	T,VE	
Sunblock Lotion	15	Lotion	B,C,SL	CB	B,C,D,F,P,SA	T,VE	
Sunblock Spray	15	Spray	B,C,SL	CB	B,C,D,F,P,SA	VE	
Lancôme							
Conquête du soleil:							
Barrier Solaire Waterproof Ultra Protection Creme	25	Cream	B,C,SL	PPG	B,C,D,E,F,P,PG	BHA,BHT,T	
Maximum Sunblock for Face and Body	23	Lotion	B,C,SL	PPG	B,C,D,E,F,P,PG	BHA,BHT,T	
Spray de Soleil Non-Gras Oil-Free Sun Spray	6	Spray	B,C	PPG	B,C,E,I,P,PG	T,VE	
Waterproof Body Sunblock	15	Lotion	B,C,PB	IS,M	F,P,PB,PG	BHA,BHT,MCZ,MZ	
Mary Kay Sun Essentials							
Sensitive Skin Waterproof Sunblock	15	Lotion	B,C,SL		E,I	T	
Super Sunblock	30	Lotion	B,C,ECD,SL		DM,P,PG	T	
Waterproof Sunscreen	8	Lotion	B,C		E,I	T	
Milopa							
Sportcream	2	Cream	C	IM,M	C,F,P,PG		†
Sun Cream	8	Cream	C	IM,M,PT	C,E,F,P,PG		
Sun Milk	4	Lotion	C	IM,M	C,F,I,P		
Neutrogena							
PABA-Free Sunblock	15	Lotion	B,C	M	B,C,P		
New Essentials							
New Essential Protection	25	Lotion	B,C,MA,SL		B,C,I,P	VE	
Physician's Formula							
Sun Shield Moisture	25	Lotion	B,PB,SL,TI	M	B,D,L,P		
Sun Shield Protection Plus	20	Lotion	B,C,SL,TI		B,D,L,P		
Swimmer's Sun Shield	20	Lotion	B,PB,SL,TI	M	B,D,L,P		
Photoplex							
Broad Spectrum Lotion	15+	Lotion	BM,PB	M,PT	I,PB		

	SPF	Form		IM,PT*	A*,D*,F,PB,Q*	MCZ*,MZ*,T*	
PreSun							
Creamy Sunscreen	4	Cream	PB		A,B,D,F,PB	MCZ*,MZ*,T*	
Creamy Sunscreen	39	Cream	B,PB		A,B,D,F,PB	MCZ,MZ,T	
Sensitive Skin Sunscreen	29	Lotion	B,C,SL		A,B,C,D	MCZ,MZ,T	+
Princess Marcella Borghese							
Termi di Montecatini Spa Solare Ageless							
Sun for Body Creme	8	Cream	B,C	M,OP,PT	B,C,E,P	VE	
Purpose							
Dual Treatment Moisturizer	12	Lotion	B,C	M,OS	B,C,P,Q	BHT	
Rachel Perry							
Aloe-Suma Advanced Treatment							
Sunblock	30	Cream	B,C,SL	CB,DO,MM	B,C,DM,E,P,PG	T,VE	
Aloe-Suma All Season Sunblock	15	Cream	B,C	CB,DO,MM	B,C,DM,E,F,P,PG	T,VE	
Sea & Ski							
Block Out Lotion	30	Lotion	B,C,PB	PGS,PPG,PT	B,C,D,F,P,PB	T	
Suntan Lotion with Collagen	4	Lotion	PB	CB,M	D,F,L,P,PB,PG	BHA,BHT,PGL,T	
Tropic Sun Dark Tanning Lotion	0	Lotion	PB	CB,M	E,F,I,L,P,PB,PG	BHA,BHT,PGL,T	+
Tropic Sun Dark Tanning Oil	0	Oil	PB	CB,M	L,PB,PG	BHA,BHT,PGL	
Stendhal							
Intensive Tan	2	Cream	B	OP,S	B,F,P,PG	VE	+
Sunscreen for Sensitive Areas	16	Compact	B,C,TI		B,C,F	VE	+
Waterproof Sun Gel	10	Cream	B,C	OP,S	B,C,F,P,PG	VE	+
Sundown							
Broad Spectrum Sunblock Cream	30	Cream	B,C,SL,TI	M	A,B,C,F,Q	VE	
Sunblock	15	Lotion	B,C,PB	M	A,B,C,F,PB,Q		
Sunblock Cream	24	Cream	B,PB	IM,M	A,B,F,I,P,PB		
Ultra	20	Lotion	B,C,PB,TI	M	A,B,C,F,PB,Q		
Tropical Blend							
Hawaii Blend Dark Tanning Oil	0	Oil	SL	CB,M,OO	F,L		
Hawaii Blend Dark Tanning Oil	2	Oil	B,PB	CB,M,OO	B,F,L,PB	VE	
Jamaica Blend Dark Tanning Oil	0	Oil	SL	CB,M,OO	F,L	VE	
Rio Blend Dark Tanning Oil	0	Oil	SL	CB,M,OO	F,L	VE	
Vaseline							
Intensive Care:							
Moisturizing Sunblock Lotion	15	Lotion	B,C	PT	B,C,DM,F,P	T,VE	
Moisturizing Sunscreen Lotion	8	Lotion	B,C	PT	B,C,DM,F,P	T,VE	
Moisturizing Suntan Lotion	2	Lotion	C	PT	C,DM,F,P	T,VE	
Moisturizing Suntan Lotion	4	Lotion	B,C	PT	B,C,DM,F,P	T,VE	

OIL-FREE SUNSCREENS CONTAINING EMOLLENT ESTERS

Product name	SPF	Form	Active sunscreen ingredients	Possible comedogenic ingredients	Possible sensitizers	Other possible sensitizers	Coal tar colors
Almay							
Sun Care:							
Moisturizing Lotion	8	Lotion	B,C,SL		B,C,I,P	T,VE	
Oil-Free Lotion	8	Lotion	B,C,MA,SL		B,C,I,P	VE	
Oil-Free Lotion	15	Lotion	B,C,MA,OC,SL		B,C,I,P	VE	
Oil-Free Lotion	20	Lotion	B,C,MA,OC,SL		B,C,I,P	T,VE	
Oil-Free Waterproof Sunblock	30+	Lotion	B,C,MA,SL,TI		B,C,I,P	VE	
Oil-Free Spray	8	Spray	B,C,SL		B,C,I,P	VE	
Oil-Free Spray	15	Spray	B,C,MA,OC,SL		B,C,I,P	VE	
Oil-Free Spray	20	Spray	B,C,MA,OC,SL		B,C,I,P	VE	
Sun Stress SPF 8 Spray	8	Spray	B,C,SL		B,C,I,P	VE	
Bain de Soleil							
Body Silkening Creme	30	Cream	B,C,PB		B,C,DM,F,I,P, PB,PG	T	
Biotherm							
Triple Protection:							
Oil-Free Sun Spray	10	Spray	B,C		B,C,F	VE	
Oil-Free Tanning Gel	8	Gel	B,C		B,C,F,I,P	T,MCZ,MZ,VE	†
Chanel							
Bronzage Progressif Protective Bronzing Lotion	8	Lotion	B,C	IN,IS,OP	B,BP,C,E,F,P,PG	VE	
Bronzage Satine Protective Bronzing Mist	4	Spray	C	DO,IN,M,OP	C,E,F,P	VE	
Protection Intense Oil-Free Sun Shelter Lotion	23	Lotion	B,C,SL	PGS	B,BP,C,E,F,P	VE	
Clinique							
Full-Service Sunblock	10	Lotion	C,MA,SL		C,E,I,P	BHT,T,VE	
Full-Service Sunblock	20	Lotion	B,C,SL		C,E,I,P	BHT,T,VE	
Coppertone							
Sun Sense Towelettes	15	Towels	B,C,SL		B,C,DM	VE	
Tan Magnifier	4	Lotion	C		C,F,I,P,PG	VE	
Elizabeth Arden							
Spa for the Sun Sunmist Oil-Free Sunscreen	15	Lotion	B,C,SL		B,C,E,F	VE	
Erno Laszlo							
Oil-Free Sun Block	25	Lotion	B,C,SL		B,C,DM,E,F,P	T,VE	

Product	SPF	Form				
Lancôme						
Conquête du Soleil:						
Ecran Solaire Waterproof Basic						
Sunblock Creme	15	Cream	B,C,SL		B,C,D,E,F,P	T
Oil-Free Sun Spray	10	Spray	B,C		B,C,I,PG	T
Spray de Soleil Non-Gras Oil-Free Sun						
Spray	18	Spray	B,C,OC,PS	PPG	B,C,E,I,P,PG	T,VE
La Prairie						
Sun Care Cream	6	Cream	PB		E,F,I,P,PB,PS	T
Nu Skin						
Sunright Spray 10	10	Spray	C,SL	OP,OS	C	VE
Sunright 25	25	Lotion	B,C,SL	OP,OS	B,C,D,P	VE
Physician's Formula						
Sun Shield Oil-Free	25	Lotion	B,PB,SL	IS	B,P,Q	
Sea & Ski						
Clear PABA-Free Tanning Lotion	4	Lotion	C,SL		C,F	
Clear Waterproof Tanning Lotion	2	Lotion	SL		F	
STRICTLY OIL-FREE SUNSCREENS						
Almay						
SPF 4 Protective Tanning Gel	4	Gel	PS		I,P	T,VE
Bain de Soleil						
Body Silkening Spray	25	Spray	B,C,PB		B,C,DM,F,I,P,PB	T
Sunblock Creme	30	Cream	B,PB		B,DM,F,I,PB	T
Ultra Sunblock Body Silkening Creme	25	Cream	B,C,PB		B,C,DM,F,I,P,PB	T
Clinique						
Oil-Free Sunblock	15	Spray	B,C,OC,SL		B,C	BHT,R
Coppertone						
Moisturizing Sunblock Lotion	45	Lotion	B,C,OC,SL		B,C,F,I,P	T,VE
Elizabeth Arden						
SunScience Oil-Free Ultra-Block	15	Gel	B,PB		F	
Estee Lauder						
Oil-Free Sunspray	10	Spray	B,C,SL		A,B,C,F	BHT,VE
Sport Bronzer	8	Cream	C		C,F,I,P,PG	+
Formula 405						
Solar Lotion	8	Lotion	C		C,P	T
Merle Norman						
Ultra Skin Protector	23	Lotion	B,C		B,C,DM,P	

Product name	SPF	Form	Active sunscreen ingredients	Possible comedogenic ingredients	Possible sensitizers	Other possible sensitizers	Coal tar colors
Nu Skin							
Sunright 4	4	Lotion	C		C,D,P,PG	T,VE	
Sunright 8	8	Lotion	B,C		B,C,D,P,PG	T,VE	
Sunright 15	15	Lotion	B,C		B,C,D,P,PG	T,VE	
Physician's Formula							
Sun Shield PABA-Free Waterproof	20	Lotion	B,C,SL,TI		B,C,D,I,P	T	

CHILDREN'S SUNSCREENS

Product name	SPF	Form	Active sunscreen ingredients	Possible comedogenic ingredients	Possible sensitizers	Other possible sensitizers	Coal tar colors
Almay							
SPF 20 Waterproof Sunblock for Kids	20	Lotion	B,C,SL		B,C,I,P	VE	
Avon							
Sunseekers:							
Children's Sunblock	15	Cream	B,C	CB	B,C,I	VE	
Children's Ultra Sunsafe Superblock	30	Cream	B,C,SL	CB	B,C,I	VE	
Banana Boat							
Baby Sunblock Lotion	29	Lotion	B,C,SL	CB	B,C,P	T,VE	
Coppertone							
Water Babies:							
Sunblock Lotion	15	Lotion	B,C	IM	B,C,F,I,P	T	
Lotion	30	Lotion	B,C,SL	M	B,C,F,I,P	T,VE	
Sunblock Lotion (oil-free)	45	Lotion	B,C,OC,SL		B,C,F,I,P	T,VE	
Sunblock Cream	25	Cream	B,C,SL		B,C,F,I,P	T,VE	
Eclipse							
Child Garde Sunblock Spray (nonaerosol) (water- & oil-free)	20	Spray	B,C,PB		B,C,PB		
Estee Lauder							
Baby Block Children's Waterproof Sunscreen	30+	Cream	B,C,SL		A,B,C,E,I,P	BHT,T,VE	
Frances Denney							
Sun Care Children's Sunblock Spray	20	Spray	B,C,PB		B,C,PB		
Johnson & Johnson							
Baby Sunblock Lotion	15	Lotion	B,C,SL,TI	II	A,B,C,F,PG,Q	BHT,VE	
Physician's Formula							
Children's Waterproof Sun Shield	20	Lotion	B,C,SL,TI		B,C,D,P	BHA,BHT	
PreSun							
Children's Sunscreen	29	Lotion	B,C,SL		A,B,C,D	MCZ,MZ,T	

EYE SUNSCREENS[1]

Product	SPF	Form	TI	PT	I,P	VE
Almay						
Sun Care Eye Protector (sunblock)		Cream				
Bain de Soleil						
Under Eye Protector	15	Cream	B,C,SL	M,OA,PT	B,C,P	BHA,VE
Clinique						
Eye Zone	25	Stick	C,SL		C,P	VE
Estee Lauder						
Sun Stick (for ears, lips, nose, and eye area)	15	Stick	B,C		B,C,E,L,P	BHT,VE
Frances Denney						
Sun Care Eye and Lip Protector	15	Compact	B,PB	IM,PT	B,F,L,PB	
Lancôme						
Conquete du Soleil:						
Baton Solaire Eye and Lip Protector	12	Stick	B,C	CB,M,OA,PT	B,C,L,P	BHA,BHT
Waterproof Eye and Lip Protector	12	Compact	B,PB	M,PT	B,L,P,PB	BHA
Waterproof Eye and Lip Protector	18	Compact	B,C	PT	B,C,E,L,P	BHA,BHT
La Prairie						
Sun Care for Lips and Eyes	15	Compact	B,PB	M,MM	B,P,PB	VE
Merle Norman						
Ultra Eye Protector	23	Compact	B,C,MA	ML,PT	B,C,L,P	BHT,VE

OIL-CONTAINING FACIAL SUNSCREENS

Product	SPF	Form	TI	PT	I,P	VE
Avon						
Sunseekers:						
Face Tanning Cream	20	Cream	B,C,TI	CB	B,C,I,P,PG	T,VE
Tanning Cream for the Face	8	Cream	B,C	CB	B,C,I,P,PG	T,VE
Tanning Cream for the Face	15	Cream	B,C	CB	B,C,I,P,PG	T,VE
Banana Boat						
Lotion for Faces	23	Lotion	B,C,PB	CB,M	B,C,F,P,PB,Q	MO,T,VE
Chanel						
Protection Extreme Sun Shelter Face Block	15	Cream	B,PB	IS,M	B,BP,E,L,P,PG	BHA,PGL,VE
Estee Lauder						
Face Block for Sensitive Skin	15	Cream	B,C,SL	IM,PGS	A,B,C,F,I,P	BHT
Sun Stick (for ears, lips, nose, and eye area)	15	Stick	B,C		B,C,E,L,P	BHT,VE
Total Face Block	25	Cream	B,C,SL		A,B,C,F,I,P	BHT,VE

[1]All of the preparations listed below are water-free.

Product name	SPF	Form	Active sunscreen ingredients	Possible comedogenic ingredients	Possible sensitizers	Other possible sensitizers	Coal tar colors
Frances Denney Sun Care Facial Sunblock	25	Lotion	B,C,SL,TI	M	A,B,C,D,P	T	
Lancôme Conquête du Soleil:							
Air Light Sun Protection for the Face	10	Lotion	B,C	IM	B,C,F,I,P	BHT,T	
Air Light Sun Protection for Face and Body	23	Lotion	B,C,SL	PPG	B,C,D,E,F,P,PG	BHA,BHT,T	
Mary Kay Sun Essentials Facial Sunblock	15	Lotion	B,C,SL		E,I	T	
Physician's Formula Sun Shield for Faces	23	Lotion	B,P,SL		B,C,D,P	BHA,BHT,MO	
Prescriptives For the Face	30	Lotion	B,C,SL	MM	B,C,I,P	BHT,VE	
Princess Marcella Borghese Termi di Montecatini Spa Solare Ageless Sun for Face Creme	15	Cream	B,C,	M,MM,PT	B,C,E,P	VE	
Shiseido UV Facial Protection Complex	8	Lotion	B,PB,TI	PT	B,F,P,PB	VE	
Stendhal Vital Face Protection	6	Lotion	B,C		B,C,F	MCZ,MZ,T,VE	†

OIL-FREE FACIAL SUNSCREENS CONTAINING EMOLLIENT ESTERS

Product name	SPF	Form	Active sunscreen ingredients	Possible comedogenic ingredients	Possible sensitizers	Other possible sensitizers	Coal tar colors
Bain de Soleil Face Creme	15	Cream	B,PB	SLS	B,DM,P,PB	T	
Coppertone Oil-Free Face Lotion	15	Lotion	B,PB	IM	B,F,I,P,PB	T	
Lancôme Conquête du Soleil: Refuge du Soleil Matte Sun Shield for the Face	18	Lotion	B,C,OC	PPG	B,C,D,E,P,PG	T	
Mary Kay Oil-Free Facial Sunblock	15	Lotion	B,C,SL		DM,P	ED	

STRICTLY OIL-FREE FACIAL SUNSCREENS

Product	SPF	Form					
Bain de Soleil							
Face Creme	6	Cream	B,PB		B,DM,P,PB,PG	T	
Face Creme	25	Cream	B,C,PB		B,C,DM,I,P,PB	T	
Clinique							
City Block Oil-Free Daily Face Protector	13	Lotion	TI		A,E,I,PG	BHT,T,VE	
Max Factor							
Pure SPF Daily Face Protector	12	Lotion	C,PS		C,D,P	T	+

OIL-CONTAINING LIP SUNSCREENS

Product	SPF	Form					
Almay							
Sun Care for Lips	15	Stick	B,C	M,PT	B,C,P	BHA,VE	
Avon							
Sunseekers Tropical Lip Block	15	Gel	B,C	CB,M,PT	B,C,F	BHA,VE	*
Clinique							
Lip Block	11	Stick	B,C	PT	B,C		
Estee Lauder							
Sun Stick (for ears, lips, nose, and eye area)	15	Stick	B,C		B,C,E,L,P	BHT,VE	
Frances Denney							
Sun Care Eye and Lip Protector	15	Compact	B,PB	IM,PT	B,F,L,PB		
Lancôme							
Conquête du Soleil:							
Baton Solaire Eye and Lip Protector	12	Stick	B,C	CB,M,OA,PT	B,C,L,P	BHA,BHT	
Waterproof Eye and Lip Protector	12	Compact	B,PB	M,PT	B,L,P,PS	BHA	
Waterproof Eye and Lip Protector	18	Compact	B,C	PT	B,C,E,L,P	BHA,BHT	
La Prairie							
Sun Care for Lips and Eyes	15	Compact	B,PB	M,MM	B,P,PB	VE	
Mary Kay							
Sun Essentials Lip Protector	15	Stick	B,C	BS,M	F,L,P	BHA,VE	†
Merle Norman							
Ultra Lip Protector	23	Stick	B,C	DO,OA	B,C,F,L	BHA,BHT	†
Prescriptives							
Protective Lip Shield	15	Stick	B,C,SL				
Revlon							
Triple Action Lip Defense	15	Compact	B,C	OP,OS	B,C,F,L,P	BHA,VE	*

SUNBLOCKS

Product	Form				
Almay					
Sun Care Eye Protector	Cream	TI	PT	I,P	VE

SUNSCREENS THAT LIST ONLY ACTIVE INGREDIENT INFORMATION

Product name	SPF	Form	Active sunscreen ingredients
Alo Sun			
Fashion Tan Sunblock Lotion	15+	Lotion	B,PB
Fashion Tan Sunblock Lotion	27	Lotion	B,C,OC,SL
Clinique			
Oil-Free Sunblock	15	Spray	B,C,OC,SL
Sunblock	20	Lotion	B,C,SL
Total Cover Sunblock	30	Cream	B,C,PB,SL
Coppertone			
Nosekote Cream	8	Cream	B,SL
Eclipse			
Cancer Garde Ultra Protection Sunblock Lotion	33	Lotion	B,C,PB,TI
Total Eclipse Spray	20	Spray	B,C,PB
Elite			
Maximal Sun Block	15	Lotion	B,C
Frances Denney			
Sun Care Children's Sunblock	33	Lotion	B,C,PB,TI
Hawaiian Tropic			
Baby Faces Sunblock Spray	25	Spray	B,C,MA,SL
Maxafil			
Cream Sunscreen for Sensitive Skin	Physical Sunblock	Cream	C,MA
Neutrogena			
Sunblock	8	Cream	C,MA
Sunblock	30	Cream	C,MA,OC
Pfeiffer			
Petroleum Jelly Lip Treatment Sunblock	15	Ointment	B,PB
Prescriptives			
Waterproof Oil-Free Mist Sunscreen	15	Lotion	B,C,SL
Waterproof Oil-Free Sunscreen	15	Lotion	B,C,SL
Waterproof Sunscreen	23	Lotion	B,C,SL
Advanced Sun Protection Stick	15	Stick	B,C,SL
Solbar			
PF Lotion	15	Lotion	B,C
Plus Cream	15	Cream	B,PB
Stendhal			
Intensive Tan	2	Gel	B
Moisturizing Body Emulsion	6	Lotion	B,C
Special Sport Waterproof Sun Gel	10	Gel	B,C
Sunscreen for Sensitive Areas	16	Compact	B,C,TI

PART FOUR

THE EYES

CHAPTER 16

Problems Unique to the Eyes

The skin near the eye and on the eyelid is thinner and less oily than other areas of the face and is therefore more likely to become dry than other facial areas. Because dry skin is a less effective barrier against the environment than normal moist skin, the skin around the eye is especially prone to inflammation caused by irritants and allergic reactions. When the skin of the eyelids becomes inflamed for any reason, the soft, elastic skin fills with fluid, which leads to puffiness.

COSMETICS AND EYE INFECTIONS

Eye infections can occur when cosmetics are used improperly around the eyes. It is absolutely essential for eye cosmetics to contain proper preservatives to prevent contamination from bacteria that can lead to infection, even though preservatives can cause allergic reactions.

Because the area around the eye can develop infection easily, eye cosmetics should never be applied using saliva, diluted with water, shared with other people, or tested in the store on the eye area (try it out on your wrist). It is also wise to discard products at home when they become discolored or dried out or when they have an unpleasant odor. Remember to use a fresh applicator each time a refillable product is refilled.

In addition, it is safest to apply mascara only to the outer two-thirds of the eyelashes. Apply eyeliner outside the lash line, keeping it away from the inside edge of the lid.

WRINKLES OF THE SKIN AROUND THE EYES

Wrinkles in the skin previously thought to be caused entirely by normal aging are largely related to the cumulative effects of the sun over time. The thin skin around the

---

EYE SHADOW AND EYE INFECTIONS

All eye products are prone to bacterial contamination and therefore should contain preservative ingredients. These are not products to buy preservative-free! They should never be applied using saliva, diluted with water, or shared with other people. Never test them on your eyes while in the store. Although there is no specific expiration date for an eye shadow product, it is wise to discard products that are discolored, dried up, or have unpleasant odors. Be sure to use a fresh applicator each time a refillable product is refilled.

---

eyes is one of the first areas where this wrinkling tends to be visible. The regular use of sunscreens can substantially slow down the development of wrinkles. In addition, many dermatologists believe that vitamin A acid (Retin-A) is effective in reversing sun-related wrinkling around the eyes; however, this has not yet been proven conclusively.

COLORS UNSAFE FOR USE NEAR THE EYES

Coloring ingredients derived from coal tar have been determined to be unsafe for use near the eyes. These coloring agents have been proven to be carcinogenic and have even caused blindness in at least one instance. Some protection is provided for the consumer by the Color Additive Amendment of 1960, which prohibits eye cosmetics from containing color additives made from coal tar. Coal tar colors are found on cosmetic ingredients labels and will be designated with the abbreviation FD&C (e.g., FD&C Red #3) or D&C (e.g., Ext. D&C or D&C Red #7). Unfortunately, many women use foundation makeup on the skin around the eyes. These products were not designed for use near the eyes and may contain coal tar–derived color additives that make them unsuitable for this purpose. Be sure to read the ingredients label carefully before using any cosmetic products near the eyes.

CHAPTER 17

Eye Shadows

Eye shadow is designed to add color and depth to the eyelids. Most cosmetologists think that eye shadow looks best when color-coordinated with the wardrobe and not with eye color. Frosted products will often accentuate wrinkles, and darker colors can accentuate any irregular skin coloration on the eyelid.

CHOOSING EYE SHADOW

A professional application of eye shadow often utilizes three different shades. A light to medium color will be used on the eyelids, a darker color on the crease, and a lighter shade under the eyebrows. Thorough blending is essential where these colors meet. Some makeup specialists can enhance the size of the eyes by redefining the crease of the eyelid at a higher point. The eyelid crease is first concealed by applying eye shadow primer and eye shadow.

> When buying eye shadow, beware of the fluorescent lighting often found at cosmetics counters. For sanitary reasons, do not apply the tester to your eyes. Use the back of your hand or the inside of your wrist and go out into the daylight to evaluate the color.

The crease is then redefined by applying a darker shade of shadow along the edge of the bone at the top of the eye socket. The outer edge of this line can be further emphasized with an even darker color to create a more dramatic effect.

Finish
Although oil-based shadows tend to have more shine, metals such as aluminum, copper, silver, tin, or bronze can also be added to create a shiny look. Ingredients such as bismuth oxychloride, mica, or fish scale are used to create frosted or pearly finishes.

Pigment
Pigment is perhaps the most important ingredient in eye shadow. The U.S. Food and Drug Administration requires that ingredients be listed in order of quantity, from most to least. Coloring agents are an exception: Manufacturers are allowed to list them at the end, with the words "May contain..." With this format, manufacturers can use the same label on all eye shadow colors and save money on printing labels.

As mentioned, color derived from coal tar cannot be used safely in eye cosmetics. Eye shadow colors are derived instead from other types of refined minerals. If the ingredients seem a lot like those of an artist's paintbox, they are. Titanium dioxide is used for white. Chromium oxide makes green. Iron oxides are used for red and brown. Lapis lazuli, which you may associate with jewelry, used to be ground up to provide the ultramarine blue for eye shadow. Now, ultramarine blue is manufactured synthetically. There's a whole family of synthetic "ultramarine" colors — green, pink, red, and violet.

Like the coloring agents used in mascara, the minerals and synthetics used in eye shadow are classified as "noncertified color additives." The FDA has determined that individual batches don't require testing.

REACTIONS TO EYE SHADOW

Although eye products can cause allergic reactions, irritation reactions are more common. It is important to realize that eye makeup is not the only cause of allergic reactions around the eyes. In fact, the most common cause is wet nail polish that comes in contact with the eyelids when a woman touches her eyes (see Chapter 24). Additives used to create a metallic or pearly shine increase the likelihood of an irritant reaction to eye shadow, and products containing these additives should be avoided by anyone who tends to get adverse reac-

tions to eye shadow. Eye shadow can also cause eye irritation for people who wear contact lenses. Always put contact lenses in the eyes before applying eye makeup.

There is also a tendency to develop more adverse reactions to dark color shades and when shadow is used too near the inner eye corner where it is likely to get washed into the eye by tears. The abrasive effect from applying eye shadow to sensitive eyelid skin also can lead to irritation. Powder eye shadow is the least abrasive of the eye shadow products.

TYPES OF EYE SHADOW

Most eye shadows wear well so wearability is not the basis on which to choose an eye shadow. The choice should depend on characteristics such as water resistance, oiliness, ease of application, and coverage.

Eyelid skin can vary from dry to slightly oily. It is rarely very oily, and acne of the eyelid is extremely uncommon. Although skin type is not as critical in the choice of shadow as it is in most other types of cosmetics, oily shadow will feel most comfortable on dry skin, whereas less oily products will feel best on oilier skin. Many shadows are available in a variety of finishes. You can choose the shadow desired by looking at the chart below.

Type of Eye Shadow	Oiliness	Application	Coverage
cream (waterproof)	very high	easy	good
stick, crayon (waterproof)	very high	fairly easy	good
pencil (waterproof)	high	sometimes difficult	good
water-based	moderate	fairly easy	moderate
powder with oil	slight to moderate	very easy	moderate
powder, oil-free	minimal	very easy	moderate

"Automatic" Eye Shadow

Automatic eye cosmetics are soft creams sold in cylindrical tubes with screw-on tops containing an applicator brush.

Waterproof Eye Shadow Creams

Waterproof eye shadows are very oily water-free creams. They will not smear or run when exposed to tears. However, they are soluble in oil and can crease (migrate) on oilier eyelid skin and appear uneven.

Since these products are oily, they are often useful for dry eyelid skin. Application is easy and they provide good coverage of discoloration and shallow wrinkles. However, these products can also shift and concentrate in deeper wrinkles leading to accentuation of these features. The eye creams are therefore not the best choice for deeper wrinkles. The use of an eye shadow setting cream can minimize the creasing problem. Some waterproof eye shadows are packaged as automatic eye shadows.

Pencil and Stick Eye Shadows

Pencil, stick, and crayon eye shadows are waterproof eye shadows with increased wax content to make them solid. They are similar in character to the waterproof eye shadows but tend to be more difficult to apply evenly because they drag on the skin. The pencil products are hardest and most apt to be troublesome in this regard. Stick eye shadows, which are packaged in a tube similar to lipstick, and crayons are less hard than pencils and create less drag on the skin.

Water-based Eye Shadow Creams

Water-based eye shadows are creams that are somewhat less oily than the waterproof eyeliners, fairly easy to apply, and provide moderate coverage. They are not waterproof, however. Most are automatic eye shadows packaged in cylindrical tubes with applicators.

Powder Eye Shadows

Powder eye shadows are either oil-containing or oil-free powders that are less oily than eye shadow creams because of the large amount of powder they contain. Most are pressed powders, but at least one loose powder eye shadow is currently on the market. Creme powders generally have more oil than other powder eye shadows. Powder eye shadows are extremely easy to apply evenly and provide moderate coverage. Oil-containing products are best for drier eyelid skin and oil-free products are best for oilier eyelid skin.

Eye Shadow Primers

Eye shadow primers or setting creams (base coats) are designed to be used under eye shadow to increase weartime and to hide wrinkles. Most are water-free, but there are a few less oily water-based products available.

USE OF REGULAR FOUNDATION MAKEUP UNDER EYE SHADOW

Many women choose to wear regular foundation makeup under eye shadow. Some foundation makeups can be safely used in this manner; however, some contain coal tar colors that are not safe near the eyes. Foundation makeup products containing coal tar colors are indicated in the charts (see Chapter 9). When using a product not listed on the charts, be sure to read the ingredients label carefully. Coal tar colors will be listed on the ingredients label and will begin with the abbreviation FD&C (e.g., FD&C Red #3) or D&C (e.g., D&C Red #7). Products containing coal tar colors should never be used near the eyes.

Chart 17–1
EYE SHADOWS

The charts are designed to help you minimize adverse reactions and choose products with the proper oil content for your skin type. If you have cosmetics-related acne, you should also choose products with the least amounts of potentially comedogenic ingredients.

Although most cosmetics contain potentially sensitizing ingredients, there is no reason to avoid any ingredient unless you are experiencing adverse reactions to cosmetic products. If you know you are allergic to certain ingredients, the charts will show you which products to avoid. If you are experiencing reactions to a certain cosmetic product, the charts can help you select alternative products that do not contain the same potentially sensitizing ingredients. To choose new products that are least likely to cause allergic reactions, keep in mind that fragrance is by far the most frequent cause of allergic reactions to cosmetics, followed by ingredients listed as "possible sensitizers." The ingredients listed as "other possible sensitizers" cause allergic reactions less frequently. Using these charts should help solve many cosmetics-related skin problems; however, if a problem persists, consult a dermatologist for advice and possible patch testing.

The products listed in these charts include many of the nationally advertised and distributed brands that have the largest market share of cosmetics sales; an extensive sampling of other brands available in the Chicago area is also included.

After locating several suitable products, use the pricing information on pages 18–19 for comparison shopping.

KEY

Possible Comedogenic Ingredients

BS — butyl stearate
DO — decyl oleate and derivatives
II — isopropyl isostearate
IM — isopropyl myristate
IN — isostearyl neopentanoate
IP — isopropyl palmitate
IS — isocetyl stearate and derivatives
LA — lanolin, acetylated
M — mineral oil
ML — myristyl lactate
MM — myristyl myristate
OA — oleyl alcohol
OP — octyl palmitate
OS — octyl stearate and derivatives
PGS — propylene glycol stearate
PPG — myristyl ether propionate
PT — petrolatum
S — sesame oil/extract
SLS — sodium lauryl sulfate

Possible Sensitizers

A — and other ingredients
BP — bronopol (2-bromo-2-nitropropane-1,3-diol)‡
C — cinnamates
D — diazolidinyl urea‡
DM — DMDM hydantoin‡

> Names of products and product lines, and ingredients, are continually changing. Read the labels carefully before purchasing any beauty or skin-care product.

E—essential oils and biological additives
F—fragrances
I—imidazolidinyl urea‡
L—lanolin and derivatives that may cross-react with lanolin
P—parabens
PB—PABA
PG—propylene glycol
PS—potassium sorbate
Q—quaternium-15‡
SA—sorbic acid

Other Possible Sensitizers

BHA—butylated hydroxyanisole
BHT—butylated hydroxytoluene
BO—bismuth oxychloride
CA—captan

CH—chlorhexidine and derivatives
CX—chloroxylenol
MCZ—methylchloroisothiazolinone
MDG—methyldibromoglutaronide
MO—mink oil
MZ—methylisothiazolinone
PGL—propyl gallate
PMA—phenylmercuric acetate
R—rosin (colophony) and derivatives
T—triethanolamine and derivatives that may cross-react
UFR—urea/formaldehyde resin
VE—vitamin E (tocopherol and derivatives)
Z—zinc pyrithione

* may contain [see column head]
‡ formaldehyde-releasing ingredients

WATERPROOF EYE SHADOW CREAMS

Product name	Possible comedogenic ingredients	Possible sensitizers	Other possible sensitizers
Adrien Arpel			
Powdery Cream Eye Shadow	BS,IN,M,OP,OS,PT	L,P	BHA,BO*
Avon			
Color Multiples	M		BHT,BO*,UFR
Colortwists	M		BHT,BO*,UFR
Coordinates Colortips			BHT,BO*
Bonne Bell			
Eye Strokes Waterproof Eye Color		P	BHA,BO*
Clarion			
Wear-Proof Eye Shadow (automatic)	M	P,Q	BHA,BO*
Clinique			
Touch Base for Eyes		P	BO*,PMA
Estee Lauder			
Eyecoloring (Liquid-to-Powder Eye Shadow)	OS		BHT,BO*,VE
Lancôme			
Les Aquatiques Waterproof Creme EyeColour	LA		BHT
Max Factor			
Satin Shadow Creme	M	I,P	BO*
Maybelline			
Creme-On Eye Shadow (automatic)		P	BHA

Product name	Possible comedogenic ingredients	Possible sensitizers	Other possible sensitizers
Pupa			
Creamy Eye Shadow	OP,PT	P	R,VE
Creamy Eye Shadow (older formulation)	IM,IP,LA,M,OS	L,P	BHA,BHT
Kajal		P	VE
Revlon			
Shadow Card	IM	P	
Shiseido			
Silky Finish Eye Shadow	M,PT	F,P	VE

WATER-RESISTANT EYE SHADOW CREAMS

Product name	Possible comedogenic ingredients	Possible sensitizers	Other possible sensitizers
Avon			
Perfect Eyes Eye Color		C,D,L,P	BHT,BO*,R

EYE SHADOW PENCILS, STICKS, AND CRAYONS

Product name	Form	Possible comedogenic ingredients	Possible sensitizers	Other possible sensitizers
Almay				
All-Day Shadow Liner	Pencil	BS,M	P	BHA,BO*
Waterproof Shadowpencil	Pencil		P	BHA,BO*
Artmatic				
Soft Eye Shadow Pencil	Pencil	M,OA	L,P	BHA
Avon				
Avon Color Luxury Pencils	Pencil	MM,OS	L	BHT,BO*
Colorsticks Pencil	Pencil	IM	P	BHT,BO*
Glimmersticks	Pencil	M		BHT,BO*,UFR
Shadowstix	Pencil	M		BHT,BO*,UFR
Ultra Wear Pencil	Pencil	OS		BO*
Aziza				
Shadow Twist Plus Liner (sold with Pencil Eyeliner)	Pencil	M	I,P	BO*
Body Shop				
Colourings: Eyeshadow Pencil	Pencil	SLS*	I,P,SA*	BO*
Shadowlight Pencil (current)	Pencil		I,P	BO*
Shadowlight Pencil (revised)	Pencil		P,SA	BO*
Chanel				
Cream Color Crayon	Crayon		P	BO*
Clinique				
Lid Stick (eyeliner and eye shadow)	Stick		P	BHA,BO*
Flame Glo				
Waterproof Creme Eye Color Crayon	Crayon		P	BHA,BO*

Product name	Form	Possible comedogenic ingredients	Possible sensitizers	Other possible sensitizers
Lancôme				
Le Crayon Waterproof Creme EyeColour	Crayon		P	BHT,BO*
Le Kohl Poudre Eye Shadow Pencil	Pencil		P	BO*,MDG
Mary Kay				
Waterproof Eye Color Crayon	Crayon		P	BO*,PGL
Max Factor				
Maxi-Soft Creamy Eye Color Pencil	Pencil	IM,M	L,P,Q	BHA,BHT
Montaj				
Jumbo Shadow Pencil	Pencil	IM,ML	P	BHA,BHT
Revlon				
Waterproof Creme Eyemarker	Pencil	OP	P	BHA,BO*

WATER-BASED EYE SHADOW CREAMS

Product name	Possible comedogenic ingredients	Possible sensitizers	Other possible sensitizers
Avon			
Color Active Eye Shadow	M	C,D,L,P	BHT,R
Ultima II			
Penultimate Lid Color (automatic)	M,SLS	L,P,PG,Q	T

OIL-CONTAINING EYE SHADOW POWDER

Product name	Possible comedogenic ingredients	Possible sensitizers	Other possible sensitizers
Adrien Arpel			
(Mix and Match) Eye Shadows:			
Disco Colors	M,OP	I,L,P	BO*
Other Colors	M	I,P	BO*
Eyeliner & Shading Shadow	M	I,P	BO*
Allercreme			
Color Sheers Eye Shadows	M	I,P	BO*
Almay			
8 Hour Eye Color	M	I,P	BO*
Eye Color Singles	M	I,P	BO*
Avon			
Avon Color Silk Finish Embossed	M	I,L,P	BHT,BO*,UFR
Coordinates Highlight 'N' Shadow	DO,M	P	BO*
Coordinates Smooth Touch Powder	M	P	BO*,UFR
Powder Eye Shadow	M,OS	L,P	BO*
Powderstix		I,P	BO*
Pure Care Eye Shadow	M	P,PB	BO*
Silk Finish Creme Powder Eye Shadow		C	BHA,BO*
Soft Dimensions	M	I,P	BO*

Product name	Possible comedogenic ingredients	Possible sensitizers	Other possible sensitizers
Ultra Wear Powder	DO,M	P	BHT,BO*,UFR
Ultra Wear Powder Restage	M	I,L,P	BHT,BO*,UFR
Youthful Visions:			
Eyecoloring System Cream Primer	M,OP,OS	C	BHT,BO*,UFR,VE
Eyecoloring System Powder	M	C,I,P	BHT,BO*,UFR,VE
Aziza			
Color & Care Moisture Lock Eye Shadow		I,P	BO*,MO,VE
Color Portfolio (sheer frost)	OP,PT	I,P	BO*
Color Series Eye Color (frost shades)	OP,PT	I,P	BHA,BO*
Color Series Eye Color (velvet shades)	M	P	BO*
Colorations for the Eyes	OP,PT	I,P	BO*
Long Wearing Chromatics	M*,OP,PT	I,P	BHA,BO*
Black Radiance			
Eyeshadow	M,OP,OS	D,P	BO*
Body Shop			
Colourings Eye Shadow (current)	M,PT		BHT
Colourings Eye Shadow (revised)	M	P	T
Colourings Tinted Eye Color	M,OP,OS	P	BHT,BO
Chanel			
Les Quatre Ombres Eye Shadow	M	BP,L,P	BO*
Ombre Facette de Chanel Dual Eye Shadow	M	BP,L,P	BO*
Charles of the Ritz			
Perfect Finish Eye Powder Pencil	M	P,SA	BO*
Christian Dior			
Two Eye Shadows	LA	L,P,SA	
Clarins			
Les Ombres Duo Eye Color Duo	M,OP,OS	E,P	BO*
Clarion			
Classic Colors for the Eyes	M	P,Q	BHA,BO*
Color Harmonies/Essential Color Collection			
Eye Shadows	M	P,Q	BHA,BO*
Creative Color Collection Eye Shadows	M	P,Q	BHA,BO*
Individual Beauty:			
Captive Color Eye Shadow (sold with base)	M	P	BHT,BO
Silk Palette Eye Shadow	M,OS	P	BHT
Clinique			
Quick Eyes Powder	M	P	BO*
Soft-Pressed Eye Shadow	II,M	P	BO*,CX
Color Me Beautiful			
Eye Shadow	IM,M	I,L,P	BHA,BHT,BO*
Color Style (Revlon)			
Long Wearing Eyecolor	M,OP	P	BO*

Product name	Possible comedogenic ingredients	Possible sensitizers	Other possible sensitizers
Cosmyl			
Perfection Eye Shadow Duo	M	I,P	BHA,BO*
Cover Girl			
Luminesse Shadow	II,M	P,Q	BHA,BO
Pro-Colors Frosted Collection	II*	P,Q	BHA,BO*
Pro-Colors Spun Satin Collection	II,M	P,Q	BHA,BO
Professional Color Match Eye Shadows	M	P,Q	BHA,BO*
Scramble Eye Tints	M	P,Q	BHA,BO*
Soft Radiants Silky Matte Eye Shadow	IS,M	P,Q	BHA,BO
Damascar			
Compact Eye Shadow	IM,M	L,P	BO*
Elizabeth Arden			
Luxury Eye Color	IM	I,P	BO*,VE
Estee Lauder			
Just Blush! Eye and Cheek Powder	II,M,PT	P	BHT,BO*,VE
Signature Eye Shadow (frosted)	PT	I,L,P	BO*,VE
Signature Eye Shadow (matte)	II	I,P	BO*,VE
Fashion Fair			
Night Time Eye Shadows		I,L,P	BHA
Shades of Beauty Eye Shadows	IP	I,L,P	BHA,BO*
Shades of Fantasy Eye Shadows	IP	I,L,P	BHA,BO*
Shades of Mardi Gras Eye Shadows	IP	I,L,P	BHA,BO*
Ultimate Eye Shadows		I,L,P	BHA
Fernard Aubry			
Eye Shadows Aubrylights/Aubryssimes	LA	BP,L,SA	
Flame Glo			
Natural Glow Long-Wearing Eye Shadow Powder (sold with cream base)	M	L,P,Q	BO*
Professional Shadow	M	L,P,Q	BO*
Flori Roberts			
Eye-Dears Eye Shadows	M	I,P	
Gold/Chromatic Eye Compact #1	M	I,P	
Frances Denney			
Moisture Silk Eye Color	IM*,M	I,L,P	BO*
Germaine Monteil			
Rich Powder Eye Shadow	IM,LA,OP	I,PG	BO*,CA,VE
L'Oreal			
Couleur Couleur 8 Hour Eye Shadows	M,OP	I,P	BO*
Mahogany Image			
Tint Set Eye Shadows	M,OP	I,L,P	BHA
Max Factor			
Maxi Colors-to-Go Eye Shadow	M	I,P	BO*
Satin Shadow Color Collection	M	I,P	BO*

Product name	Possible comedogenic ingredients	Possible sensitizers	Other possible sensitizers
Maybelline			
Blooming Colors Eye Shadow	M	I,P	BO
Colour Wand II Powder Shadow	M	I,P	BHA,BHT
Colour Wand Powder Eye Shadow	M	I,P	BO*
Expert Eyes Eye Shadow	M	I,P	BO
Powder Eye Pearls	M	I,P	
Shadow Slims	M	I,P	BO*
Shine Free Colorribbon Eye Shadow	M	I,P	BO
Naomi Sims			
Eye Enhancer Pressed Powder Eye Shadows		I,P	BO*,VE
Natural Wonder			
Shadow Co-Stars Powder Eye Shadow	M	L,P	BHA,BO*
Shadow Stars Powder Eye Shadow	OA	P,Q	BHA,BO*
New Essentials			
Eye Color Duo	M	I,P	BO*
Orlane			
Eye Shadow	M	P	
Physician's Formula			
Gentle Light Shadow	M	I,L,P	BO*
Prescriptives			
Eye Shadow Powder	II,OS	P	BO*
Princess Marcella Borghese			
Perlati Colour Brilliance for Eyes, Cheeks and Lips (loose)	II,OS	P	BO*
Perlati Colour Pastello for Eyes, Cheeks and Lips (pressed)	IM,PT	F,P,Q	BO*,CH,VE
Shadow Milano (new formula)	II,M,OS	P	BO*
Shadow Milano Eye Shadow (old formula)		F,P,Q	BO*,CH,VE
Pupa			
Compact Eye Shadow	OS	L,P	
Eye Shadow	IM,IP	BP,L,SA	BO*
Revlon			
Custom Eyes Shadow	M	P	BO*
Eye Shadow Prisms	M	P	BO*
Eye Shaper—Highlighter (sold with liner)	IS,M,OS	P	BO*
Sisley			
Botanical Eye Shadow		C,E,P,PG	BO,MCZ,MZ
Ultima II			
3 Shot Eye Color	M	P	BHA,BO*
Color Cassette Eye Shadow	M,OP,PGS	P,Q	BHA,BO*
Patina Eye Shadows	IM,M	L,P	BO*
THE Colors Eyecolor	OS	D,P	BO*

Product name	Possible comedogenic ingredients	Possible sensitizers	Other possible sensitizers
Wet 'N' Wild			
Silk Finish Creative Eye Shadows	M,OP,OS	D,P	BO*
Yves Saint Laurent			
Eye Shadow Powder	IM,IN,M	L,P,PG	BHA,BO*,PGL

OIL-FREE EYE SHADOW POWDER CONTAINING EMOLLIENT ESTERS

Product name	Possible comedogenic ingredients	Possible sensitizers	Other possible sensitizers
Alexandra de Markoff			
Professional Palette Eye Shadow	OS	P	BO*
Artmatic			
Soft Blend Eye Shadow	IN,OS	I,P	BO*
Aziza			
Contact Lens Eye Color	IN,OP	I,P	BO*
Bonne Bell			
Hi-Lites Eye Shadows	II	I,P	BO*
Charles of the Ritz			
Perfect Finish Eye Color		D,P	BO*
Christian Dior			
5-Couleurs Eye Shadow Compact	OS	P,SA	BHT,PGL
Clientele			
Eye Color Treatment	OP	P,PG	
Elizabeth Arden			
Colour Dynamics Powder Perfection for Eyes	IN	P	BO*
Fashion Fair			
Eye Shadow Duo	IS	I,P	BHA
Lancôme			
Colour Gift Coffrette Maquillage Eye Shadows	OS	P,SA	BHT,PGL
Maquiriche Creme Powder Eye Colour	OP	I,P	BO*
Mary Kay			
Eye Shadow	IN	I,P	
Powder Perfect Eye Color		I,P	BO*
Max Factor			
Designer Eyes Satin Shadow	OS	I,P	BO*
Multi-Press Eye Shadow	OS	I,P	BO*
Quick Stroke Eye Color	OS	I,P	BO*
Visual Eyes Picture Perfect Shadows	OS	I,P	BO*
Merle Norman			
Dual Performing Eye Shadow Duet	OP	I,P	BHT,BO*
Revlon			
Custom Eyes Matte Eye Shadow	OS	D,P	BO*
Overtime Shadows	OP	P	BO*
Stagelight			
Pressed Eye Shadows	OS	I,P	BO*

Product name	Possible comedogenic ingredients	Possible sensitizers	Other possible sensitizers
Stendhal			
Eye Shadow Powder	IM	BP,P	BO*
Ultima II			
Color Shots for Eyes	IN,OS	P	BHA,BO*
Matte + Eye Colors	OS	D,P	BO*
The Nakeds Eye Color	OS	D,P	BO*

STRICTLY OIL-FREE EYE SHADOW POWDER

Avon			
Sungleamers		P	BO*
Chanel			
Ombre Couture Eye Color		BP,P	BO*
Mahogany Image			
Eye Dust			
Stagelight			
Matte Eye Powder[1]		I,P	
Sparkle Eye Powder			

WATER-FREE EYE SHADOW PRIMERS

Aziza			
Color Fix Eye Color Primer	PT	P	BO
Crease Resistant Base	M	P	BO
Clarion			
Individual Beauty Captive Color Eyeshadow Base (sold with eye shadow)	PPG	P	VE
Cover Girl			
Professional Shadow Primer (base)	PT	P,Q	
Estee Lauder			
Shadow Stay Eyelid Foundation (stick)	M,ML	P	PMA
Flame Glow			
Natural Glow Long-Wearing Eye Shadow Cream Base (sold with powder)	IN	E,P	BHT,VE
Merle Norman			
Automatic Shadow Base	ML,OP,PT	L	BO
Revlon			
Color Lock Lid Perfecting Shadow Base	M,OP	L,P	BHA
Super Wear Eye Shadow Base	M,OP	L,P	BHA
Wear and Care Shadow Base	M,OP	E,L,P	BHA,VE

WATER-BASED EYE SHADOW PRIMERS

Adrien Arpel			
Moisturizing Shadow Undercoat	IP,M	F,L,P,PG,PS	BO,T

[1]This product may contain coal tar colors.

Product name	Possible comedogenic ingredients	Possible sensitizers	Other possible sensitizers
Almay			
Wear Extending Eye Shadow Primer	M	I,P	BO
Chanel			
Ombre Base Pour Paupieres			
Eye Shadow Base	M,OP,PGS	BP,L,P,PG	T
Elizabeth Arden			
Visible Difference Eye-Fix Primer		A,I,P	
Max Factor			
Professional Eye Shadow Base	IS,S	E,I,L,P	BHA,T
Merle Norman			
Crease Resistant Shadow Base	IN,OP	I,P,PG	T
Princess Marcella Borghese			
Eye Duetta Eye Primer	M,PGS,PT	L,P,PG,Q	
Eye Shadow Base	IM,M,PGS,PT	L,P,PG,Q	
Pupa			
Shadow Base	IM,M	F,I,P	BHA,T
Ultima II			
Moisturizing Eye Shadow Base	M,PGS,PT	L,P,PG	

OIL-FREE EYE SHADOW PRIMERS CONTAINING EMOLLIENT ESTERS

Color Me Beautiful			
Eye Shadow Base	DO,MM	I,P,PG	T

CHAPTER 18

Eyeliners

Eyeliners are designed to highlight the entire eye by placing a line of color along the eyelash margins. There are liquid, pen, powder, and pencil types. They can be used either above or below the upper or lower eyelashes. Eyeliner should be color-coordinated to the eye shadow and often is chosen to blend into the lashes. In general, a darker color will bring more attention to the eyes than a lighter shade.

TYPES OF EYELINERS

Automatic Liquid Eyeliners

Some eyeliners packaged in cylindrical tubes with an applicator are called automatic eyeliners. Automatic liquid eyeliners are either waterproof (water-free), water-resistant (oil-based), or regular (water-based or oil-free). In general, the more waterproof varieties are oilier and harder to remove but are useful when other eyeliners tend to smear or run. However, the solvent in these eyeliners, the need to use removal products, and the friction necessary to remove these eyeliners can cause irritation in some people. Irritation and difficulty with removal are less of a problem with regular (nonwaterproof) liquid eyeliners but they are more prone to running. Liquid eyeliners require significant application skill to apply in a cosmetically appealing manner but when applied properly can give a thin, sharply defined line.

Bottled Regular Liquid Eyeliners

Bottled regular liquid eyeliners are either water-based or oil-free products and are similar to regular automatic eyeliners in terms of usage.

Pen Eyeliners

Pen eyeliners are automatic liquid eyeliners packaged in a marking pen and are otherwise similar to other automatic liquid eyeliners. They may be somewhat easier to use than automatic eyeliners that have a brush. Both require a very steady, careful hand to avoid a heavy, theatrical look.

Powder Eyeliners

Powder eyeliners are pressed powders that are similar to regular automatic liquid eyeliners but do not contain water. They are prone to running and caking, which can irritate the eyes.

Pencil Eyeliners

Pencil eyeliners are oil-based with wax added to solidify the product. They are by far the most popular type of eyeliner because they are easy to apply, relatively water-resistant, and if soft will create the smudged effect that is currently in style. Many women hold a match or lighter to the pencil point briefly to soften the tip before use. On oilier eyelid skin, pencil eyeliners can spontaneously spread across the eyelid as the day progresses, and a regular liquid eyeliner may be a better choice. Smudging can particularly be a problem under the eyes if an oily under-eye cover-up is used. Alternatively, an eye shadow setting cream can be used prior to applying eyeliner pencil and may help the pencil to adhere and remain in place.

Kohl Eyeliner Pencils

A kohl eyeliner pencil is one that specifically achieves a smoky finish. These products have similar properties to other eyeliner pencils.

ALLERGIC AND IRRITANT REACTIONS TO EYELINERS

Some women have allergic and irritant reactions to eyeliners. Allergic reactions are more common when the eyeliner is used on the inside of the eyelashes (immediately bordering the eye). This is especially true when eyeliner is used inside the lower eyelid, because tears will wash the eyeliner into the eyes. All women, even if not subject to eye irritations, should avoid placing eyeliner inside the eyelash line.

The more waterproof forms of liquid eyeliner are more likely to cause irritation. However, all liquid eyeliner is more apt to cause this problem than pencil eyeliner.

Eyeliners and Eye Infections

Eyeliners can cause eye infections. To help prevent eye infections, eyeliners should never be applied with saliva, shared with other people, or tested on the eyes in the store. Powder eyeliners should not be diluted with water. Liquid or powder eyeliners should be discarded if they are discolored, dried out, or have an unpleasant odor.

Chart 18–1
EYELINERS

The charts are designed to help you minimize adverse reactions and choose products with the proper oil content for your skin type. If you have cosmetics-related acne, you should also choose products with the least amounts of potentially comedongenic ingredients.

Although most cosmetics contain potentially sensitizing ingredients, there is no reason to avoid any ingredient unless you are experiencing adverse reactions to cosmetic products. If you know you are allergic to certain ingredients, the charts will show you which products to avoid. If you are experiencing reactions to a certain cosmetic product, the charts can help you select alternative products that do not contain the same potentially sensitizing ingredients. To choose new products that are least likely to cause allergic reactions, keep in mind that fragrance is by far the most frequent cause of allergic reactions to cosmetics, followed by ingredients listed as "possible sensitizers." The ingredients listed as "other possible sensitizers" cause allergic reactions less frequently. Using these charts should help solve many cosmetics-related skin problems; however, if a problem persists, consult a dermatologist for advice and possible patch testing.

The products listed in these charts include many

of the nationally advertised and distributed brands that have the largest market share of cosmetics sales; an extensive sampling of other brands available in the Chicago area is also included.

After locating several suitable products, use the pricing information on pages 18–19 for comparison shopping.

> Names of products and product lines, and ingredients, are continually changing. Read the labels carefully before purchasing any beauty or skin-care product.

KEY

Possible Sensitizers

BP—bronopol (2-bromo-2-nitropropane-1,3-diol)‡
D—diazolidinyl urea‡
DM—DMDM hydantoin‡
E—essential oils and biological additives
F—fragrances
I—imidazolidinyl urea‡
L—lanolin and derivatives that may cross react with lanolin
P—parabens
PG—propylene glycol
PS—potassium sorbate
Q—quaternium-15‡

Other Possible Sensitizers

BHA—butylated hydroxyanisole
BHT—butylated hydroxytoluene
BO—bismuth oxychloride
CH—chlorhexidine and derivatives
MDG—methyldibromoglutaronitrile
PGL—propyl gallate
PMA—phenylmercuric acetate
R—rosin (colophony) and derivatives
T—triethanolamine and derivatives that may cross-react
VE—vitamin E (tocopherol and derivatives)

*may contain [see column head]
‡formaldehyde-releasing ingredients

WATERPROOF AUTOMATIC EYELINERS

Product name	Possible sensitizers	Other possible sensitizers
Maybelline Ultra-Liner (waterproof)	P	BHA
Merle Norman Waterproof Eyeliner	I,P	
Yves Saint Laurent Automatic Eye-Lighter	F,P	

WATER-RESISTANT AUTOMATIC EYELINERS

Product name	Possible sensitizers	Other possible sensitizers
Max Factor Linemaker Waterproof Eyeliner	F,P,Q	BHA

REGULAR AUTOMATIC EYELINERS

Product name	Form	Possible sensitizers	Other possible sensitizers
Alexandra de Markoff Lasting Luxury Eyeliner	Oil-free	P,PG	

Product name	Form	Possible sensitizers	Other possible sensitizers
Almay			
Eye-Defining Liquid Liner	Water-based	I,P,PG	BO*
Skip-Proof Eyelining Pen	Oil-free	P*,Q*	BHA,MDG
Avon			
Colorglide Liquid Eyeliner	Oil-free	I,P,PG	
Fine Line Eye Pen (all shades except blue)	Oil-free	P,Q	BHT
Fine Line Eye Pen (blue)	Oil-free	P,Q	BHT
Glimmersticks for Eyes	Water-free		BHT
Ultra Wear Liquid Eyeliner	Oil-free	I,P,PG	
Aziza			
Color & Care Eyeglider Pen (black/brown)	Oil-free	P,Q	BHA,MDG,T
Color & Care Eyeglider Pen (blue)	Oil-free	Q	BHA,MDG,T
Perfect Performing Penliner	Oil-free	P,PG,Q	
Soft Liner (Fine Line Brush)	Oil-free	P,PG,Q	
Body Shop			
Colourings Eyeliner Pen	Water-based	P,Q	BHT,MDG,T*
Chanel			
La Ligne Fluide de Chanel Instant Eyeliner	Oil-free	E,P	CH,VE
Clarion			
Precision Liquid Liner	Oil-free	P,Q	
Cover Girl			
Extremely Gentle Soft Liner	Water-based	P,PG	
Liquid Pencil Soft Precision Liner	Oil-free	D,P,PG	
Damascar			
Silk Protein Eyeliner	Oil-free	F,P	BHA
Elizabeth Arden			
Luxury Eyeliner Pen	Oil-free/Ester	P,Q	BHA,MDG,T
Fernand Aubry			
Eyeliner	Oil-free	P,PG	
Flame Glo			
Fine Stroke Liquid Eyeliner	Oil-free	I,P,PG,PS	BO*,T
No Mistake Eyeliner Pen	Oil-free	P,Q	BHA,T
Lancôme			
Liner Plume Eyelining Pen	Oil-free	P,Q	BHA,MDG
Liner Precis Automatic Eyelining Pen	Oil-free	D,P,PG	
Max Factor			
Quick Draw Magic Eyeliner Pen	Oil-free	P,Q	BHA
Maybelline			
Line Works Felt Tip Eyeliner	Water-based	DM*,P,Q	
Perfect Pen Eyeliner	Water-based	P,Q	
Merle Norman			
Automatic Eyeliner	Water-based	I,L,P	PMA,T

Product name	Form	Possible sensitizers	Other possible sensitizers
Princess Marcella Borghese			
Eyeliner Automatico	Water-based	P,PG	BO*,T
Revlon			
Micropure Precision Eyelining Pen	Oil-free	P,Q	BHA,T
Stagelight			
Liquid Eyeliner	Oil-free/Ester	F,I,P,PG	T
Stendhal			
Stendhalmatic Eyeliner	Water-based	E,F,P,PG	R
Ultima II			
Advanced Formula Liquid Eye Pencil	Water-based	L,P,PG	
Penultimate Line Color	Oil-free	P,Q	BHA,T

BOTTLED REGULAR LIQUID EYELINERS

Product name	Form	Possible sensitizers	Other possible sensitizers
Mary Kay			
Eyeliner	Oil-free	P,PG	PMA,T,VE
Maybelline			
Liquid Eyeliner	Oil-free	P,PG,Q	T
Revlon			
Fabuliner	Water-based	P,PG	T
Smudgeproof Fabuliner	Water-based	P,PG	

POWDER EYELINERS

Product name	Possible sensitizers	Other possible sensitizers
Avon		
Ultimate Effect Cake	D,P	BO*
Princess Marcella Borghese		
Lumina Cream Kohl Eyeliner		BO*
Revlon		
Eye Shaper-Liner (sold with highlighter)	D,P	BO*
Ultima II		
Double Effects Lid & Brow Definer Powder	P	BO*
Wet 'N' Wild		
Kohl-Kajal Eyeliner Soft Crayon	P	BHA,BHT

PENCIL EYELINERS

Product name	Possible sensitizers	Other possible sensitizers
Adrien Arpel		
Dark Eyes Soft Eyeliner Pencil	P	BHA
Kohl Eye Rimmers	P	BHA,BO*
Alexandra de Markoff		
Pencil Colour for the Eyes	P	BHA,BO*

Product name	Possible sensitizers	Other possible sensitizers
Allercreme		
Eyebrow/Eyeliner Pencil	P	BHA,BHT
Soft Eye Pencil	P	BHA,BHT
Almay		
Easy Eyes Self-Sharpening Eye Pencil	P	BHT,BO*
Kohl Formula Eyeliner Pencil	P	BHA,BO*
Artmatic		
Eyebrow and Eyeliner Pencils	P	BHA,BHT
Professional Eyeliner Pencil	P	BHA,BHT
Avon		
Avon Color Pencil	P	BHT,BO*
Coordinates Brow and Liner Pencil	P	BHT,BO*
Luxury Eye Lining Pencil	L,P	BHT,BO*
Ultra Wear Pencil	P	BHT,BO*
Aziza		
Eye Brightener Pencil	P	BHA
Contact Lens Eyeliner	P	BHA,BO*
Shadow Twist Plus Liner (sold with Shadow Pencil)	P	BHA,BHT,BO*
Silklining Pencil	P	BHA
Black Radiance		
Eyeliner Pencil (black)	P	VE
Eyeliner Pencil (blue)	P	BHA,BHT
Body Shop		
Colourings Eye Definer	P	BHA,BO*
Bonne Bell		
Eye Pencil	P	BHT,BO*
Kohl Eye Pencil	P	BHA,BHT
Precision Kohl Eye Pencil Code A	P	BHA,BHT,BO*
Precision Kohl Eye Pencil Code C	D,P	BHT,BO*,VE
Chanel		
Smudge Eyeliner	P	
Charles of the Ritz		
Perfect Finish Eyelining Pencil	L,P	BHA,BO*
Christian Dior		
Kohl Eyeliner Pencil	P	BHA
Clarion		
Eye Definer Lining Pencil	P	BHA,BHT
Individual Beauty Pensilks	P	BHT
Clinique		
Eye Shading Pencil	P	BHA,BHT,BO*
Lid Stick (eyeliner and eye shadow)	P	BHA,BO*
Quick Eyes Eyelining Pencil	P	BHA,BHT,BO*

Product name	Possible sensitizers	Other possible sensitizers
Color Me Beautiful		
Smudgeliner Eye Pencil	P	BHA,BHT,BO*
Cosmyl		
Eye Accenter	P	BHA
Coty		
Optical Illusion Eye Rimming Pencil	P	BHA,BO*
Cover Girl		
Eyebrow and Liner Pencils	L,P	BHA,BHT
Pro-Lining Perfect Blend Eye Pencils	P	BHA,BHT
Pro-Lining Perfect Point Eye Pencils	P	BHA,BHT
Pro-Lining Ultra-Precise Eye Pencils	P	BHA,BHT
Soft Radiants Sheer Color Eye Definer	L,P	BHA,BHT
Elizabeth Arden		
Creative Coloring Pencil Slenderliner for Eyes	P	BHA,BO*
Slenderliner for Eyes	P	BHA,BO*
Estee Lauder		
Eye Contouring Pencil	P	BHA,BHT,BO*
Eye Definer Duo	P	BO*
Signature Automatic Pencil for Eyes	P	VE
Fashion Fair		
Eye Color Pencil	P	BHA,BHT
Fernand Aubry		
Eyeliner Aubryissmes	I,P,PG	
Flame Glo		
Define & Dazzle Eyeliner	P	BHA,BO*
Natural Glow Soft Look Eye Pencil	P	BHT
No Skip Eye Liner[1]	P	BHT,BO*
Perfect Kohl Eye Definer	P	BHA,BO*
Professional Eyeliner	P	BHA,BHT
Flori Roberts		
Eye Contour Pencil (older formulation)	D,P	BHT,VE
Eye Contour Pencil (newer formulation)	BP,P	BHA,BHT
Opalescent Eye Contouring Pencil	P	BHA,BHT
Frances Denney		
Kohl Pencil	P	BHA,BHT
L'Oreal		
Le Grand Kohl	P	BHA,BO*
Lancôme		
Le Crayon Kohl Pencil	P	BHA
Mahogany Image		
Liner	P	BHA,BHT,BO*

[1]This product contains coal tar colors.

Product name	Possible sensitizers	Other possible sensitizers
Mary Kay		
Eye Defining Pencil (made in Great Britain)		
Eye Defining Pencil (made in West Germany)	I,P	BO*
Max Factor		
Eyebrow and Eyeliner Pencil	L,P	BHA,BHT
Featherblend Kohliner	P,Q	BHA,BO*
Maxi ColorKohl Liner	P,Q	BHA,BO*
Maxi Color on Color Eye Luster Pencil	L,P,Q	BHA,BHT,BO*
Splish Splash Underwater Eye Pencil	L,P	BHT,BO*
Maybelline		
Automatic Sharpener Brow and Liner Pencil	P	
Blooming Colors Eye Pencil	P	BHA,BHT,BO*
Brow and Liner Pencil	L,P	BHA,BHT
Colour Wand Powder Shadow Pencil	I,P	
Colour Wand II Eyeliner Pencil	P	BHA,BHT
Expert Eyes Brow and Liner Pencil	P	
Eye Styler Pencil	P	BHA,BHT,BO*
Natural Accent Eye Pencil	L,P	BHA,BHT
Performing Color Eyeliner	L,P	BHA
Turning Point Eyeliner	P	BHA,BHT
Merle Norman		
Trimline Eye Pencil	P	BHA,BO*
Trimline Eye Pencil Duo	P	BHA
Trimline Split Color Eye Pencil	P	BHA
Montaj		
Slim Eyeliner Pencil	P	BHA,BHT
Natural Wonder		
Finer Liner Waterproof Eye Pencil	P	BHA,BO*
New Essentials		
Eye Liner Pencil	P	BHA,BO*
Orlane		
Extraordinary Eye Pencil	P	BHA,BO*
Physician's Formula		
Fine Line Eye Pencil	P	BHA,BHT
Gentle Wear Eye Pencil (waterproof)	P	
Posner		
Eyeliner Pencil	P	BHA,BHT
Prescriptives		
Eye Coloring Pencil	P	BHA,BO*
Princess Marcella Borghese		
Eye Accento Kohl Pencil	P	BHA,BO*

Product name	Possible sensitizers	Other possible sensitizers
Revlon		
Eyebrow and Eyeliner Pencil	L,P	BHA,BHT
Micropure Slimliner for Sensitive Eyes	P	BHA,BO*
Special Eyes Micropure Slimliner	P	BHA,BO*
Waterproof Eye Shaper	L,P	BHA,BO*
Shiseido		
Eyeliner Pencil Crayon		VE
Simply Satin		
Kohl Eyeliner Pencil	P	BHA*,VE*
Sisley		
Botanical Eyeliner Pencil	E,P	PGL
Stagelight		
Color Stick	L,P	BHA
Liner Stick[2]	P	BHA,BHT
Ultima II		
Double Effects Lid & Brow Definer Pencil	P	BHA,BHT,BO*
Opalescent Kohl Eye Pencil:		
Amethyst & Pearl	P	BHA,BO*
Charcoal & Pearl	P	BHA,BO*
Wet 'N' Wild		
Kohl Kajal Eyebrow & Eyeliner Crayon	P	BHA,BHT
Yves Saint Laurent		
Eye Pencil	P	PGL

[2]This product may contain coal tar colors.

Eyebrow Makeup

Eyebrow makeup is designed to improve the appearance of the eyebrows by filling in sparse areas or reshaping the line of the brow. It should be chosen in a color that closely matches hair color.

TYPES OF EYEBROW MAKEUP

Eyebrow makeup includes pencils, sticks, crayons, pens, powders, and sealers. Eyebrow pencils are water-free products with wax added to solidify the product. Some pencils are designed for use both as eyeliner and eyebrow pencil, but this is not a good idea. People with seborrhea have yeast organisms on the eyebrows that can be transferred to the eyelids by these pencils, causing inflammation of the eyelids. Eyebrow sticks and crayons are similar to eyebrow pencils but will produce a less defined line. The same effect can be obtained by using a pencil and smudging the line. Eyebrow pens are liquid eyebrow makeup products packaged as pens that will also create a well-defined line. Eyebrow powders or cake-on brows are oil-containing or oil-free pressed powders that will also create a less defined brow line. Eyebrow sealer is merely a hair grooming product for unruly eyebrows. Hairspray on a brow brush will serve the same purpose. Spray just a tiny bit onto your palm, dip/rub the brow brush into it, and brush the brow hairs into whatever shape/direction you wish. It's invisible and it's cheaper because you're using a product you already have, and it works all day.

Chart 19–1
EYEBROW MAKEUP

The charts are designed to help you minimize adverse reactions and choose products with the proper oil content for your skin type. If you have cosmetics-related acne, you should also choose products with the least amounts of potentially comedogenic ingredients.

Although most cosmetics contain potentially sensitizing ingredients, there is no reason to avoid any ingredient unless you are experiencing adverse reactions to cosmetic products. If you know you are allergic to certain ingredients, the charts will show you which products to avoid. If you are experiencing reactions to a certain cosmetic product, the charts can help you select alternative products that do not contain the same potentially sensitizing ingredients. To choose new products that are least likely to cause allergic reactions, keep in mind that fragrance is by far the most frequent cause of allergic reactions to

Names of products and product lines, and ingredients, are continually changing. Read the labels carefully before purchasing any beauty or skin-care product.

cosmetics, followed by ingredients listed as "possible sensitizers." The ingredients listed as "other possible sensitizers" cause allergic reactions less frequently. Using these charts should help solve many cosmetics-related skin problems; however, if a problem persists, consult a dermatologist for advice and possible patch testing.

The products listed in these charts include many of the nationally advertised and distributed brands that have the largest market share of cosmetics sales; an extensive sampling of other brands available in the Chicago area is also included.

After locating several suitable products, use the pricing information on pages 18–19 for comparison shopping.

KEY

Possible Comedogenic Ingredients

II—isopropyl isostearate
IP—isopropyl palmitate
M—mineral oil
ML—myristyl lactate

O—oleic acid
OP—octyl palmitate
OS—octyl stearate and derivatives
PGS—propylene glycol stearate

Possible Sensitizers

DM—DMDM hydantoin‡
E—essential oils and biological additives
I—imidazolidinyl urea‡
L—lanolin and derivatives that may cross-react with lanolin
P—parabens
PG—propylene glycol
PS—potassium sorbate
Q—quaternium-15‡
SA—sorbic acid

Other Possible Sensitizers

BHA—butylated hydroxyanisole
BHT—butylated hydroxytoluene
BO—bismuth oxychloride
CH—chlorhexidine and derivatives
T—triethanolamine and derivatives that may cross-react
VE—vitamin E (tocopherol and derivatives)
Z—zinc pyrithione

*may contain [see column head]
‡formaldehyde-releasing ingredients

EYEBROW PENCILS, PENS, STICKS, AND CRAYONS

Product name	Possible comedogenic ingredients	Possible sensitizers	Other possible sensitizers
Adrien Arpel Two-Tone Brow Pencil	ML	P	BHA,BHT,BO*
Alexandra de Markoff Soft Effect Brow Pencil	M	P	BHA
Allercreme Eyebrow/Eyeliner Pencil		P	BHA,BHT
Almay Professional Soft Brow Color (pencil)	M	P	BHA,BO*
Artmatic Eyebrow and Eyeliner Pencils		P	BHA,BHT

Product name	Possible comedogenic ingredients	Possible sensitizers	Other possible sensitizers
Avon			
Coordinates Brow and Liner Pencil		P	BHT
Glimmersticks for Brows	M	P	BHT
Ultra Wear Brow Pencil		L,P	BHT
Chanel			
Crayon à Sourcils Eyebrow Groomer	OS	P	BO*
Cover Girl			
Eyebrow and Liner Pencils		L,P	BHA,BHT
Estee Lauder			
Natural Line Brow Pencil		P	BHA,BHT,BO*
Signature Automatic Pencil for Brows		L,P	VE
Fashion Fair			
Eyebrow Pencil			BHT,T
Fernand Aubry			
Eyebrow Pencil	IP	L,P	BHT
Frances Denney			
Quickbrow Pencil	M	P	
Germaine Monteil			
Brow Liner (pencil)		P	BHA,BHT
Lancôme			
Le Crayon Brow Definer	OS	P	BHA,BO*
Mary Kay			
Eyebrow Pencil		L,P	BHA,BHT,BO*
Max Factor			
Eyebrow and Eyeliner Pencil		L,P	BHA,BHT
Maybelline			
Automatic Sharpener Brow and Liner Pencil	M	P	
Brow and Liner Pencil		L,P	BHA,BHT
Expert Eyes Brow and Liner Pencil	M	P	
Revlon			
Color Up Stick for Brows (waterproof)	M,ML	L,P	BHA,BHT
Eyebrow and Eyeliner Pencil		L,P	BHA,BHT
Fineline Natural Brow Pencil		P	BHA
Powder Pencil for Lids and Brows		P,SA	BO*
Waterproof Eyebrow Pencil		L,P	BHA,BHT
Ultima II			
Double Effects Lid & Brow Definer Pencil	M	P	BHA,BHT,BO*
Penultimate Brow Color Pen (oil-free)	O	P,Q	BHA,T
Wet 'N' Wild			
Kohl Kajal Eyebrow & Eyeliner Crayon		P	BHA,BHT

EYEBROW POWDERS

Product name	Possible comedogenic ingredients	Possible sensitizers	Other possible sensitizers
Body Shop			
Colourings Eyebrow Makeup (current) (contains oil)	M	P	
Colourings Eyebrow Makeup (revised) (contains oil)	M	P	T
Charles of the Ritz			
Kohl+Kohl (oil-free)		I,P	BO*
Perfect Brow Color (contains oil)	IP,M	I,L,P	
Clinique			
Brow Shaper (oil-free)		PS	BO*,VE,Z
Color Me Beautiful			
Brow Color (contains oil)	M	I,P	
Elizabeth Arden			
Brow Makeup (contains oil)	M	I,P	
Estee Lauder			
Eyebrow Color (contains emollient ester)		PS	BO*,VE,Z
Signature Eyebrow Color (oil-free)			BO*,VE,Z
Max Factor			
Brush and Brow Eyebrow Color (contains oil)	M	L,P,Q	
Merle Norman			
Only Natural Brush-On Eyebrow Color (contains oil)	M		
Revlon			
Natural Brows Color and Style System (contains oil)	II,M,OP	P	BHA,BO*

EYEBROW SEALERS

Product name	Possible comedogenic ingredients	Possible sensitizers	Other possible sensitizers
Adrien Arpel			
Eyebrow Thickener (water-based)	PGS	I,P	T
Chanel			
Forme Sourcils Brow Shaper (oil-free)		E,P	CH,T,VE
Color Me Beautiful			
Brow Fixative (oil-free)		I,P	T
Estee Lauder			
Brow Gel (water-based)		P,PG	
Max Factor			
Brow Tamer (water-based)		I,P	
Merle Norman			
Tinted Brow Sealer (oil-free)		DM,P	T
Stagelight			
Hibrow (oil-free)		I,P	

CHAPTER 20

Mascara

Mascaras provide color, thickness, and/or length to the eyelashes. The color *intensity* of mascara looks best when equivalent to the color intensity of the hair; for example, brown or navy would be appropriate for lighter hair. However, black mascara is the biggest seller and will look attractive on most women.

TYPES OF MASCARAS

There are no specific types of mascaras for different skin types, because these products are applied to hair, not skin. The choice of mascara is largely a matter of personal preference; however, mascaras differ in ease of removal and tendency to run when exposed to tears. In general, the more waterproof varieties are harder to remove.

THE ALL-IMPORTANT BRUSH
Consumer Reports (February 1991) reported that a volunteer panel judged the applicator/brush to be an important factor in how they rated mascara. The applicators the panelists most often preferred had straight brushes with narrowly spaced bristles. But brush preference is a very individual matter. If possible, look at the brush supplied before purchasing a mascara.

This feature may be a disadvantage except for persons who tend to perspire, tear more than average, or swim frequently. Most nonpowder mascaras are packaged in cylindrical tubes with an applicator and are called automatic mascaras.

Waterproof Mascaras
Waterproof mascaras are water-free products. These products are completely waterproof but are more difficult to remove than other mascaras. The solvent in waterproof mascaras, the need to use mascara removal products, and the friction necessary to remove these mascaras can cause irritation in some women. On the other hand, these products are not as prone to bacterial contamination as other mascaras and are less likely to lead to eye infections, since their petroleum-based solvents are inhospitable to microbes.

Water-Resistant Mascaras
Water-resistant mascaras are water-in-oil products. Compared to waterproof mascara, they are a little less waterproof, easier to remove, and less likely to cause irritant reactions. However, they are slightly more likely to lead to bacterial contamination and eye infections.

Regular Mascaras

Regular mascaras are water-based mascaras or oil-free mascaras. They are very easy to remove but some may be prone to running. Oily eyelid skin may cause regular mascara to smear unless carefully applied; in which case, waterproof mascara that is allowed to dry thoroughly is probably a better choice.

Regular mascaras are least likely to irritate the skin but can still cause eye irritation in some women. This can be caused either by the emulsifiers found in these products or by the occasional tendency of these products to cake. Mascara that cakes on the eyelashes can flake into the eye and cause irritation in contact lens wearers. The water-based mascaras are also most prone to bacterial contamination and can cause eye infections. In fact, there are some women who will develop irritation from water-based mascara but will tolerate waterproof mascara without a problem. In general, the opposite is usually true.

Some mascaras on the market clearly contain more water than oil and are therefore regular mascaras. Unfortunately, this cannot always be determined accurately from the ingredients label, because the total amount of several oily ingredients may exceed the amount of water present even if water is listed as the primary ingredient. It is possible therefore that some of the mascaras listed as regular may actually be water-resistant products. Products with water as the primary ingredient but labeled water-resistant are listed as water-resistant in this book.

Gel-based and Other Oil-free Mascaras

Some oil-free mascaras are available; these have properties similar to other regular mascaras.

Mascaras for Lengthening or Thickening Eyelashes

Some mascaras contain protein that attaches to the hair and/or moisturizing ingredients to temporarily thicken the hair shaft. These products act in the same way as protein hair conditioners for the scalp. Some mascaras designed to lengthen lashes often contain artificial fibers such as nylon or rayon; these products are available in colored or uncolored forms.

Lash Primers, Conditioners, and Top Coats

Lash primers are products designed to be applied to eyelashes as a base coat under mascara. They may decrease the tendency for mascara to run. Lash conditioners are products designed to thicken eyelashes through the use of moisturizing ingredients or protein (which attaches to and temporarily thickens the hair shafts). Eyelash conditioners use the same approach as thickening mascaras to thicken the eyelashes. Lash top coats are products that are used either to eliminate smudges or to put a protective coat over mascara.

Always put in contact lenses before applying eye makeup. Care should be taken not to place mascara too close to the inner corner of the eye where it can get washed into the eye by tears and lead to eye irritation.

The colorants used in mascara are inorganic mineral pigments (iron oxide in black mascara) that belong to a Food and Drug Administration category of "noncertified color additives." This means they are approved for cosmetic use without special safety testing.

REACTIONS TO MASCARAS

Irritation reactions are more common than allergic reactions to mascaras. The more waterproof forms of mascara are more likely to cause irritation; however, some women will be more irritated by water-based mascaras.

If irritation develops with one type of mascara, it is worth trying another type to see if it is better tolerated. The artificial fibers in the lengthening mascaras can end up in the eye and cause problems for wearers of contact lenses. Water-based and powder forms are more likely to cause problems because they tend to cake more easily.

Avoiding Eye Infections Caused by Mascara

Mascaras are especially prone to bacterial contamination and therefore should contain preservative ingredients. Do not buy mascara that does not contain preservatives. Never apply mascara with saliva, share mascara with other people, or test mascara on eyelashes in the store. Apply mascara only to the outer two-thirds of the eyelashes. Although the water-based mascaras are the most easily contaminated, all mascaras can become contaminated by bacteria. You should therefore discard all mascaras after about three months. Waterproof mascaras are recommended for people who experience repeated eye infections. If this does not solve the problem, there are disposable mascaras available that are packaged for short-term use.

Chart 20–1
MASCARAS

The charts are designed to help you minimize adverse reactions and choose products with the proper oil content for your skin type. If you have cosmetics-related acne, you should also choose products with the least amounts of potentially comedogenic ingredients.

Although most cosmetics have potentially sensitizing ingredients, there is no reason to avoid any ingredient unless you are experiencing adverse reactions to cosmetic products. If you know you are allergic to certain ingredients, the charts will show you which products to avoid. If you are experiencing reactions to a certain cosmetic product, the charts can help you select alternative products that do not contain the same potentially sensitizing ingredients. To choose new products that are least likely to cause allergic reactions, keep in mind that fragrance is by far the most frequent cause of allergic reactions to cosmetics, followed by ingredients listed as "possible sensitizers." The ingredients listed as "other possible sensitizers" cause allergic reactions less frequently. Using these charts should help solve many cosmetics-related skin problems; however, if a problem persists, consult a dermatologist for advice and possible patch testing.

The products listed in these charts include many of the nationally advertised and distributed brands that have the largest market share of cosmetics sales;

> Names of products and product lines, and ingredients, are continually changing. Read the labels carefully before purchasing any beauty or skin-care product.

an extensive sampling of other brands available in the Chicago area is also included.

After locating several suitable products, use the pricing information on pages 18–19 for comparison shopping.

KEY

Possible Sensitizers

BP—bronopol (2-bromo-2-nitropropane-1,3-diol)‡
D—diazolidinyl urea‡
DM—DMDM hydantoin‡
E—essential oils and biological additives
F—fragrances
I—imidazolidinyl urea‡
L—lanolin and derivatives that may cross-react with lanolin

P—parabens
PG—propylene glycol
PS—potassium sorbate
Q—quaternium-15‡

Other Possible Sensitizers

BHA—butylated hydroxyanisole
BHT—butylated hydroxytoluene
BO—bismuth oxychloride
CX—chloroxylenol
DHA—dihydroabietyl alcohol
MCZ—methylchloroisothiazolinone
MDG—methyldibromoglutaronitrile
MO—mink oil
MZ—methylisothiazolinone
PGL—propyl gallate
PMA—phenylmercuric acetate
R—rosin (colophony) and derivatives
T—triethanolamine and derivatives that may cross-react
TH—thimerosol
VE—vitamin E (tocopherol and derivatives)

*may contain
‡formaldehyde-releasing ingredients

WATERPROOF MASCARAS

Product name	Possible sensitizers	Other possible sensitizers
Almay		
Wetproof Mascara	P	BHA
Aziza		
Really Waterproof Mascara	DM,P	
Clarion		
Perfect Waterproof Mascara	P	BHA
Cover Girl		
Extension Waterproof Mascara	P	BHA
Lasting Performance Gel-based Mascara	P	BHA
Marathon Mascara	P	BHA
Elizabeth Arden		
Twice as Thick Two Brush Mascara	DM,I,P	T
Lancôme		
Aquacils Waterproof Mascara with Keratin		BHT
Mary Kay		
Waterproof Mascara	I,P	BHA

Product name	Possible sensitizers	Other possible sensitizers
Max Factor		
Comb-On Lash Maker Mascara	F,P,Q	
Splish Splash Lash (underwater mascara)	P,Q	BO*
Super Lash Maker Mascara	F,L,P,Q	BHA,BHT
Maybelline		
Cake Mascara	P	BHA,T
Dial-A-Lash Waterproof Mascara	L,P	BHA
Expert Eyes Mascara	P	BHA,DHA
Fresh Lash Waterproof Mascara	L,P	BHA
Magic Mascara	P	BHA
Shine Free Waterproof Extra Thickening Mascara	L,P	BHA
Ultra Big Ultra Lash Mascara	P	BHA
Ultra Lash Mascara	P	BHA,DHA
Ultra Lash Waterproof Mascara	P	BHA
Ultra Thick Ultra Lash Waterproof Mascara	L,P	BHA
Merle Norman		
Waterproof Mascara	D,L,P	
New Essentials		
Very Waterproof Mascara	P	BHA
Princess Marcella Borghese		
Volumino Lash Colour	DM,P,PG	R
Revlon		
Super Rich Mascara (waterproof)	L,P,PG	BHA

WATER-RESISTANT MASCARAS

Product name	Possible sensitizers	Other possible sensitizers
Allercreme		
Waterproof Mascara	I,P,PG	
Avon		
Advanced Wear Waterproof Mascara	I,P,PG	BHA
Chanel		
Cils Magiques Aqua Resistant Instant Waterproof Mascara	E,P,PG	PGL,VE
Luxury Waterproof Mascara	I,P,PG	BHA,PGL,PMA
Christian Dior		
Dior-Matic Waterproof Mascara	P	
Clinique		
Swimmer's Mascara	P,PS	R
Cover Girl		
Clean Lash Mascara	L,P,PG,Q	BHA
Extremely Gentle Sensitive Eyes Mascara	L,P,PG,Q	BHA
Elizabeth Arden		
Lavish Lash Waterproof Mascara	P	CX

Product name	Possible sensitizers	Other possible sensitizers
Estee Lauder		
Precision-Lash Waterproof Mascara	I,P	CX,R
Flame Glo		
Lush Lash Mascara with Keratin	I,P	BHA,BO*,PMA
Germaine Monteil		
Acti-Vita Emollient Mascara	I,P	DHA,T,VE
L'Oreal		
Miracle Wear Mascara	P,PG	TH
Max Factor		
Legendary Lash Mascara	D,P,PG	BO*
Natural Wonder		
Extra Long Big Lash Mascara	DM,P,PG	BHA
Physician's Formula		
Gentle Wear Mascara	D,P,PG	BHA
Princess Marcella Borghese		
Lumina Luxuriant Mascara	P,PG	BHA,PMA
Pupa		
Creamy Mascara	I,P,PG	T
More Lash Mascara	I,P,PG	T
Revlon		
Super Waterproof Mascara	E,L,P,PG	BHA
Water-Tight Mascara	L,P,PG	BO*
Shiseido		
Waterproof Mascara	F,P	
Stendhal		
Stendhalmatic Mascara	I,P,PG	BHA

REGULAR MASCARAS

Adrien Arpel		
Super Brush Conditioning Mascara	I,L,P	TH
Alexandra de Markoff		
Lash Colour	I,P	R,VE
Allercreme		
Conditioning Mascara	D,P	R,T
Almay		
Conditioning Mascara	I,P,Q	
Longest Lashes Mascara	I,P,Q	
Mascara Plus . . .	I,P,Q	VE
One Coat Mascara	I,P,Q	
Perfect Mascara	I,P,PG	BO*
Super Rich Mascara	I,P,Q	

Product name	Possible sensitizers	Other possible sensitizers
Artmatic		
Clear Mascara	I,P	T
Protein Rich II Mascara	I,P,Q	
Avon		
A Little Color Mascara (colors)	I,P,PG	BO*,T
A Little Color Mascara (clear)	I,P,PG	T
Body Workout Mascara	I,P,PG	BHT,BO*,T
Colorcreme Mascara	I,P,PG	BHT,BO*,T
Coordinates Mascara	I,P,PG	BHT,BO*,T
Curl and Color Mascara	I,P,PG	BHA,T
Lash Paint Mascara	I,P,PG	BHT,BO*,T
Lash Selector Mascara	I,P,PG	BHT,BO*,T
Lots o' Lash Mascara	I,P,PG	BHT,BO*,T
Nutra Lash Mascara	I,P,PG	BHT,BO*,T
Pure Care Mascara	I,P,PG	BHT,BO*,T
Pure Care Mascara for Contact Lens Wearers	D,P,PG	BO*,T
Rich Coat Mascara	I,P	T
Ultra Wear Washable Mascara	I,P,PG	
Aziza		
Color & Care Nutri-Lash Mascara	DM,E,I,P	VE
Contact Lens Mascara (flake-proof)	DM,P,Q	T
Exceptional Eyes Mascara	DM,P,Q	T
Extra Length Mascara with Sealer	DM,P,Q	T
Lasting Elegance Mascara	DM,P,Q	T
Lasting Elegance Mascara (smudge-proof)	DM,P,Q	T
Mega Mascara	DM,I,P	VE
Mink Coat Mascara	I,P	MO
Soft and Silky Mascara	I,P,Q	
Black Radiance		
Lash Lengthening Mascara	D,P	BO*,T
Body Shop		
Colourings Mascara (current)	PG	VE
Colourings Mascara (revised)	P	T
Bonne Bell		
Clean Color Mascara	I,P	T
Clean Color Sensitive Formula Mascara	I,P,Q	
Wash-Off Waterproof Mascara	L,P,Q	
Chanel		
Cils Magiques Instant Lash Mascara	E,P,PG	PGL,T,VE
Luxury Cream Mascara	P,PG	BHA,R,T
Charles of the Ritz		
High Density Lash Mascara	D,P,PG	
Perfect Lash Mascara	I,P,PG	
Perfect Water-Resistant Mascara	I,P,PS,Q	

Product name	Possible sensitizers	Other possible sensitizers
Christian Dior		
Thickening Lash Care	F,P	R,T
Clarion		
Lash Booster Mascara	P,PG,Q	T
Lash Magnifier Mascara	L,P,PG,Q	BHA
Lash Multiplier Mascara	P,Q	T
Luxurious Lash Mascara	P,Q	
Pure Lash Mascara	L,P,PG,Q	BHA
Clinique		
Glossy Brush-On Mascara	I,P,PG	
Color Me Beautiful		
Mascara (water-resistant)	I,P	TH
Sensitive Eyes Mascara	I,P,PG	T
Cosmyl		
Expressive Eyes Mascara	I,P	
Coty		
Airspun Powderessence Mascara	D,P,PG	BHA,T
Disposable Mascara	I,P,PG	BO*,T
Thick 'N' Healthy Mascara	I,P,PG	BO*,T
Cover Girl		
Long 'N' Lush Mascara	P,Q	
Natural Lash Clear Mascara	D,E,P	T
Professional Mascara	P,PG,Q	T
Thick Lash Mascara	P,PG,Q	T
Damascar		
Mascara Cream	I,P,PG	T
Elizabeth Arden		
Proven Performance Mascara	P,Q	DHA,PGL,R,T
Two Brush Mascara	I,P,Q	
Twice as Long Two Brush Mascara	I,P	R,T
Erno Laszlo		
pHelityl Luxury Mascara	I,P	MO
Estee Lauder		
Luscious Cream Mascara	I,P,PG	BO*
More Than Mascara	I,P,PG	BO*
Fashion Fair		
Regular Automatic Mascara	E,I,P	
Fernand Aubry		
Mascara	I,P,PG	T
Flame Glo		
Double Take Two Brush Mascara	I,P,Q	
Gentle Performance Mascara	I,L,P	PMA,T
Natural Glow Longer Look Mascara	I,P,PG	BO*,R,T
Power Mascara	I,P,PG	BO*,R,T
Waterwear Waterproof Washable Mascara	L,PG,Q	MDG

Product name	Possible sensitizers	Other possible sensitizers
Flori Roberts		
Lash Set Mascara	I,P	TH
Frances Denney		
Protein Lash Color	I,P,PG	
Germaine Monteil		
Luxe Premier Mascara	D,P	BO*
Plus de Couleur Color Intensive Mascara	DM,P,PG	R
Kelemata		
Mascara	E,I,P,PG,Q	BHA,R,T
L'Oreal		
Formula Riche Mascara	P	R,T,TH
Lash Out Lash Extending Mascara	I,P,PG,PS	R,T,TH
Lancôme		
Definicils High Definition Mascara	I,P	T
Immencils Gentle Lash Thicknener	P	R,T,TH
Keracils Mascara with Keratine	I,P	R,T
Maquacils Automatic Mascara	I	TH
Mary Kay		
Conditioning Mascara	I,P,Q	
Flawless Mascara	I,P,PG	T
Max Factor		
For Your Eyes Only Mascara	D,P	BO*,T
Maxi ColorKohl Mascara	I,P	BO*
No Color Mascara	I,P	T
Stretch Mascara	D,P,PG	BO*
2000 Calorie Mascara	D,P,PG	BO*
Maybelline		
Blooming Colors Mascara	DM,P	BHA,MO,T
Dial-A-Lash Mascara	P,PG,Q	T
Expert Eyes Mascara	P,PG,Q	T
Great Lash Mascara	P,PG,Q	T
Illegal Lengths Mascara	P,PG,Q	BHA,T,VE
No Problem Mascara	P,PG,Q	
Perfectly Natural Mascara	I,P,PG	
Performing Mascara	P,PG,Q	
Shine Free Baby Lash Gentle Mascara	I,P,PG	
Shine Free Extra Thickening Mascara	P,PG,Q	T
Shine Free Thickening Mascara	P,PG,Q	T
Merle Norman		
Creamy Flo-Matic Mascara	I,L,P	PMA
Montaj		
Mascara	P	R,T,TH
Naomi Sims		
Mascara	P,Q	BO*

Product name	Possible sensitizers	Other possible sensitizers
Natural Wonder		
Extra Thick Big Lash Mascara	DM,P,PG	R
Lash Mania Mascara	DM,P,PG	R
New Essentials		
Lash Increasing Mascara	I,P,Q	
Orlane		
Mascara	P	T
Physician's Formula		
Gentle Care Mascara	I,P	
Vital Lash Conditioning Mascara	D,P,PG	MO
Prescriptives		
Basic Black Mascara	P,PG	BHA
Princess Marcella Borghese		
Lash Stravagante	DM,I,P,PG	R
Lumina Luxuriant Mascara	P	
Maximum Mascara for Sensitive Eyes	DM,P,PG	R,VE
Revlon		
Fabulash Mascara	P,PG	R
Long and Lustrous Mascara	P,PG	BHA
Long Distance Mascara	D,P,PG	BO*
Micropure Mascara for Sensitive Eyes	DM,P,PG	R
Quick Thick Mascara	DM,P,PG	R
Sheer Tints Mascara	I,P,PG	R
Special Eyes Micropure Mascara	DM,L,P,PG	R
Super Lustrous Mascara (smudge-proof)	L,P,PG	BHA
Shiseido		
Mascara	F,P	
Sisley		
Botanical Mascara	P	MCZ,MZ,T
Stagelight		
Stagelight Mascara	I,P	TH
Stendhal		
Stendhalmatic Mascara Creme	P	R,T,VE
Stendhalmatic Waterproof Roll-On Mascara	BP,P,PG	T
Ultima II		
Advanced Formula Mascara	P,PG	BHA
Double Shots Mascara	DM,P,PG	R
Extra Full Mascara for Sensitive Eyes	P	R
Wet 'N' Wild		
Silk Finish Protein Mascara	P	BHA,BO*,R,TH
Yves Saint Laurent		
Automatic Mascara	F,P,PG	MO,T

GEL AND OTHER OIL-FREE MASCARAS

Product name	Possible sensitizers	Other possible sensitizers
Cover Girl Anti-Smudge Mascara (oil-free)	P,Q	
Max Factor Some Color Mascara (clear gel)	I,P	BO*

LASH PRIMERS, CONDITIONERS, AND TOP COATS

Product name	Form	Possible sensitizers	Other possible sensitizers
Adrien Arpel Every Other Layer Lash Thickener, Conditioner, and Separating Creme	Water-based	I,P	
Alexandra de Markoff Lash Amplifier		P	R,VE
Almay Lash Perfection Mascara Corrector (stick)	Water-based Water-free	I,P P	 BHA,BHT
Avon Lash Primer and Conditioner	Water-based	I,P	T
Aziza Conditioning Lash Primer	Oil-free gel	E,P	T
Estee Lauder Lash Primer	Water-based	I,P,PG	
Kelemata Eyelash Balm (conditioner)	Water-free		BHT
Lancôme Forticils Fortifying Lash Conditioner	Water-based	I,P	R,T
Max Factor The Waterproofer (top coat)	Water-free	D,P	
Revlon Lash Repair (conditioner)	Oil-free gel	P	T

PART FIVE

THE LIPS

CHAPTER 21

Problems Unique to the Lips

SUN DAMAGE

Many women are aware that excessive sunlight causes considerable damage to the skin but do not realize that it can cause similar damage to the lips. Excessive sun exposure can lead to dryness, cracking, and wrinkles at the corners of the mouth. More important, excessive sun exposure can lead to skin cancers on the lips. In particular, squamous cell carcinoma of the lips is a relatively common cancer and is more aggressive on the lips than on most other areas of the skin. The earliest sign of excessive sun exposure on the lips is often the development of precancerous patches of white skin called *actinic chelitis.*

Protection from the Sun

It is very important for women who have significant sun exposure to protect the lips adequately. All lipsticks have some ability to block sunlight because of their opacity. More opaque lipsticks will give greater protection because they contain an increased

> When a white area or a skin growth of any type develops on the lips, consult your dermatologist for advice.

> The combination of smoking and excessive sun exposure is particularly worrisome, and it is advisable for smokers to be especially careful to use lip sunscreens.

amount of titanium dioxide, which acts as a sunblock. However, the best protection is provided by lipsticks and lip moisturizers with added sunscreen ingredients. These products will have a sun protection factor (SPF) number that indicates how much protection from the sun the product will provide. Sunscreen can also minimize flare-ups of cold sores triggered by the sun.

DAMAGE CAUSED BY SMOKING

Smoking causes damage to the lips very similar to that caused by excessive sunlight. Heavy smokers often develop dried, cracked lips with wrinkles at the corners of the mouth referred to as "smoker's lines." In addition, smoking can lead to brownish-yellow discoloration of the lips. Heavy smoking, like excessive sun exposure, also predisposes a person to the development of white precancerous areas (in this case called *leukoplakia*) and squamous cell carcinoma of the lips.

UNSAFE COLORING AGENTS

Certain coloring ingredients derived from coal tar have been determined to be cancer risks when used on the lips. The Color Additive Amendment of 1960 requires that certain color additives made from coal tar can only be put in products for external use. These ingredients will be on the ingredients label and will contain the abbreviations D&C and Ext. (e.g., Ext. D&C Violet #2). Although these ingredients will not be found in cosmetics designed for the lips, many women use foundation makeup for the face on their lips. These products were not designed for the lips and may contain "external use only" coal tar–derived color additives that make them unsuitable for this purpose. It is important to read cosmetics ingredients labels carefully before using cosmetic products on the lips that are not especially designed for the lips.

CHAPTER 22

Lipsticks and Related Products

Lipstick should be color-coordinated with the wardrobe, blusher, and nail polish color. Lip liners should be chosen in a shade a little darker than the lipstick they accompany. Color is most accurately chosen when viewed in natural sunlight. Darker colors will give more coverage on lips with uneven color. A blue tone to a lipstick can make teeth appear whiter, whereas orange colors can make teeth appear unpleasantly yellow.

TYPES OF LIP COSMETICS

Although regular lipstick is most practical most of the time, lip crayons, lip gloss, lip creams, and liquid lip products are also useful for certain purposes.

Lip products vary in several ways. First, the firmness of the product can vary. Regular lipstick is intermediate in firmness. Lip crayons are firmer, while lip gloss and lip creams are softer. There are also liquid lip products. Most lip products are oil-containing products that are water-free (except for nonglossy liquid lip products). Stick and crayon products have wax added to make them more solid.

Second, lipstick coverage can vary: there are sheer and more opaque products. Most products are not sheer unless listed as such on the charts.

Third, the finish can vary from matte to frosted to glossy. Lip crayons and most regular lipsticks will have a somewhat matte finish while oilier regular lipsticks, lip glosses, and lip creams will have a glossy finish. Frosted products have a pearly appearance that is achieved by adding fish scale, mica, or bismuth oxychloride.

Lip Crayons

Lip crayons contain firmer wax and less oil than classic lipsticks, thus creating a matte finish. These products are hard and some may be difficult to apply. They are useful for women who develop pimples when using regular lipsticks or if lipsticks become uneven after application because of color migration caused by skin oiliness. They are also useful if lipsticks migrate into lip wrinkles to create an uneven appearance.

Lip Gloss and Lip Creams

Lip gloss and lip creams are very oily products that will add a glossy look to the lips. They are sometimes also used over regular lipstick to give a shinier look to the lips.

Gloss products are usually sheer in coverage and may be creams, very soft sticks that look like regular lipstick, or liquids. Lip creams usually come in jars and have a frosted (pearly) finish. Since lip gloss and creams are soft, they may migrate into wrinkled lip areas, giving an uneven appearance. Because these products are very oily, they may smear during wear if the surrounding skin is oily. They will work best on younger women with dry to normal skin.

Liquid Lip Products

There are a few products available that are lip coloring agents in liquid form. They will color the lips but provide very little coverage. Some of these products will give a glossy finish; these are listed in the charts as lip gloss.

Lip Powders

Lip powders are oil-containing pressed or loose powders for the lips. Most of these products contain a considerable amount of oil to make them very creamy in consistency in order to be pleasant when applied to the lips. They vary in finish from matte to glossy, depending on the relative amounts of oil and powder in the product. They are sometimes sold in a compact that also contains a clear gloss or sealer that is applied over the powder.

Lip Liners

Lip liners are essentially oil-containing (water-free) products with wax added to make a pencil. These products will add a defining line to the border of the lips. For longer wear, they can also be used as primers to shade the entire lip prior to using lipstick. Lip liners will help prevent migration of lipstick or lip crayon onto surrounding skin or wrinkles. They should be chosen in shades slightly darker than the lipstick that accompanies them.

Lip Coats

A lip coat is a product designed to go over lipstick as a shiny top coat. These products are essentially clear lip gloss products.

Lip Sealants and Lip Foundations (Primers)

Lip sealants and lip foundations are water-free or water-based products used to increase wearing time and coverage or to minimize smearing of lipstick. These products will also help prevent migration of lipstick or lip crayon onto surrounding skin or wrinkles.

Chart 22–1
LIPSTICKS AND RELATED PRODUCTS

The charts are designed to help you minimize adverse reactions and choose products with the proper oil content for your skin type. If you have cosmetics-related acne, you should also choose products with the least amounts of potentially comedogenic ingredients.

Although most cosmetics have potentially sensitizing ingredients, there is no reason to avoid any

> Names of products and product lines, and ingredients, are continually changing. Read the labels carefully before purchasing any beauty or skin-care product.

ingredient unless you are experiencing adverse reactions to cosmetic products. If you know you are allergic to certain ingredients, the charts will show you which products to avoid. If you are experiencing reactions to a certain cosmetic product, the charts can help you select alternative products that do not contain the same potentially sensitizing ingredients. To choose new products that are least likely to cause allergic reactions, keep in mind that fragrance is by far the most frequent cause of allergic reactions to cosmetics, followed by ingredients listed as "possible sensitizers." The ingredients listed as "other possible sensitizers" cause allergic reactions less frequently. Using these charts should help solve many cosmetics-related skin problems; however, if a problem persists, consult a dermatologist for advice and possible patch testing.

The products listed in these charts include many of the nationally advertised and distributed brands that have the largest market share of cosmetics sales; an extensive sampling of other brands available in the Chicago area is also included.

After locating several suitable products, use the pricing information on pages 18–19 for comparison shopping.

KEY

Possible Comedogenic Ingredients

BS—butyl stearate
CB—cocoa butter
DO—decyl oleate and derivatives
II—isopropyl isostearate
IM—isopropyl myristate
IN—isostearyl neopentanoate
IP—isopropyl palmitate

IS—isocetyl stearate and derivatives
LA—lanolin, acetylated
L4—laureth-4
M—mineral oil
ML—myristyl lactate
MM—myristyl myristate
OA—oleyl alcohol
OP—octyl palmitate
OS—octyl stearate and derivatives
PPG—myristyl ether propionate
PT—petrolatum
S—sesame oil/extract

Possible Sensitizers

B—benzophenones
BP—bronopol (2-bromo-2-nitropropane-1,3-diol)‡
C—cinnamates
D—diazolidinyl urea‡
E—essential oils and biological additives
F—fragrances
I—imidazolidinyl urea‡
L—lanolin and derivatives that may cross-react with lanolin
P—parabens
PB—PABA
PG—propylene glycol
Q—quaternium-15‡
SA—sorbic acid

Other Possible Sensitizers

BHA—butylated hydroxyanisole
BHT—butylated hydroxytoluene
BO—bismuth oxychloride
CH—chlorhexidine and derivatives
HQ—hydroquinone and derivatives
MO—mink oil
PGL—propyl gallate
R—rosin (colophony) and derivatives
T—triethanolamine and derivatives that may cross-react
VE—vitamin E (tocopherol and derivatives)

*may contain [see column head]
†does contain (coal tar colors)
‡formaldehyde-releasing ingredients

LIPSTICKS

Product name	Finish type	Possible comedogenic ingredients	Possible sensitizers	Other possible sensitizers	Coal tar colors
Adrien Arpel					
Lipstick	Regular			BO	†
Powder Cream Lipstick	Regular	IP,LA	F,P	BHA	*
Alexandra de Markoff					
Lip Colour	Regular	M,OA,PT,S	F,L,P	BHA,BO*	*
Allercreme					
Lipstick	Regular		C,E,P	BHA,BO*	*
Almay					
Lasting Finish Lipcolor	Regular		P	BHA,BO*	*
Artmatic					
Magic Color Lipstick with Vitamin E	Regular	IM	F,L,P,PG	BHA,PGL,VE	*
Moisturizing Long Lasting Lip Color with Vitamin E	Regular	IM	F,L,P,PG	BHA,PGL,VE	*
Avon					
Color Rich Lipstick	Regular	IN	F,L,PB	BHA	
Color Rich Super Frost Lipstick	Frosted	IN	F,L,PB	BHA	*
Satin Moist Lipstick	Glossy	LA,OP	F,L,PB	BHA,BO*	*
Black Radiance					
Lip Moisturizer	Regular	M,OA,PT		VE	*
Perfect Tone Lip Color	Regular	M,OA,PT		BO*,VE	*
Body Shop					
Colourings Lipstick	Regular	OA,PT	B,E,F,PB	VE	*
Bonne Bell					
	Frosted				
Frosty Gloss Lipstick		M,LA,S	PG	BHA,PGL,VE	*
Frosty Gloss Lipstick SPF 6	Frosted	M,S	B,C,PG	BHA,PGL,VE	*
Light 'N' Shiny Lipstick	Glossy	OA,OP	F,PG	BHA,BO*,PGL	*
Chanel					
Brillant Soleil Sheer Brilliance Lipstick SPF 8	Regular	OA	F,L,P,PG	PGL,VE	*
Levres Douceur Protective Lip Color Control	Regular	LA,M	F,P,PB,PG	PGL	*

Product name	Finish type	Possible comedogenic ingredients	Possible sensitizers	Other possible sensitizers	Coal tar colors
Rouge a Levres					
Super Hydra Base					
Creme Lipstick	Regular	IP,OA,PT	F,L,P,PG	BHA,PGL	*
Rouge Extreme Lip					
Rouge	Regular	OA,PT	F,PG	PGL	*
Sheer Brilliance					
Lipstick SPF 8	Regular	LA,OA	C,F,L,P,PG	BHA,PGL	*
Super Hydrabase					
Creme Lipstick	Regular	IP,LA,OA,PT	F,L,P,PG	BHA,PGL	*
Charles of the Ritz					
Opulent Color					
Lipstick	Regular	M,OA,PT	F,L,P,PB	BHA,BO*,VE	*
Christian Dior					
Lipstick	Regular	BS,LA,M,ML	C,F,P,PG	BHT,VE	*
Clarion					
Cream Lipstick	Regular	IP,OA	P	VE	*
Cream Lipstick with					
SPF 15	Regular	DO,OA*,OS,PT	C,P	VE	*
Frost Lipstick with					
SPF 15	Frosted	DO,OA*,OS,PT	C,P	VE	*
Lasting Color					
Lipstick	Regular	IP,ML,OA	P	VE	*
Precision Lip Color	Regular	DO,OA*,OS,PT	C,P	VE	*
Sheer Cream					
Lipstick with SPF					
15	Regular	OA,OS,PT	C,P	VE	*
Soft Color Lip Silks					
(SPF 15/sheer)	Regular	OA,OS,PT	C,P,PG	VE	*
Clientele					
Lip Color Treatment					
Lip Color	Regular	IM,M	E,L,P	MO	*
Clinique					
Almost Lipstick					
(sheer)	Regular		P	BO*,VE	*
Different Lipstick	Regular	IM,LA,ML	L,P	BO*,VE	*
Re-Moisturizing					
Lipstick	Regular	IP,LA	L,P	BO*,VE	*
Semi-Lipstick	Glossy	LA,ML	L,PB	BO*,VE	*
Sunner's Lipstick					
SPF 8	Regular	M,ML,MM	C,P	BHA	*
Color Me Beautiful					
Classic Lipstick	Regular	OA	F,L,P,PB	BHA,BO*,VE	*
Lipstick (Soft					
Colors)	Regular		F,P,PB	BHA	*

Product name	Finish type	Possible comedogenic ingredients	Possible sensitizers	Other possible sensitizers	Coal tar colors
Color Style (Revlon)					
Color Enriched Lipstick	Regular	OP	C,F,L,P	BHA,BO*	*
Cosmyl					
Cream Plus Lip Color	Regular	BS,M	F,L	BO*,VE	*
Coty					
"24" Creme Lipstick	Regular	OA	F,L,PG	BHA,PGL	*
"24" Luminescent Lipstick	Regular		F,P,PG	BHA,BO*,PGL	*
Sheer 'N' Sweet Glosstick	Glossy		L,P,PB,PG	BHA,BO*,PGL	*
Sheer to Stay 6 Hour Lip Color	Glossy		F,L,P,PB,PG	BHA,BO*,PGL	*
Slick Stick Lipstick	Regular	OA	BP*,E,F,L,P,PB,PG	BHA,BO*,PGL,VE	*
Cover Girl					
Continuous Color Lipstick (creme/frost)	Regular	LA,OS	C,F,L,P	BO,R,VE	*
Continuous Color Gloss Lipstick	Glossy	II,LA,OS	F,P	VE	*
Luminesse Lipstick	Glossy	LA,OA	F,P	VE	*
Remarkable Lipcolor Lipstick (creme/frost)	Regular	OS	C,L,P,PG	BO,VE	*
Soft Radiants Light Lipstick Creme	Regular	LA,OA*	F,PG	VE	*
Damascar					
Glossy Lipstick	Glossy	IM	C,F,L,P	BHA,R,VE	*
Eboné					
Extended Wear Lipstick	Regular	IM,M	F,L	BO*,VE	*
Elizabeth Arden					
Luxury Lip Sheer	Regular	IP,LA	C,F,P	BHA,BO*,VE	*
Luxury Lipstick	Regular	BS,M	F,L	BO*,VE	*
Spa for the Sun Lip Spa Sun Shade Lipcolor SPF 15 Pink Ginger	Regular	IP	C,E,F,L,PG	BHT,VE	†
Estee Lauder					
All-Day Lipstick	Regular	BS,M	F,L,P	BO*,VE	*
Featherproof Lipstick	Regular		E,F,P	BO*,VE	*
Perfect Lipstick	Regular	LA,M,OA	C,L,P	BHA,BO*,VE	*

Product name	Finish type	Possible comedogenic ingredients	Possible sensitizers	Other possible sensitizers	Coal tar colors
Polished Performance Lipstick	Regular	IM,ML	F,L,P,PB	BO*,VE	*
Fashion Fair					
Fragrance-Free Lipstick	Regular	OP	F,PG	BHA,PGL	*
Lipstick	Regular		L	PGL,VE	*
Fernand Aubry					
Lipstick Aubrylights	Glossy	M	F,L,SA	BHT	*
Lipstick Aubryssimes	Regular	M	F,L,P	BHT	
Flame Glo					
Hours Longer Cream Lipstick	Regular	IP,M	F,L,P,PB	BHA,VE	*
Hours Longer Frosted Lipstick	Frosted	IP,M,ML,OA,PT	F,L,P,PB	BHA,VE	*
Natural Glow Sheer Lip Color	Regular	IM,PT	F,L,P,PB	BO*,VE	*
Flori Roberts					
Gold/Hydrophylic Lipstick (older formulation)	Regular	S	F,P,PB	BHA,MO,VE	*
Gold/Hydrophylic Lipstick (newer formulation)	Regular	IP,PT,S	L,P	BO*,MO,PGL	*
Lipstick	Regular	OA,PT	F,L,P	PGL	*
Frances Denney					
FD-29 Lip Color Formula SPF 15	Regular		B,C,L,P	BHA,VE	*
Moisture Silk Lip Color	Regular	IP	F,L,P,PB	BHA	*
Moisture Silk Lip Color	Frosted		F,P,PB	BHA,BO*	*
Germaine Monteil					
Treatment Lipstick	Regular	LA,M,OA,PT	B,L,P,PB	BO*,VE	*
L'Oreal					
Colour Supreme Long Wear Lipstick	Regular		F,L,P,PG	BHA,BO*,PGL,VE	*
Creme Riche Lipstick	Regular	IP	F,P,PG	BHA,BO*,PGL	*
Lip Accents (creme)	Regular	OP	F,PG	BHA,PGL	*
Lip Accents (perle)	Frosted	OP	F,PG	BHA,BO*,PGL	*

Product name	Finish type	Possible comedogenic ingredients	Possible sensitizers	Other possible sensitizers	Coal tar colors
Lancôme					
Hydra Riche Hydrating Creme Lip Colour	Regular	IP,LA	C,F,L,P	BHA,BO*,VE	*
Maquiglace Emollient Rich Lip Colour	Regular	IP,LA	F,L,P	BHA	*
Rouge a Levres Satine Satin Lip Colour	Regular	OP	F,L,P	BHA,BO*	*
Rouge Superbe Matte Lip Colour	Regular	OP,OS	C,F,P	BHA,BHT,VE	*
Rouge Superbe Sheer Lip Colour	Regular		C,E,F,L,P	BHT,VE	*
Mahogany Image					
Lipstick	Regular	IM,OA,OP,PT	F,L,PG	BHA,BO*,PGL	*
Mary Kay					
Intensity Controller Lip Color Enhancer	Regular	IP	F,L,P	BHA	*
Lasting Color Lipstick	Regular	BS,M	F,L,PG	BHA,BO*,PGL,VE	*
Lip Color	Regular	IP	F,L,P	BHA	*
Max Factor					
Color Gloss Lipstick	Glossy		C,F,L,P	BHA	*
Lasting Color Lipstick	Regular	LA,PT	F,L,P	BHA,BO*	*
Maxi-Moist Not Quite Lipstick	Regular	M,MM	F,P	BHA,BO*	*
Maxi-Soft Lustre Long Lasting Lipstick	Regular		F,L,P	BHA,BO*	*
Moisture Rich Lipstick	Regular	LA	F,L,P	BHA,BO*	*
Maybelline					
Color Fresh Lipstick	Glossy	LA,OA	F,L,P,PG	BHA,BO*,PGL,VE	†
Glossy Clear Lipstick	Glossy	LA,M	F,L,P,PG	BHA,PGL	†
Long Wearing Lipstick	Regular	LA,OA	F,L,P,PG	BHA,BO*,PGL	*
Moisture Whip Lipstick with Sunscreen	Regular	LA	F,L,P,PG	BHA,BO*,PGL,VE	*
Moisture Whip Nourishing Lipstick	Regular	LA	F,L,P,PG	BHA,BO*,PGL,VE	*

Product name	Finish type	Possible comedogenic ingredients	Possible sensitizers	Other possible sensitizers	Coal tar colors
Revitalizing Color Lipstick	Frosted	OP,OS	C,E,F,L,P	BHA,BO*,PGL,VE	*
Revitalizing Color Lipstick	Regular	OP,OS	C,E,F,L,P	BHA,BO*,PGL,VE	*
Sheer Accents Lipstick SPF 8	Frosted	M	C,E,F,L,P	BHA,BO*,PGL,VE	*
Sheer Accents Lipstick SPF 8	Regular	M	C,E,F,L,P	BHA,BO*,PGL,VE	*
Shine Free Color Soft for Lips	Regular	LA	F,L,P,PG	BHA,BO*,PGL,VE	*
Slim Elegance Lipstick	Regular	LA,OA	F,L,P,PG	BHA,BO*,PGL	*
Slim Elegance Lipstick (Creamy Satin Color)	Regular	LA,OA	F,L,P,PG	BHA,BO*,PGL	*
Merle Norman					
Moist Lip Color	Glossy	PT	F,I,L,P	BHA,BHT	*
Performance Lipstick	Regular	BS,M	F,L,P	BHA,BHT,BO*,VE	*
Regular Lipstick	Regular	DO,LA,PT	F	BHA,BHT,BO*	*
Moon Drops					
Luminesque Lipstick	Frosted	OP,OS	F,L,P,PB	BHA,BO*,VE	*
Luminesque Lipstick	Regular	OP,OS	F,L,P,PB	BHA,BO*,VE	*
Moisture Creme Lipstick	Regular	IP,MM,OP,OS,S	F,L,P,PB	BHA,BO*,VE	*
Naomi Sims					
Lipstick	Regular	OP	F,PG	BHA,BO*,PGL	*
Natural Wonder					
Shiny Lips Lipstick	Glossy	OP	P,PB	BHA,VE	*
New Essentials					
Lip Color	Regular		P	BHA,BO*	*
Orlane					
Lipstick	Regular	OP,OS	B,C,F,P	BHA	*
Physician's Formula					
Creme Lipstick	Regular	M*,ML*,OP,OS		BHA,BHT,BO*	*
Frost Lipstick	Frosted	OP,OS		BHA,BHT,BO*	*
Lipstick	Regular	M,ML,OP,OS		BHA,BHT,BO*	*
Posner					
Extra Rich Custom Creme Lip Color	Regular	LA,ML	BS,C,F,P	BHA,BO*,VE	*
Moisturizing Lip Color	Regular	CB,IM,LA,M	F,L,P,PG	BHA,BO*,PGL	*

Product name	Finish type	Possible comedogenic ingredients	Possible sensitizers	Other possible sensitizers	Coal tar colors
Prescriptives					
Classic Lipstick	Regular	IS,LA,ML	L,P,PB	BO*,VE	*
Princess Marcella Borghese					
Lumina Lipstick	Regular	M,OA	F,L,P	BHA	*
Pupa					
Lipstick	Regular	LA,M,PT	F,P	R,VE	*
Revlon					
Color Shine Lipstick Creme	Glossy	LA,OA,OP	F,L,P	BHA	*
Super Lustrous Lipstick Creme	Regular	OP	F,L,P	BHA,BO*	*
Super Lustrous Lipstick Creme	Frosted	OP	F,L,P	BHA,BO*	*
Super Lustrous Sheer Lip Color	Regular	OP	C,F,P	BHA,BO*	*
Velvet Touch Lipstick	Regular		F,L,P	BHA,BO*	*
Shades of You (Maybelline)					
Lipstick	Regular	OA	L,P	BHA,BO*	*
Shiseido					
Lipstick	Regular		B,F,L	VE	*
Simply Satin					
Long Lasting Lipstick	Regular		F,L,P	BHA	*
Sisley					
Natural Plant Extract Lipstick	Regular	OP	E,F,L		*
Stagelight					
Stagelight Lipstick	Regular	PT	L,P,PG	BHA,PGL	*
Stendhal					
Moisture Protective Lipstick	Regular	M	F,L,P	BHA,BHT,HQ,PGL	*
Ultima II					
Coutre Lip Colors	Regular		F,L,P,PB	BHA	*
Lipchrome	Regular	OA	E,F,L,P	BHA,VE	*
Matte + Lipchrome	Regular		F,P	BHA	*
Super Luscious Sheer Lipstick	Regular	OA	C,F,L,P	BHA,BO*	*
The Nakeds Lipchrome	Regular	OA	E,F,L,P	BHA,VE	*

Product name	Finish type	Possible comedogenic ingredients	Possible sensitizers	Other possible sensitizers	Coal tar colors
Wet 'N' Wild					
Lip-Tricks Mood Lipstick	Regular	BS,M,ML	F,L,P	BHA	*
Silk Finish Lipstick	Regular	M,OA	F,PB,PG	BHA,PGL,VE	*
Ultra Performing Lip Color	Regular	BS,M,MM,PT	E,F,P,PB	BHA,BO*,VE	*
Yves Saint Laurent					
Lipstick	Regular	M,OA,PT	F,L,P,PG	BHA,BO*,PGL	*

LIP CRAYONS

Product name	Possible comedogenic ingredients	Possible sensitizers	Other possible sensitizers	Coal tar colors
Alexandra de Markoff				
Lasting Luxury Lipstick	M,OA,PT	F,L,P	BO*,VE	*
Charles of the Ritz				
Powderful Lipstick	LA	F,L,P	BHA,BO*	*
Mary Kay				
Waterproof Lip Color Crayon	ML,OP,OS	F,L,P	BO*,PGL	*

LIP CREAMS AND GLOSSES

Product name	Possible comedogenic ingredients	Possible sensitizers	Other possible sensitizers	Coal tar colors
Alexandra de Markoff				
Lasting Luxury Lip Gloss	M	F,L,P	BHA,BO*	*
Artmatic				
Wet Lips (liquid)	IP*	F,L,P		*
Avon				
Tri-Color Lip Gloss	IP	F,L,P	BHA	†
Body Shop				
Colourings Tinted Lip Color	OA,PT	B,C,E,	VE	*
Bonne Bell				
Lip Gloss with Vitamin E and SPF 4	IM,LA,M	F,L,PB,PG	BHA,PGL,VE	*
Lip Smacker Flavored Lip Gloss	M,S	PG	BHA,PGL	*
Chanel				
French Lip Gloss SPF 8 (pen)	IP,LA,M,OA	F,L,P,PB	BHT	*
Christian Dior				
Brilliant Lip Gloss	IP,M,OA	F,L,P	BHT,PGL,VE	*
Clientele				
Lip Color Treatment Lip Gloss	IP,M,PT	E,L,P	MO	*
Clinique				
Lip Gloss	IP	C,L,P	BO*,VE	*

Product name	Possible comedogenic ingredients	Possible sensitizers	Other possible sensitizers	Coal tar colors
Coty				
Sheer 'N' Clear Gloss Stick		F,L,P,PB		†
Water Splash Lip Color	CB,M	D,F,L,P		*
Cover Girl				
Lip Slicks Lip Gloss	LA,OA,PT	F,L,P,PG	VE	*
Elizabeth Arden				
Luxury Lip Gloss (compact)	IP,PT	C,F,L,P	BHA,BO*	*
Estee Lauder				
Just A Kiss (High Performance Lipshine SPF 4)	OA	C,L,P	BHT,BO*,VE	*
Fashion Fair				
Lip Gloss		F,L,PG	BHA,PGL	*
Flame Glo				
Natural Glow Automatic Lip Gloss	M,S	E,P		
Natural Glow Glossy Lip Balm	PT,S	B,P	VE	*
Natural Glow Lip Gloss Sticks	IM,PT,S	E,L,P	BO*,VE	*
Natural Glow Roll On Lip Gloss	M,S	E,P		
Flori Roberts				
Lip Polish (compact solid cream)	ML,PT	F,L,P		*
Liquid Lip Gloss (older formulation)	IP,PT	L,P		*
Liquid Lip Gloss (newer formulation)	ML,PT	L,P		*
Frances Denney				
Truly Natural Lip Gloss		L,PB,PG,SA	BHA,MO,PGL	*
Lancôme				
Hydra Riche Hydrating Creme Lip Colour	IP	C,F,L,P	BHA,VE	*
Rouge Superbe Lasting Creme Lip Colour		C,F,L,P	BHT,VE	*
Sorbet de Lancôme Fondant a Levres Lip Gloss	M	F,L,P	BHT	*
L'Oreal				
Glossique Lip Gloss	M	C,F	BO*	*
Mahogany Image				
Lip Gloss	ML,PT	L,P		*
Mary Kay				
Lip Gloss (natural or pearl)	IP,M	F,L,P	VE	†
Max Factor				
X-Rated Lip Gloss	M,OA	F,P	BHA,BHT	*
Maybelline				
Kissing Koolers (flavored lip gloss)	M	L,P,PG	BHA,PGL	*
Kissing Slicks	M	P	BHA	*
Liquid Lip Pearls		F,L,P,PG	BHA,BO*,PGL	†
Merle Norman				
Lip Makeup	DO,OA	F,L	BHA,BHT,BO*	*

Product name	Possible comedogenic ingredients	Possible sensitizers	Other possible sensitizers	Coal tar colors
Montaj				
Lip Gloss	M	F,L,P	BO*	*
Natural Wonder				
Keep Shining 5 Hour Lip Luster (+ aloe)		F,L,P	BHA	*
Physician's Formula				
Gloss Guard Protective Shine for Lips SPF 15	M*,PT	B,P,PB	BHA,BHT,BO*	*
Lipstick Glazes	OP,OS		BHA,BHT,BO*	*
Prescriptives				
Glossing Stick		C,L,P	BO*,VE	*
Princess Marcella Borghese				
Lip Gloss Fluido (liquid)	M	F,L,P	BHA,BO*	*
Lumina Mini Lip Gloss		C,F,L,P	BHA,BO*	*
Pupa				
Gloss Balsam	IM,M,PT	C,P	BHA,R	†
Lip Cream	M,PT	F,L,P	R,VE	*
Quencher				
Moisturizing Lipshine	IM,LA,PT	F,L,P,PB	BHA,BO*,VE	*
Moisturizing Lipshine SPF 15	M,S	B,PB,PG	BHA,BO*,PGL,VE	*
Revlon				
Powder-On Lip Color	OP,OS,PT	F,P	BO*,VE	*
Shiseido				
Lip Gloss		B,F,L	VE	*
Stagelight				
Lip Gloss Pot	ML,PT	L,P		*
Wet 'N' Wild				
High Gloss Liquid Lip Color	PT	F,L,P,PB,PG	BHA,PGL,VE	*
Yves Saint Laurent				
Automatic Lip Gloss	M	F,L,P,PB	VE	*

LIQUID LIP PRODUCTS

Product name	Possible comedogenic ingredients	Possible sensitizers	Other possible sensitizers	Coal tar colors
Artmatic				
Liquid Lipstick	IM,IP	F,L,P,PG	BHA,PGL,VE	*
Body Shop				
Colourings Lip Tint	IM*,M*,PT*	B,F,P		*
Estee Lauder				
Automatic Lipshine SPF 4	IP	B,F,L,P,PB	BO*,VE	*
Fashion Fair				
Automatic Lip Color	IP,PT	F,L,P	BHA	*
Max Factor				
Rosewater Lip Blush (oil-free transparent tint)		D,P		*

Product name	Possible comedogenic ingredients	Possible sensitizers	Other possible sensitizers	Coal tar colors
Quencher Lip Quencher Moisture Charged Color for Lips with Vitamin E & Sunscreen	IP,PT	F,L,P,PB	BO*,VE	*
Ultima II Penultimate Lip Color Pen (waterproof)	M	F,L,P,SA	BHA	*
Wet 'N' Wild Liquid Lip Color	PT	F,L,P,PB,PG	BHA,PGL,VE	*

LIP POWDERS

Product name	Possible comedogenic ingredients	Possible sensitizers	Other possible sensitizers	Coal tar colors
Cover Girl Lip Advance Powder (sold with sealer) (pressed)		P	BO*,VE	*
Damascar Compact Lip Powder Powder Lip Color	IM,M IM,M	L,P F,L,P	BO* BO*	* *

Princess Marcella Borghese
Lip Colour Superlativo (pressed)
Perlati Colour Brilliance for Eyes, Cheeks
   and Lips (loose)
Perlati Colour Pastello for Eyes, Cheeks and
   Lips (pressed)
	IM,OS,PT
	
	II,OS
	
	IM,PT
		F,P
		
		P
		
		F,P,Q
			BO*,VE
			
			BO*
			
			BO*,CH,VE
				*
				
				*

Pupa Lip Powder	OS	F,L,P		*
Stagelight Lip Powder (pressed)		I,P		*

LIP LINER PENCILS

Product name	Possible comedogenic ingredients	Possible sensitizers	Other possible sensitizers	Coal tar colors
Adrien Arpel Wear with Everything Lipliner		P	BHA,BHT,BO*	*
Alexandra de Markoff Pencil Colour for Lips	BS,MM,PT	P	BHA,BO*	*
Almay Lipcolor Pencil	M	P	BHA,BO*	*
Artmatic Professional Lip Liner Pencil		P	BHA,BHT	*
Black Radiance Lipliner Pencil		P	BHA*,BHT	*
Body Shop Colourings Lipliner	IM	P	BHA,BO*	*
Bonne Bell Lip Pencil Precision Lipliner Pencil		P P	BHT,BO* BHA,BHT,BO*	* *

Product name	Possible comedogenic ingredients	Possible sensitizers	Other possible sensitizers	Coal tar colors
Chanel				
Crayon Contour des Levres Lip Liner	MM	P	PGL	*
Christian Dior				
Lip Liner Pencil	M	P	BHA,BO*	*
Clinique				
Lip Pencil		P	BHT,BO*	*
Color Me Beautiful				
Lip Pencil	BS,IM,M	P	BHA	*
Cosmyl				
Lip Accenter	BS,M	P	BHA	*
Coty				
Stop It! Anti-Feathering Lipliner	PPG	I,P	BO*	*
Elizabeth Arden				
Creative Coloring Pencil Slenderliner Lip Pencil	IM	P	BHA	*
Estee Lauder				
Perfect-Line Lip Pencil		P	BHA,BHT,BO*	*
Signature Automatic Pencil for Lips		P	BO*,VE	*
Fashion Fair				
Lip Liner Pencils		P	BHA,BHT	†
Fernand Aubry				
Lip Pencil	IP	L,P	BHT	*
Flame Glo				
Natural Glow Soft Look Lip Definer		P	BHT	*
No Skip Lip Liner	PPG	P	BHT,BO*	*
Professional Lip Liner		P	BHA,BHT	*
Shape and Hold Lipliner Duo	BS,M	P	BHA	*
Flori Roberts				
Lip Contour Pencil		P	BHA,BHT	*
Frances Denney				
Lip Liner Pencil		P	BHA,BHT	*
Germaine Monteil				
Lip Ligne Liner	M	L,P	BHA,BO*	*
Lancôme				
Le Crayon Contour des Levres Lip Contour	M	P	BHA	*
Mary Kay				
Lip Liner Pencil	IM	P	BHA	*
Max Factor				
Lip Definer	MM	P	BHA,BHT	*
Maybelline				
Precision Lipliner	PPG	P	BHA,BHT	*

Product name	Possible comedogenic ingredients	Possible sensitizers	Other possible sensitizers	Coal tar colors
Merle Norman				
Lip Pencil Plus-1/3 Lip Liner	M,OA	P	BHA,BO*	*
Lip Pencil Plus-2/3 Lip Color	IP,LA,M,MM	P	BHA,BO*	*
Trimline Lip Pencil	M	P	BHA,BO*	*
Prescriptives				
Lip Coloring Pencil	M	L,P	BHA,BO*	*
Princess Marcella Borghese				
Perfetta Lip Pencil		P	BHA,BO*	*
Pupa				
Lip Pencil		P	VE	*
Revlon				
Waterproof Lip Shaper	IN	P	BHA,BO*	*
Quencher				
Precision Color Pencil for Lips	IM,LA,PT	F,L,P,PB	BHA,BO*,R,VE	*
The Treatment Lipliner		P	BHA,BHT	*
Sisley				
Botanical Lip Liner	MM	E,P	PGL	*
Ultima II				
Super Luscious Lip Liner	IM	P	BHA,BO*	*
Wet 'N' Wild				
Creme Lip Liner		P	BHA,BHT	*

LIP COATS

Product name	Possible comedogenic ingredients	Possible sensitizers	Other possible sensitizers	Coal tar colors
Bonne Bell				
Lip-Lites (Alone or Over Lipstick) (water-free)	LA,M	P	BHA	*
Coty				
Nature's Lip Tint (glossy) (water-free)		F,L,P,PB		†
Estee Lauder				
Perfect Lipstick Perfect Conditioner (water-free)	M,OA	C,L,P	BHA,VE	
Fashion Fair				
Crystal Clear Lip Gloss (compact/water-free)		F,L,P,SA	BHA,PGL	†
Flame-Glo				
Lush Lips Lip Polish (oil-based)	M	P		
Flori Roberts				
Lip Oil Stick (water-free)	BS	F,P		*
Germaine Monteil				
Demi-Tient Continuelle Protective Lip Tint SPF 6 (water-free)	OP	B,C,E,P	BHA,BO*	*

Product name	Possible comedogenic ingredients	Possible sensitizers	Other possible sensitizers	Coal tar colors
Maybelline				
Kissing Potion (flavored/roll-on) (water-free)	M	P	BHA	
Merle Norman				
Lip Moisture (compact/water-free)		F,L	BHA,BHT	†
Stagelight				
Lipstick Fixative (water-free)	IM	E		

LIP SEALANTS

Product name	Possible comedogenic ingredients	Possible sensitizers	Other possible sensitizers	Coal tar colors
Elizabeth Arden				
Lip-Fix Creme	IM,M	P	BC,CH	
Adrien Arpel				
Lipstick Lock (water-free)	BS,IP,PT	P	BHA	
Cover Girl				
Lip Advance Sealer (water-free) (sold with powder)	OA,OS	L,P,PG	VE	†
Alexandra de Markoff				
Undercover for Lips	M,PGS	E,F,P	BHA,BHT,VE	
Fashion Fair				
Perfect Primer Lip Balancer (water-free)	OP	F,PG	BHA,PGL	*
Flori Roberts				
Lip Base Coat (stick) (water-free)	OA,PT	F,L,P	PGL	*
Max Factor				
Lip Renew Conditioning Primer (water-based)	OP	E,I,P	T	
Stay Put! Anti-Fade Lip Base (water-free)	OA	F,L,P	BHA,VE	
Merle Norman				
Lip Stay Lip Treatment Cream (water-based)	IP,LA,M,MM	D,P		
Revlon				
Lip Zone Perfector:				
Roll Away (water-free)	IS	I,P		
Fill-In (water-based)	IN,IS,PT	C,E,I,P	VE	†
Stagelight				
Lipstick Fixative (water-free)	IM	E		
Top Billing				
Top Billing Sealed Lips (water-free)	IM	E		

PART SIX

THE NAILS

CHAPTER 23

Nail Structure and Problems of the Nails

The nail is a specialized structure made of the same material as the outer layer of the skin. New nail is formed in the nail matrix found at the base of the nail. Part of the nail matrix is visible on the surface as a white crescent called the lunula; the matrix also extends beneath the skin at the base of the nail. A thin protective skin layer called the cuticle forms over the lunula.

NAIL GROWTH AND CARE

The nails grow continuously outward from the matrix toward the end of the finger, forming the nail plate. Although the nail plate is white, it appears pink where attached to the skin because of the rich blood supply of the underlying nailbed.

Fingernails grow approximately one-eighth inch each month on the average; however, slightly faster growth takes place during summer, during pregnancy, or after injury. Slower growth occurs with illness or old age. Toenails grow considerably more slowly than fingernails.

Splitting of the Nails

A number of factors can lead to split or chipped nails. First, cutting or filing nails improperly can lead to splitting. In general, nails are less likely to split when the corners are left relatively square rather than rounded. Nail clippers have been designed to round the tips of the nails but to leave the corners squared; therefore, they will properly and more easily cut nails than will scissors. Filing the nails frequently is actually the best way to care for nails, since the trauma associated with cutting them can cause splitting.

Some nails split because they are brittle and dry. Women who frequently have their hands in water, detergents, or household cleaners can develop dry, brittle nail plates that break more easily. This can largely be

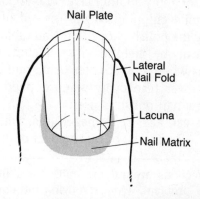

Nail Plate

Lateral Nail Fold

Lacuna

Nail Matrix

Top view of fingertip showing nail structures

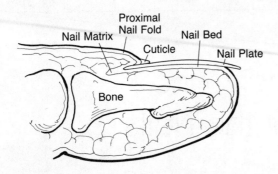

Nail Matrix
Proximal
Nail Fold
Cuticle
Nail Bed
Nail Plate
Bone

Cross-section through a fingertip showing nail structures

avoided by wearing gloves when doing housework. The use of moisturizers on the nails after the hands have been in water is also often effective. Moisturizers will work best when applied directly to the nail plate, but it is unclear how effective these products are when applied over nail polish. Nail polishes are plastic acrylic or polyester films that may act as barriers against nail moisturizers.

Overuse of nail enamel removers can also lead to dry, brittle nails. To minimize this, use nonacetone removers that are less drying, or apply another layer of nail polish when mild chipping occurs instead of removing the polish altogether. Nail moisturizers can be helpful in reducing nail dryness when applied after using nail polish remover (especially when applied before new nail polish is used).

Nails can also be damaged and split by trauma, chemicals, or by removal of artifi-

> If infections around the nails are a frequent problem, avoid removing the cuticles.

cial nails. Wearing gloves while doing housework and handling harsh chemicals will decrease splitting significantly.

Nail Hardeners
If other approaches to damaged nails are not effective, nail hardeners can be tried. These products are nail base coats with high concentrations of resins designed to increase the strength of brittle nails. Some of these products contain nylon or other artificial fibers to reinforce the nails further. Almost all nail hardeners have now been reformulated without formaldehyde, which was found to cause frequent allergic reactions.

Gelatin and Brittle Nails
Although gelatin added to the diet has been widely used for years to treat brittle nails, there is currently no persuasive evidence that it is effective for this purpose.

INFECTIONS AROUND THE NAILS AND CUTICLE REMOVAL

The skin around the base of the nails can sometimes become infected. Although many women and manicurists believe that nail appearance is improved by removing the cuticles, this protective skin layer is important in preventing infections. Most dermatologists do not recommend using cuticle removers or cutting away the cuticles. In addition, cuticle removal products dissolve the cuticle through the use of chemicals, such as 2 percent to 5 percent sodium or potassium hydroxide, that have a strong basic pH and can be significantly irritating to the surrounding skin when applied for too long.

Nail Polish and Other Routine Nail-Care Products

Nail polish is used to improve the cosmetic appearance of nails. The best manicurists use three thin coats of polish. The first coat is a base coat that is essentially a foundation designed to increase the adherence of the second layer. The second layer is the actual nail polish. The third layer is a top coat that is designed to increase gloss and prevent chipping. This is often just clear polish. Some products are designed to be used as both base coat and top coat. The use of three coats is not absolutely necessary but keeps the nails looking optimal for a longer period of time. Products listed in the charts as "quick-dry nail products" can be used on top of other nail products to give a glossy finish. These products contain mostly moisturizing ingredients.

TYPES OF NAIL POLISH

Most nail polishes have a similar composition, but the appearance of nail polish can be modified by adding various ingredients. Frosted nail polishes contain ingredients such as fish scales, guanine, or mica to give a pearly shine. Sheer nail polish can be made creamy by adding titanium dioxide to increase coverage.

ALLERGIC REACTIONS TO NAIL POLISH

Allergic reactions to nail polish are usually seen not on the fingers but near the eyes or other areas of the face touched by the fingers while nail polish is still wet. Dried nail polish rarely causes allergic reactions. Allergic reactions are almost always caused by an ingredient called *toluene sulfonamide/formaldehyde resin.* Some nail polishes that have substituted polyester resin for this ingredient rarely cause allergic reactions; however, these products are more prone to chipping.

TYPES OF NAIL POLISH REMOVER

Nail polish must be removed either with acetone or with nail polish removers (which contain acetone or other solvents). Solvents, especially acetone, may sometimes irritate the skin surrounding the nail. There are nail polish removers that do not contain acetone and may be less irritating to those who cannot tolerate this ingredient. Acetone-based polish removers will remove artificial nails or nail "tips"; therefore, only acetone-free products should be used when removing polish from them.

Chart 24–1
NAIL POLISH AND RELATED NAIL-CARE PRODUCTS

Although almost all cosmetics have potentially sensitizing ingredients, there is no reason to avoid any ingredient unless you are experiencing adverse reactions to cosmetic products. If you know you are allergic to certain ingredients, the charts will show you which products to avoid. If you are experiencing reactions to a certain cosmetic product, the charts can help you select alternative products that do not contain the same potentially sensitizing ingredients. To choose new products that are least likely to cause allergic reactions, keep in mind that toluene sulfonamide/formaldehyde resin is the cause of almost all allergic reactions to nail products (other than nail polish removers and nail moisturizers) and that most of these reactions occur at distant sites such as the eyes and face that come in contact with wet nail products. If an allergic reaction to nail products is suspected, choosing a product without toluene sulfonamide/formaldehyde resin should be the first thing to try. However, nail products without toluene sulfonamide/formaldehyde resin tend to chip more easily.

Using the charts should help solve many cosmetics-related skin problems; however, if a problem persists, consult a dermatologist for advice and possible patch testing.

The products listed in these charts include many of the nationally advertised and distributed brands that have the largest market share of cosmetics sales; an extensive sampling of other brands available in the Chicago area is also included.

After locating several suitable products, use the pricing information on pages 18–19 for comparison shopping.

> Names of products and product lines, and ingredients, are continually changing. Read the labels carefully before purchasing any beauty or skin-care product.

KEY

Possible Sensitizers

B—benzophenones
E—essential oils and biological additives
F—fragrances
FO—formaldehyde
L—lanolin and derivatives that may cross-react with lanolin
P—parabens
PG—propylene glycol
TSF—toluene sulfonamide/formaldehyde resin

Other Possible Sensitizers

BHA—butylated hydroxyanisole
BO—bismuth oxychloride
ER—epoxy, epoxy resin
PGL—propyl gallate
T—triethanolamine and derivatives that may cross-react
VE—vitamin E (tocopherol and derivatives)

* may contain [see column head]
† does contain (coal tar colors)

NAIL POLISH			
Product name	Possible sensitizers	Other possible sensitizers	Coal tar colors
Alexandra de Markoff Lasting Luxury Nail Lacquer	TSF	BO*	*
Almay Nail Enamel	B	BO*	

Product name	Possible sensitizers	Other possible sensitizers	Coal tar colors
Avon			
Color Last Plus Nail Enamel	B,TSF	BO*	*
Chanel			
Creme Nail Enamel	TSF		*
Charles of the Ritz			
Perfect Finish Nail Lacquer	B,TSF	BO*	*
Christian Dior			
Nail Enamel	B*,TSF		*
Clarion			
Clarion Nails	B,TSF	BO*	*
Pure Performance Nail Color	B,TSF	BO*	*
Clinique			
Glossy Nail Enamel	B	BO*	*
Color Me Beautiful			
Nail Color		BO*	*
Color Style (Revlon)			
Nail Enamel		BO*	*
Cosmyl			
Creme Plus Nail Lacquer	B*,TSF		*
Coty			
Limited Edition Nail Enamel	B,TSF	BO*	*
Cover Girl			
Luminesse Satin Finish Nail Color	B,TSF	BO*	*
Nail Slicks	B,TSF	BO*	*
Nail Slicks Sun Slicks	B,TSF	BO*	*
Nail Slicks Transparencies	B,TSF	BO*	*
Professional One Coat Nail Color	B,TSF		*
Cutex			
Color Quick Nail Enamel	B,TSF	BO*	*
Perfect Color	B,TSF	BO*	*
Nail Polish	B,TSF	BO*	*
Strong Nail (strengthening)	B,TSF	BO*	*
Damascar			
Nail Polish	B,TSF		*
Elizabeth Arden			
Luxury Nail Color	B	BO*	*
Estee Lauder			
Perfect Finish Nail Lacquer	B,TSF	BO*	*
Fashion Fair			
Perfect Polish	TSF	BO*	*
Fernand Aubry			
Nail Enamel Aubryssimes	TSF		

Product name	Possible sensitizers	Other possible sensitizers	Coal tar colors
Finger Mates			
Formula 10	TSF	BO*	*
Flori Roberts			
Nail Enamel	B,TSF	BO*	*
Germaine Monteil			
Lasting Nail Lacquer	B,TSF	VE	*
L'Oreal			
Cream Nail Polish	B,TSF	BO*	*
Grow Strong Restructuring Nail Color	B,FO,TSF	BO*	*
Perle Nail Enamel	B,TSF	BO*	*
Lancôme			
Nail Lacquer	B,TSF	BO*	*
Mahogany Image			
Nail Enamel			*
Mary Kay			
Color Shield	B,TSF	BO*	*
Max Factor			
Creme Nail Enamel	B,TSF	BO*	*
Diamond Hard Formula Nail Enamel (creme)	B,TSF	BO*	*
Diamond Hard Formula Nail Enamel (perle)	B,TSF	BO*	*
Maxi Endless Shine Nail Enamel	B,TSF	BO*	*
Maxi One Coat Nail Enamel	B,TSF	BO*	*
Perle Nail Enamel	B,TSF	BO*	*
Maybelline			
Long Wearing Nail Color with Glyoxal	B,TSF	BO*	*
Revitalizing Color for Nails	B	BO*,VE	*
Shine Free Color Tough for Nails	B	BO*	*
Merle Norman			
Nail Glaze (contains mineral oil)	TSF	BO*	*
Natural Wonder			
Super Nails	B,TSF	VE	*
New Essentials			
Nail Color	B	BO*	*
Nouvage			
Nail Enamel	B,TSF	BO*	*
Orlane			
Nail Lacquer	TSF	BO*	*
Orly			
French Manicure Nail Polish Kit	B,TSF	BO	†
Nail Paint	TSF	BO	†
Princess Marcella Borghese			
Lumina Radiant Finish Nail Lacquer	B,TSF		*
Protettivo Protective Nail Lacquer	B,TSF	BO*	*

Product name	Possible sensitizers	Other possible sensitizers	Coal tar colors
Pupa			
Nail Enamel	TSF		*
Nail Varnish	B,TSF		*
Revlon			
Cream Nail Color	B,TSF	BO*	*
Nail Enamel Creme	B,TSF		*
Nail Enamel Crystalline	B,TSF	BO*	*
Sally Hansen			
Hard as Nails	B*,TSF	BO*	*
Hard as Nails (with nylon)	B,TSF	BO*	*
Liquid Silk Wrap	B,TSF		*
New Lengths Liquid Fiber-Wrap Kit Step 2-Satin			
Smooth	B,TSF		†
New Lengths Micro Fiber Strengthener	B*,TSF	BO*,VE	*
New Lengths with Vitamin Calcium Complex	B,TSF	VE	*
Shiseido			
Nail Lacquer	B*	VE	*
Stagelight			
Color War Nail Lacquer[1]	TSF	BO*	*
Stendhal			
Nail Polish	TSF	BO*	*
Wet 'N' Wild			
Nail Color	TSF	BO*	*
Yves Saint Laurent			
Nail Lacquer	TSF		*

NAIL BASE COATS

Product name	Possible sensitizers	Other possible sensitizers	Coal tar colors
Almay			
Ridge Filler and Sealer	B		
Strengthening Base Coat	B		†
Chanel			
Base Protinee Protein Base Coat	TSF		
Brillant Durcisseur Pour les Ongles Nail Glaze	B,TSF		
Christian Dior			
Base Speciale Pour Ongles Fragiles Special Base Coat			
for Fragile Nails			
Extra Strength Base Specials for Nails[1]	TSF		*
Clarion			
Extra-Smooth Base Coat	B		
Fortifying Base Coat	B		
Clinique			
Base Coat for Nails	B		

[1]Product contains an ingredient listed as "UV absorber #1." It is possible that this may be benzophenone-1. Benzophenones (primarily benzophenone-1) are found in a large number of nail products.

Product name	Possible sensitizers	Other possible sensitizers	Coal tar colors
Cosmyl			
First Touch Base Coat	TSF		
Smooth Touch Ridge Filler	TSF		
Cover Girl			
10 Terrific Nails Color Cling Primer	TSF		
Cutex			
Double Magic Basecoat/Topcoat	B,TSF		†
Nail Ridgefilling Basecoat	B,TSF		†
Stain-Free Adhering Basecoat	B,TSF		†
Delore			
Instant Nail Protector (base/top coat)	B		†
Silk Ridge Filler	B		†
Estee Lauder			
Perfect Base Coat	B,TSF		†
Fashion Flair			
Perfect Polish Base Coat	TSF	BO*	
L'Oreal			
Grow Strong Primer Base Coat	B,FO,TSF		*
Miracle Base Coat	B,TSF		
Ridge Filling Base Coat	B,TSF		†
Mahogany Image			
Nail Hardener			*
Mary Kay			
Binder	B,TSF		
Mavala			
002 Protective Base Coat	B,TSF		†
Nylon Fiber Base	B,TSF		
Ridge Filler	TSF		
Max Factor			
Diamond Hard Base and Top Coat	B,TSF		
Merle Norman			
Protective Base and Top Coat	B,TSF		*
Orlane			
Nail Fortifier (base coat and top coat)	TSF		*
Orly			
Bonder Base Coat	TSF	BO	†
One Step Strengthening Base Coat	TSF		†
Pupa			
Base and Top Coat	B		*
Revlon			
Color Lock Super Wear Base Coat	B		†

Product name	Possible sensitizers	Other possible sensitizers	Coal tar colors
Professional:			
Double-Twist Instant Base and Top Coat	B,TSF		
No. 61 Clear Lustrous Nail Coat	B,TSF		
Stain Guard Anti-Stain Base Coat	B,L,TSF	VE	†
Wonder Wear Adhesive Base Coat	B,TSF		
Sally Hansen			
Dries Instantly Moisture Rich Base Coat		VE	†
Moisturizing Base Coat	B,TSF		†
New Lengths Base and Top Coat	B,TSF	VE	*
New Lengths Stain Proof Base Coat	B,TSF	VE	†
Smooth Nails Ridge Filling Base Coat	B,TSF		†
Super Strong Micro-Fiber Base Coat	B,TSF		†
Wet 'N' Wild			
Nail Complex Matte Finish Base Coat	B,TSF		

NAIL TOP COATS

Product name	Possible sensitizers	Other possible sensitizers	Coal tar colors
Almay			
Ridge Filler and Sealer	B		
Protective Shield Top Coat	B		†
Barielle			
Clearly Noticeable Nail Thickener[2]			†
Chanel			
Brillant Transparent Top Coat	TSF		
Christian Dior			
Top Coat for Nails	TSF		
Clarion			
Strengthening Shiny Top Coat	B		
Clinique			
Daily Nail Saver (top coat protector)	B		†
Top Glaze for Nails	B		†
Cosmyl			
Finishing Touch Top Coat	B,TSF		
Cutex			
Double Magic Basecoat/Topcoat	B,TSF		†
Flash Finish Quick Drying Top Coat	B		†
Maximum Life Chip Resistant Top Coat	B,TSF		†
Polish Sealer Brilliant Shine Top Coat	B,TSF		†
Strong Nail Maximum Life Chip Resistant Top Coat	TSF		†
Delore			
Instant Nail Protector (base/top coat)	B		†
Elizabeth Arden			
Luxury Nail Protector	B		†

[2]Product contains an ingredient listed as "UV absorber #1." It is possible that this may be benzophenone-1. Benzophenones (primarily benzophenone-1) are found in a large number of nail products.

Product name	Possible sensitizers	Other possible sensitizers	Coal tar colors
Estee Lauder			
Perfect Finish Top Coat	B,TSF		†
Fashion Fair			
Perfect Polish Top Coat	TSF	BO*	
Finger Mates			
Formula 10 Light	B		†
Formula 10 Seal and Shield	B,TSF		
Germaine Monteil			
Sechage Rapide Quick Dry Top Coat			†
L'Oreal			
Chip Resistant Glossy Sealer	B,TSF		*
Grow Strong Protective Top Coat	B,FO,TSF		*
Super Dry Top Coat	B,TSF		
Mahogany Image			
Clear Glaze Top Coat Nail Enamel			
Mary Kay			
Protector	B,TSF		
Satin Finish Protector	B,TSF	BO*	*
Mavala			
Color Fix Strong Flexible Super Gloss Top Coat	B,TSF		†
Protective Sealer	B,TSF		
Max Factor			
Diamond Hard Base and Top Coat	B,TSF		
Shine and Shield Top Coat			†
Maybelline			
Performance 10 Beautiful Nails with Glyoxal	B,TSF		†
Merle Norman			
Protective Base and Top Coat	B,TSF		*
Nu-Tress			
Proteinail Wet Look Super Hi-Gloss Acrylic Nail Glaze	B		†
Orlane			
Nail Fortifier (base coat and top coat)	TSF		*
Orly			
Glosser Fast Dry Top Coat[3]	TSF		†
Pupa			
Base and Top Coat	B		*
Revlon			
Calcium Gel Nail Protector with Vitamins		VE	†
Color Lock No Chip Sealer	TSF		†
Professional Double-Twist Instant Base and Top Coat	B,TSF		
Professional Extra Life Brilliant Top Coat	B,TSF		
Professional Maximum Shine Top Coat	B,TSF		†

[3]Product contains an ingredient listed as "UV absorber #1." It is possible that this may be benzophenone-1. Benzophenones (primarily benzophenone-1) are found in a large number of nail products.

Product name	Possible sensitizers	Other possible sensitizers	Coal tar colors
Sally Hansen			
New Lengths Base and Top Coat	B,TSF	VE	*
No Chip Acrylic Top Coat	B,TSF		
No More Peeling Nail Bonding Shield	B,TSF		†
Super Shine Shiny Top Coat	B,TSF		†
Wet 'N' Wild			
Crystalic One Coat Glaze	B,TSF	BO*	*
Nail Complex Clear Nail Protector	B,TSF		†
Nail Complex No Chip Top Coat	B,TSF		†

QUICK-DRY NAIL PRODUCTS

Product name	Possible sensitizers	Other possible sensitizers	Coal tar colors
Clarion			
Quick Dry Finish			†
Cosmyl			
Fast Touch Quick Dry	F		
Cover Girl			
10 Terrific Nails Dry Fast			
Cutex			
Smudge Proofer Fast Finish Nail Dry			
Delore			
Organic Nail Hardener and Instant Nail Polish Dryer		VE	
Germaine Monteil			
Sechage Rapide Quick Dry Top Coat			†
Mary Kay			
Quick Dry			
Mavala			
Mava-Dry	F		
Mava-Dry Nail Enamel Dryer (aerosol)	F		
Max Factor			
Quick Set Nail Dry	P		
Revlon			
Professional Liquid Quick Dry	P		
Professional Quick Dry Spray	F,L	BHA	
Sally Hansen			
Dry-Kwik			
New Lengths Smudgeproof Nail Dry		VE	
No More Smudges	B		†
Wet 'N' Wild			
Nail Complex Flash Dry Nail Set	P		†

ACETONE-BASED NAIL ENAMEL REMOVERS

Product name	Possible sensitizers	Other possible sensitizers	Coal tar colors
Christian Dior			
Dissolvant Doux Gentle Polish Remover	B,F		†

Product name	Possible sensitizers	Other possible sensitizers	Coal tar colors
Cosmyl			
Smearproof Polish Remover	F		†
Cutex			
Lemon and Lanolin Strong Nail Polish Remover	F,L		†
Moisturizing Polish Remover	F,L,P,PG	BHA,PGL,T	†
Strong Nail:			
Aloe with Lemon Scent Polish Remover	F		†
Instant Polish Remover with Knox Gelatin	F		†
Regular Polish Remover	F		†
Vitamin E with Clean Scent Polish Remover	F,PG	VE	†
Max Factor			
Quick and Clean Nail Enamel Remover	B,F,L		†
Revlon			
Extra Fast Nail Enamel Remover	B,F		†
Professional Moisture Treatment Nail Enamel			
Remover	F		†
Sally Hansen			
Kwik-Off Apricot Extract Nail Color Remover (with			
Vitamin E)	F,L	VE	
Kwik-Off Nail Glue Remover	F		†
Nail Color Remover with Calcium	B,F		†
Nail Color Remover with Gelatin	F	VE	†
Nail Color Remover with vitamin E	F	VE	†
Nail Polish Remover	B,F	VE	†
Remove 'N' Smooth Nail Color Remover Pads	F	VE	

ACETONE-FREE NAIL ENAMEL REMOVERS

Product name	Possible sensitizers	Other possible sensitizers	Coal tar colors
Almay			
Conditioning Formula Nail Enamel Remover			†
Nail Enamel Remover Pads	P	VE	
Vitamin Enriched Nail Enamel Remover Gel		VE	†
Cosmyl			
Extra Gentle Polish Remover Acetone-Free	B,F		†
Nail Polish Corrector			
Finger Mates			
Formula 10 Jele Polish Remover	F	T	
Mary Kay			
Advanced Nail Color Remover	B,F		†
Nail Care Thinner			
Mavala			
Extra-Mild Nail Polish Remover	E		†
Thinner			
Merle Norman			
Nail Enamel Remover	F,L		

Product name	Possible sensitizers	Other possible sensitizers	Coal tar colors
Pupa			
Nail Enamel Remover		VE	†
Revlon			
Extra Gentle Nail Enamel Remover	B,F		†
Extra Moisturizing Nail Enamel Remover	B,F		†
Professional Enamel Solvent Instant Nail Enamel Thinner			
Professional Extra Gentle Nail Enamel Remover	B,F		†
Sally Hansen			
Kwik-Off Acetone-Free Nail Enamel Remover	B		†
Manicure Corrector			
Nail Color Remover	B		†
Nail Color Thinner			

NAIL HARDENERS

Product name	Possible sensitizers	Other possible sensitizers	Coal tar colors
Almay			
Nail Fortifier	B		†
Barielle			
Clearly Noticeable Nail Thickener[4]		VE	
Instant Liquid Nail Hardener[4]		BO,VE	†
Bonne Bell			
Diamond Formula Nail Hardener	TSF		
Ceramic Glaze			
Professional Nail Strengthener	TSF		†
Professional Nail Treatment	TSF		†
Christian Dior			
Durcisseur Pour les Ongles Nail Hardener	TSF		
Cosmyl			
Active Plus Intensive Nail Hardener	FO,TSF		
Nail Plus Acrylic Hardener	TSF		
Silk Fiber Weave Strengthener	TSF		†
Cover Girl			
10 Terrific Nails Acrylic Strengthener	TSF		†
10 Terrific Nails Nail Bond Hardener	TSF		
Cutex			
Nail Developer Nail Fitness System/Fortifier		VE	†
Nail Saver Calcium Fiber Fortifier	B,TSF		
Strong Nail Nail Strengthener	B,TSF	BO*	*
Delore			
Organic Nail Hardener and Instant Nail Polish Dryer (contain oleic acid)		VE	
Finger Mates			
Formula 10 Gold Organic Nail Strengthener (contains oleic acid)		VE	

[4]Product contains an ingredient listed as "UV absorber #1." It is possible that this may be benzophenone-1. Benzophenones (primarily benzophenone-1) are found in a large number of nail products.

Product name	Possible sensitizers	Other possible sensitizers	Coal tar colors
Flori Roberts			
Forever Nails Protective Nail Hardener	FO,TSF	VE	
Germaine Monteil			
Ellonge Traitement Fortifiant Nail Fortifier	B,FO,TSF		
L'Oreal			
Acrylic Nail Hardener	B,TSF		*
Grow Strong Nail Strengthener	B,FO,TSF		†
Mahogany Image			
Nail Hardener			*
Mary Kay			
Fortifier	B,TSF		†
Mavala			
Scientifique Penetrating Nail Hardener	E,F,FO		†
Max Factor			
2'nd Nail Nail Saver	B,TSF		†
Nail Thick	B,TSF		
Maybelline			
Revitalizing Conditioning Clear	B	VE	†
Shine Free Color Tough for Nails	B	BO*	†
Nu-Tress			
Proteinail Silk System Liquid Silk Wrap			
Orly			
Romeo Fiber Nail Builder	TSF		
Pupa			
Nail Hardener	TSF		†
Revlon			
Calcium Gel Nail Builder	B,TSF		
Calcium Gel Nail Revitalizer with Zinc			
Liquid Nail Wrap Strengthener (calcium)	B,TSF	BO*	*
Liquid Nail Wrap Strengthener (calcium/epoxy)	B,TSF	BO*,ER	*
Sally Hansen			
Be-Long Nail Strengthener with Nylon Fibers	TSF		
Hard as Nails	B*,TSF	BO*	*
Hard as Nails (with nylon)	B,TSF	BO*	*
Maximum Growth	B,TSF		*
Mend-A-Nail	B		†
Nail Protex	B,TSF	VE	*
New Lengths Grow Long Nails Nail Strengthener		VE	†
New Lengths Liquid Nail Fiber-Wrap Kit Step 1			
Fiber-Firm	B*,TSF	BO*,VE	*
New Lengths Micro Fiber Strengthener	B*,TSF	BO*,VE	
No More Breaks Restructuring Strengthener	B,TSF		†

Abrasive scrubber   A rough object such as a pumice stone or loofah or a cream with rough granules that removes superficial skin scales.

Absorption base   A skin-care product containing no water but containing compounds such as cholesterol or lanolin to improve water absorption capacity.

Acne   A skin condition found in teenagers and some adults, characterized by recurring episodes of pimples.

Acne cosmetica   A condition in which acne pimples are caused by the use of cosmetics that are either too oily for a person's skin type or that contain ingredients that cause pimples.

Acnegenic   A product or ingredient known to create pimples when applied to the skin of some people.

Allergen   A substance capable of causing allergic contact dermatitis.

Allergic contact dermatitis   A specific immune reaction to a foreign substance that causes dermatitis.

Astringent   A product or substance that causes temporary tightening of the skin.

Atopic dermatitis   A hereditary skin condition often aggravated by but not caused by irritating substances.

Atopic eczema   Same as atopic dermatitis.

Atopy   An inherited medical condition that makes a person prone to eczema, respiratory allergy, asthma, and/or hives.

Automatic mascara   Mascara that comes in a cylindrical tube with a cap that has an attached applicator wand.

Base   The mixture of ingredients in a skin-care product that determines the product form (cream, lotion, solution).

Base coat   A type of nail enamel designed to be worn under nail polish to help the polish adhere better.

Benzalkonium chloride   A disinfectant ingredient added to some cosmetics.

Benzophenone   A type of sunscreen ingredient in some cosmetic products (e.g., oxybenzone).

BHA (butylated hydroxyanisole)   A preservative ingredient in some cosmetics.

BHT (butylated hydroxytoluene)   A preservative ingredient in some cosmetics.

Bismuth oxychloride   An ingredient added to cosmetics to give a frosted effect or pearly shine.

Blackhead   A small pimple (comedo) characterized by a black plug at the surface of a skin pore.

Bleeding   Migration of a cosmetic product to a site away from where it was actually applied, usually into or through fine lines or wrinkles in the skin.

Blemish   An area of skin that is irregular in color or contour.

Blush   A reddish cosmetic applied to the cheeks to add color to the face and simulate a natural flush.

Blusher   Same as blush.

Bronopol   A preservative ingredient in some cosmetics.

Bronzer   A makeup intended to give the skin a suntanned appearance or glow.

Buffer   A powder used to help makeup blend in naturally with the color of the surrounding skin.

Cake   A pressed powder cosmetic.

Cells   The basic living structural unit of the body (the body is made up of millions of live cells).

Chemical sunblock   A skin-care product containing chemicals that absorb sunlight and prevent some sunlight from striking the skin.

Chlorhexidine   A disinfectant ingredient that is added to some cosmetics.

Chloroxylenol   A disinfectant ingredient that is added to some cosmetics.

Cinnamates   Sunscreen ingredients in some cosmetic products (e.g., octyl methoxycinnamate).

Coal tar colors   Color ingredients derived from petroleum byproducts.

Collagen   The primary structural component of the dermis, the deep layer of skin. When damage occurs to collagen in the skin, wrinkling occurs.

Colophony   Same as rosin.

Color drift   A change in the color of a cosmetic that occurs while the product is on the skin.

Color wash   A liquid cosmetic that leaves a light amount of color on the skin.

Combination skin   Skin that is drier on the periphery of the face but oilier than average on the mid-face.

Comedo   A blackhead or whitehead (two types of pimples) caused by plugging of a skin pore.

Comedogenic   A product or ingredient known to cause comedones when applied to the skin of some people.

Comedones   More than one comedo.

Contact allergy   Same as allergic contact dermatitis.

Contact dermatitis   Dermatitis caused by external contact with an aggravating substance.

Cosmetic   A product designed to improve appearance.

Cover-up   A cosmetic designed to mask a skin blemish or dark under-eye circles.

Coverage   The ability of a cosmetic to mask skin blemishes or to even out a somewhat mottled complexion.

Cream   An opaque semisolid emulsion of water and lipids that is designed to be applied to the skin.

Cream/powder   An oily compressed powder cosmetic.

Cuticle   A thin layer of tissue that grows at the base of the nails.

Cyst   A sac beneath the surface of the skin filled with skin secretions. Cysts can occur alone or may occur as part of acne.

Dandruff   The common name for a mild case of the scaly scalp condition called seborrheic dermatitis.

Dermatitis   Inflammation of the skin. Dermatitis is characterized by patches of indistinctly bordered red scaly skin with fissures, erosions, or crusts. There are numerous types of dermatitis, including contact dermatitis. Dermatitis is the same as eczema.

Dermis   The layer of skin below the epidermis but above the subcutaneous fat.

Detergent   A synthetically manufactured surfactant used in skin cleansers.

Diazolidinyl urea   A preservative ingredient in some cosmetics.

Dioxybenzone   A sunscreen ingredient in cosmetic products.

DMDM hydantoin   A preservative ingredient in some cosmetics.

Dye   A coloring agent.

Eczema   Same as dermatitis.

Elastin   A component of the deep skin layer called the dermis that is responsible for the elasticity of the skin.

Emollient   A product or ingredient that softens the skin.

Emollient ester   Ingredients that are not oils but are mildly oil-like in consistency. They are often used in cosmetics to add moisturizing ability without using oils.

Emulsion   The dispersion of one substance in a second substance in which it will not dissolve. An example is a water-in-oil emulsion.

Epidermis   The surface layer of the skin.

Essential oils   Fragrance ingredients made from plant extracts.

Excoriation   Scratch marks on the skin.

Eye shadow   Colored cosmetic products to be worn on the eyelids.

Eyeliner   Colored cosmetics designed to produce a thin line on the eyelids.

Finish   The sheen imparted by a cosmetic product that ranges from matte (dull) to shiny.

Formaldehyde   A preservative ingredient in some cosmetics.

Foundation   Colored cosmetic products (i.e., makeup) applied to the entire face.

Fragrance   Ingredients designed to impart a pleasant odor to a skin-care product.

Fragrance-free   Products with no fragrance ingredients.

Glyceryl thioglycolate   An ingredient found in permanent-wave hair products.

Hair follicle   A pore in the skin through which hairs grow and through which sebum is transported to the surface of the skin.

Highlighter   Colored cosmetic products used to accentuate a facial feature.

Humectant   A non-oily ingredient that holds water in the skin.

Hyaluronic acid   The most prevalent substance forming the "ground substance" of the dermis.

Hydrocarbons   Organic substances usually derived from petroleum.

Hydrophobic   Repels, or is repelled by, water.

Hypoallergenic   A product containing no allergens capable of causing allergic reactions in large numbers of people. The term is virtually meaningless since almost all skin-care products on the market fit this definition. Furthermore, most products claiming to be hypoallergenic are capable of causing allergic reactions in some individuals.

Imidazolidinyl urea   A preservative ingredient in some cosmetics.

Immiscible   When two substances cannot be dissolved in one another.

Immune reaction   A reaction of the body's defense system (the immune system) to a specific foreign substance.

Inflammation   The body's response to injury of the skin, characterized by red, irritated skin.

Irritant contact dermatitis   Dermatitis caused by direct toxic effects of various substances on the skin. This is different from an allergic reaction to one specific substance.

Keratin   A hard substance produced by the outer layer of the skin that helps the skin form a protective barrier.

Lanolin   A moisturizing ingredient in some cosmetics.

Lentigo   One type of flat discolored area of skin.

Lesion   Any abnormality of the skin.

Lipids   Organic substances soluble in organic solvents but not in water. Lipids include oils, fats, waxes, sterols, fatty acids, and emollient esters.

Lip liner   A cosmetic product designed to outline the lips, allowing the user to "correct" the shape of the lips if desired. Lip liners can also help prevent "bleeding" of lipstick.

Liver spot   The common name for a solar lentigo.

Lotion   An opaque liquid that is an emulsion of water and lipids.

Lubricant   A substance that decreases friction.

Lunula   The white crescent visible at the base

of the nails that is part of the nail matrix (the region where new nail is formed).

Macule A skin discoloration that is not raised.

Makeup A pigmented cosmetic product, most commonly used to refer to foundation.

Manicure Grooming of the fingernails.

Mascara Pigmented cosmetic products for the eyelashes.

Mask An opaque skin-care product designed to be put on the face for a short period of time and then removed.

Matte A dull finish.

Melanin The pigmented substance in the skin that is responsible for skin color.

Melanocyte Skin cells in the epidermis that produce melanin.

Methylchloroisothiazolinone A preservative ingredient in some cosmetics.

Methylisothiazolinone A preservative ingredient in some cosmetics.

Milia A small cyst near the surface of the skin that is often seen in individuals with acne.

Moisturizer A product or ingredient that adds moisture to the skin.

Mole The common name for a nevus pigmentosum.

Mousse An aerosolized lotion that forms a foam.

Mucopolysaccharide Substances found in large amounts in the dermis of the skin.

Nailbed The skin beneath the nails to which the nails are attached.

Nail hardener A product that forms a hard coat on the nail to protect it and decrease nail breakage.

Nail matrix The area at the base of the nail where new nail is formed.

Nail polish An enamel applied to the nail to improve nail appearance.

Nevus (plural: nevi) An excess of a particular type of cell in the body. However, the term is most commonly used as a short form of nevus pigmentosum, or mole.

Nevus pigmentosum An excess of pigment-containing cells in an area of skin.

Nonacnegenic An ingredient or product that has not produced acne when applied to normal skin (usually rabbit ear skin in the laboratory).

Noncomedogenic An ingredient or product that has not produced comedones when applied to normal skin (usually rabbit ear skin in the laboratory).

Octyl dimethyl PABA A sunscreen ingredient in cosmetic products (Padimate O).

Oil Any of a wide variety of substances made up of triglycerides and fatty acids. Usually oils are liquid at room temperature. In cosmetics, the definition may be expanded to include other substances that behave like oil when placed on the skin, such as greasy hydrocarbons and waxes.

Oil-based A skin-care product primarily made up of oil with a smaller amount of water, in addition to other ingredients.

Oil-control foundation A foundation containing oil and an increased amount of powder to absorb oil.

Oil-free A skin-care product containing no oil.

Oil-in-water emulsion A skin-care product consisting of a small amount of oil dispersed in a larger amount of water. Same as water-based.

Ointment A nonwater-containing semisolid preparation that is designed to be applied to the skin.

Opaque A substance through which light will not pass.

Oxybenzone A sunscreen ingredient in cosmetic products (benzophenone-3).

PABA A sunscreen ingredient in cosmetic products (para-aminobenzoic acid).

Padimate O A PABA-derivative sunscreen ingredient in cosmetic products (octyl dimethyl PABA).

Papule A small raised skin lesion, such as the

raised red pimples seen in most types of acne.

Parabens A preservative ingredient in some cosmetics.

Paraphenylenediamine An ingredient in permanent hair dye products.

Patch test The testing technique used to identify contact allergy.

Pearlescent Substances imparting a sparkling quality or sheen to cosmetics, such as mica, fish scale, mother-of-pearl, or bismuth oxychloride.

Pencil A cosmetic product packaged inside a wooden cylinder (similar to a writing pencil) and used to produce thin lines.

Perfume Same as fragrance.

pH The 0–14 scale used for measuring acidity and alkalinity. Acids have a pH less than 7 and alkaline substances have a pH more than 7.

Phospholipid One type of substance found in the epidermis that helps the skin form a barrier of protection from outside substances.

Photoaging Discoloration, wrinkling, or other skin damage caused by the cumulative effects of sun exposure over a lifetime.

Physical sunblock An opaque substance acting as a sunblock by not allowing sunlight to pass through.

Pigment A substance that imparts color to another substance or mixture.

Pimple An acne skin lesion caused by plugging of the hair follicles usually on the face and/or upper trunk. May be used to refer to comedones, papules, pustules, and/or acne-related cysts.

Pomade An oily hair-care product.

Pore An opening in the skin, such as the opening of a hair follicle.

Powder A finely ground solid.

Propylene glycol An ingredient used as a humectant and/or solvent in some cosmetic products.

Propyl gallate A preservative ingredient in some cosmetics.

Pruritis Itching.

Pustule A small raised skin lesion filled with pus, such as the raised red pimples with white tops seen in many types of acne.

Quaternium-15 A preservative ingredient in some cosmetics.

Refiner A skin-care product that is a solution of water and humectants and/or fragrance.

Retinoids Substances derived from vitamin A that are very different from vitamin A in terms of their medical properties.

Rosacea An adult skin disorder with acne blemishes on the mid-face and enlargement of blood vessels leading to persistent redness in this area of the face.

Rosin An ingredient in some cosmetics that can sometimes cause allergic reactions.

Rouge Same as blush.

Sealant (primer) A cosmetic product designed to be put on the lips or eyelids prior to lipstick or eyeshadow to help these cosmetics adhere better.

Sebaceous glands Glands in the skin that produce skin secretions called sebum.

Seborrheic dermatitis A condition that produces redness and oily scale predominantly on the scalp and mid-face. On the scalp, milder cases are commonly called dandruff.

Sebum Fatty skin secretions that are produced by sebaceous glands.

Semimatte A makeup finish between matte (dull) and shiny.

Sensitization The elicitation of a specific immune response from an initial exposure to an allergen. Once this has occurred, subsequent exposure to the same allergen will cause an allergic reaction.

Shake lotion Powder suspended in a liquid that must be shaken to mix the contents before use.

Sheer A thin translucent product providing a slight amount of coverage.

Shiny A bright reflective finish.

Skin cells The individual basic living structures of the skin (the skin is made up of millions of live skin cells).

Soap A specific type of surfactant used as a skin cleanser made from fatty acids and alkali derived from plants or animals.

Solar lentigo A flat discolored area of skin caused by the cumulative effect of years of sun exposure. Same as liver spot.

Solute A substance that is dissolved in another substance.

Solution A mixture containing a solute dissolved in a solvent.

Solvent A substance in which another substance is dissolved.

Sorbic acid A preservative ingredient in some cosmetics.

Spray A liquid aerosol.

Stick A cylindrical wax cosmetic product in a tube.

Subcutaneous fat The deepest layer of the skin comprised largely of fat.

Sun protection factor (SPF) A number that indicates how much additional sun exposure can be tolerated when using a sunscreen. A person who can stay in the sun unprotected for 15 minutes before burning will be able to stay in the sun 15 times longer ($15 \times 15 = 225$ minutes) when wearing an SPF-15 sunscreen. The higher the SPF, the more protection is provided. The same person could remain in the sun only 30 minutes (2×15) with an SPF-2 sunscreen.

Sunblock Products or ingredients whose opacity blocks the sunlight.

Sunscreen A skin-care product that absorbs and thus prevents some sunlight from reaching the skin.

Surfactant A substance capable of dissolving oily and non-oily substances. Soaps and detergents are types of surfactants used in skin cleansers.

Thimerosal A preservative ingredient in some cosmetics.

Toluene sulfonamide/formaldehyde resin An ingredient found in most nail polishes.

Toner Same as an astringent.

Top coat A clear enamel used over nail polish to prevent chipping.

Translucent A transparent product providing slight (sheer) coverage.

Transparent A see-through product.

T-zone The oiliest areas of the face: the forehead and the mid-face.

Ultraviolet light (UV) An invisible part of sunlight divided into UVA (ultraviolet A light), UVB (ultraviolet B light), and UVC (ultraviolet C light). UVB is responsible for most sun-related skin cancers and sunburn. UVA is responsible for most sun-related allergic skin conditions. Protection against UVC is believed to be of little importance.

Undercover A cosmetic used under foundation for better coverage of blemishes and discolorations and to ensure longer wear.

Unpigmented Without color.

Unscented Having no smell. An unscented product may have a masking fragrance designed to hide the natural odor of the product. Therefore, unscented does not mean fragrance-free.

UVA Ultraviolet A light. This part of sunlight is responsible for sun-related allergic skin conditions in a small number of people. There are currently only a few sunscreens designed to provide significant broad spectrum protection against UVA light.

UVB Ultraviolet B light. This is the part of sunlight most responsible for sunburn and sun-related skin cancers. The amount of protection provided by a sunscreen product against UVB is indicated by the sun protection factor.

Vitamin C and vitamin E   Ingredients added to some cosmetic products as anti-oxidants.

Water-based   A skin-care product that is primarily water with a smaller amount of oil.

Water-free   A skin-care product containing no water.

Water-in-oil emulsion   A skin-care product consisting of a small amount of water dispersed in a larger amount of oil.

Weartime   The amount of time a cosmetic can be worn while retaining optimal appearance.

Whitehead   A small pimple (comedo) characterized by a pinpoint raised white lesion at the surface of a skin pore.

Wool wax alcohol   Same as lanolin alcohol, a moisturizing ingredient in some cosmetic products.

Wool wax   Same as lanolin.

Xerosis   Excessive dryness of the skin.

Adams, R. M., and H. I. Maibach. 1985. A five-year study of cosmetic reactions. *Journal of the American Academy of Dermatology* 13:1062–69.

Arndt, K. A. 1987. *Manual of Dermatologic Therapeutics.* 4th ed. Boston: Little, Brown.

Blank, I. H., and R. J. Scheuplein. 1964. "The Epidermal Barrier." In *Progress in the Biological Sciences in Relation to Dermatology.* Vol 2, eds. A. J. Rook and R. H. Champion. Cambridge: Cambridge University Press.

Brumberg, E. 1986. *Save Your Money, Save Your Face.* New York: Harper & Row.

Coldiron, B. M. 1992. Thinning of the ozone layer: Facts and consequences. *Journal of the American Academy of Dermatology* 27:653–62.

Cosmetic, Toiletry, and Fragrance Association, Inc. 1991. *Cosmetic Industry on Call.* 3d ed. Washington: Cosmetic, Toiletry, and Fragrance Association, Inc.

Cronin, E. 1980. *Contact Dermatitis.* Edinburgh: Churchill Livingstone.

de Groot, A. C., and J. W. Weyland. 1992. Contact allergy to methyldibromoglutaronitrile in the preservative Euxyl K 400. *American Journal of Contact Dermatitis* 2(1):31–32.

Dermatology Times. 1990. New allergens develop as use of latex products and cosmetics rises. *Dermatology Times* 11(11):34.

Draelos, Zoe D. 1992. Cosmetics designed for men. *Cosmetic Dermatology* 5(11):14–16.

———. 1990. *Cosmetics in Dermatology.* New York: Churchill Livingstone.

———. 1992. Evaluation of cosmetic marketing claims—Part 1: What do they really mean? *Cosmetic Dermatology* 5(9):14–16.

Elson, M. L. 1992. The utilization of glycolic acids in photoaging. *Cosmetic Dermatology.* 5(1):12–15.

Estrin, N. F., P. A. Crosley, and C. R. Haynes. 1982. *CTFA Dictionary.* 3d ed. Washington: Cosmetic, Toiletry, and Fragrance Association, Inc.

Fenske, N. A., and C. W. Lober. Structural and functional changes of normal aging skin. 1986. *Journal of the American Academy of Dermatology* 15:571–85.

Fisher, A. A. 1986. *Contact Dermatitis.* 3d ed. Philadelphia: Lea and Febiger.

———. 1992. Sunscreen dermatitis: Para-aminobenzoic acid and its derivatives. *Cutis* 50(3):190–92.

———. 1992. Sunscreen dermatitis: Part II—The cinnamates. *Cutis* 50(4):253–54.

———. 1992. Sunscreen dermatitis: Part III—The benzophenones. *Cutis* 50(5)331–32.

———. 1992. Sunscreen dermatitis: Part IV—The salicylates, the anthranilates, and physical agents. *Cutis* 50(6):397–98.

Fitzpatrick, T. B. 1992. "Gearing up" for the effects of high-intensity solar UVB. *Dermatologic Capsule & Comment* 14(3):1–4.

Frosch, P. J., and A. M. Kligman. 1979. The soap chamber tests: A new method for assessing the irritancy of soaps. *Journal of the American Academy of Dermatology* 1:35–41.

Fulton, J. E., Jr., S. R. Pay, and J. E. Fulton III. 1984. Comedogenicity of current therapeutic products, cosmetics, and ingredients in the rabbit ear. *Journal of the American Academy of Dermatology* 10:96.

Ghadially, R., L. Halkier-Sorenson, and P. M. Elias. 1986. Effects of petrolatum on stratum corneum structure and function. *Journal of the American Academy of Dermatology* 26:387–96.

Gilman, A. G., L. S. Goodman, and A. Gilman, eds. 1985. *The Pharmacologic Basis of Therapeutics.* 7th ed. New York: Macmillan.

Jackson, E. M. 1992. Moisturizers. What's in them? How do they work? *American Journal of Contact Dermatitis* 3(4):162–68.

Journal of the American Academy of Dermatology. 1989. American Academy of Dermatology invitational on comedogenicity. *Journal of the American Academy of Dermatology* 20:272–77.

Kligman, A. M., G. L. Grove, R. Hirose, and J. J. Leyden. 1986. Topical tretinoin for photoaged skin. *Journal of the American Academy of Dermatology* 15:836–59.

Kligman, A. M., and O. H. Mills. 1972. Acne cosmetica. *Archives of Dermatology* 106:843.

———. 1975. Acne detergecans. *Archives of Dermatology* 111:65–68.

Larsen, W. G., E. M. Jackson, M. D. Barker, et al. 1992. A primer on cosmetics. *Journal of the American Academy of Dermatology* 27:469–483.

Levy, S. B. 1992. Dihydroxyacetone-containing sunless or self-tanning lotions. *Journal of the American Academy of Dermatology* 27:989–93.

Lupo, M. L. 1992. Knowledge of facial masks important to dermatologists. *Cosmetic Dermatology* 5(5):16–22.

Mullins, J. D. 1980. "Medicated applications." In Remington's *Pharmaceutical Sciences.* 16th ed., ed. A. Osol. Easton, Pa.: Mack Publishing Company.

Nater, J., A. de Groot, and D. H. Liem. 1985. *Unwanted Effects of Cosmetics and Drugs Used in Dermatology.* 2d ed. New York: Elsevier.

Natow, A. J. 1986. Aloe vera: Fiction or fact? *Cutis* 37(2):106–107.

———. Talc: Need we beware? *Cutis* 37(5):328–29.

Nelson, F. P., and J. Rumsfield. 1988. Cosmetics: Content and function. *International Journal of Dermatology* 27:665–72.

Pathak, M. A., T. B. Fitzpatrick, F. J. Greiter, and E. W. Kraus. 1985. Principles in sunburn and suntanning, and topical and systemic photo protection in health and diseases. *Journal of Dermatologic Surgery and Oncology.* 11(6)575–79.

Plewig, G., J. E. Fulton, and A. M. Kligman. 1974. Pomade acne. *Archives of Dermatology* 101:580.

Rhodes, A. R., M. A. Weinstock, T. B. Fitzpatrick, et al. 1987. Risk factors for cutaneous melanoma: A practical method of recognizing predisposed individuals. *Journal of the American Medical Association* 258:3146–54.

Rietschel, A. L., J. R. Nethercott, E. A. Emmett, et al. 1990. Methylchloroisothiazolinone-methylisothiazolinone reactions in patients screened for vehicle and preservative hypersensitivity. *Journal of the American Academy of Dermatology* 22:734–38.

Sauer, Gordon C. 1980. *Manual of Skin Diseases.* 4th ed. Philadelphia: J. B. Lippincott.

Sauermann, G., A. Doerschner, U. Hoppe, and P. Wittern. 1986. Comparative study of skin care efficiency and in-use properties of soap and surfactant bars. *Journal of the Society of Cosmetic Chemists* 37:309–27.

Schaefer, H., A. Zesch, and G. Stutten. 1982. *Skin Permeability.* Berlin: Springer-Verlag.

Scheman, A. J. 1992. *Pocket Guide to Medications Used in Dermatology.* 3d ed. Baltimore: Williams & Wilkins.

Scher, R. K. 1982. Cosmetics and ancillary preparations for care of the nails. *Journal of the American Academy of Dermatology.* 6:523–28.

Schoen, L. A., and P. Lazar. 1989. *The Look You Like.* New York: Marcel Dekker.

Sendagorta, E., J. Lesiewicz, and R. B. Armstrong. 1992. Topical isotretinoin for photodamaged skin. *Journal of the American Academy of Dermatology* 27:S15–S18.

Shalita, A. R. 1989. Comparison of a salicylic acid cleanser and a benzoyl peroxide wash in the treatment of acne vulgaris. *Clinical Therapy* 11(2):264–67.

Shelley, W. B., and E. D. Shelley. 1986. Chapstick acne. *Cutis* 37:459–60.

Stenberg, C., and O. Larkö. 1985. Sunscreen application and its importance for the sun protection factor. *Archives of Dermatology* 121:1400–1402.

Stern, R. S., M. C. Weinstein, and S. G. Baker. 1986. Risk reduction for nonmelanoma skin cancer with childhood sunscreen use. *Archives of Dermatology* 122:537–45.

Strauss, J. S. 1987. "Sebaceous Glands." In *Dermatology in General Medicine.* 3d ed., eds. T. B. Fitzpatrick, A. Z. Eisen, K. Wolff, et al. New York: McGraw-Hill.

Tolman, E. L. 1985. "Acne and Acneiform Dermatoses." In *Dermatology.* 2d ed., eds. S. L. Moschella and H. J. Hurley. Philadelphia: W. B. Saunders.

Van Scott, E. J., and R. J. Yu. 1989. "Alpha hydroxy acids: Therapeutic potentials. *Canadian Journal of Dermatology.* 1(5):108–12.

Weiss, J. S., C. N. Ellis, J. T. Headington, et al. 1988. Topical tretinoin improves photoaged skin. *Journal of the American Medical Association* 259:527–32.

Wilkinson, J. B., and R. J. Moore. 1982. *Harry's Cosmeticology.* 7th ed. New York: Chemical Publishing.